Trends and Prospects in Metacognition Research across the Life Span

Despina Moraitou • Panayiota Metallidou
Editors

Trends and Prospects in Metacognition Research across the Life Span

A Tribute to Anastasia Efklides

Springer

Editors
Despina Moraitou
School of Psychology
Aristotle University of Thessaloniki
Thessaloniki, Greece

Panayiota Metallidou
School of Psychology
Aristotle University of Thessaloniki
Thessaloniki, Greece

ISBN 978-3-030-51672-7 ISBN 978-3-030-51673-4 (eBook)
https://doi.org/10.1007/978-3-030-51673-4

This Springer imprint is published by the registered company Springer Nature Switzerland AG.
The registered company address is: Gewerbestrasse 11, 6330 Cham, Switzerland

Preface and Tribute to Anastasia Efklides

In the book *Trends and Prospects in Metacognition Research* (Efklides and Misailidi 2010), there were two main parts, the first presenting basic research on the nature and functioning of metacognition and the second one the development of metacognition and educational implications of metacognition research. Since then, research on metacognition has progressed and offered solid evidence on the mechanisms underlying the functioning of metacognition as well as the effectiveness of metacognitive regulation in learning. Yet, there is also growing awareness that metacognitive monitoring is often inaccurate and metacognitive regulation ineffective. Thus, new questions arise and metacognition research faces new challenges.

Ten years later, in this volume, some of the trends already featuring then are still present, but there is a major shift of interest from metacognition per se to metacognition and its interactions with affect. Also, metacognitive regulation is now seen as a constituent of self- and co- and/or shared regulation, which stresses, firstly, the interactions between metacognition, motivation, and emotions, and, secondly, that metacognition and metacognitive regulation is not a purely individual phenomenon but has a strong social nature. Such a social perspective on metacognition has implications for education and the role of teacher and peers as sources of feedback that impact metacognitive monitoring and control. The development of metacognition is also viewed through the lens of affect and social influences. Looking at development as a lifelong process, it becomes clear that changes in metacognition take place in the lifespan and interactions of metacognition with motivation and affect are evident in self-regulation from early childhood to old age. This has implications for the construction of intervention programs for young students but also older adults who see their cognitive efficiency to decrease. Finally, another domain in which metacognition has not been extensively studied is creativity, which, along with giftedness, is another challenge for research in metacognition. This overview of the field does not cover other also important research developments such as the neuroscience of metacognition. The focus of this volume, however, was inspired by the work of Anastasia Efklides, professor emerita of psychology in

Aristotle University of Thessaloniki, Greece, and one of the editors of the volume published in 2010.

Thus, the aim of this volume was, besides bringing to the fore trends and prospects in metacognition research in the last ten years, to also offer a tribute to Anastasia Efklides, a mentor of the editors of this volume and many young researchers in the field, and a theorist who has foreseen in her work some of the developments taking place in metacognition research in the last decade. Specifically, Anastasia Efklides' research was inspired by Flavell's (1979) seminal article that posited three facets of metacognition, namely, metacognitive experiences, metacognitive knowledge, and metacognitive strategies (skills). She, particularly, focused on metacognitive experiences (feelings, judgments, online metacognitive knowledge) (see Efklides 2006, 2008) but with an emphasis on the feeling of difficulty and the estimate (or judgment) of effort, which both have a metacognitive but also a motivational and an affective character. This perspective allowed her to integrate in her theorizing different research traditions and theoretical frameworks ranging from metamemory to motivation and affect as sources of feeling of difficulty, estimate of effort, and confidence.

Studying metacognitive feelings led her in two theoretical directions: one, an enriched model of metacognition (Efklides 2008) that expanded the one proposed by Nelson (1996), and the other, a model of self-regulated learning that posited relations between metacognition, motivation, and affect [the Metacognitive and Affective Model of Self-Regulated Learning (MASRL); Efklides 2011]. Specifically, the enriched model of metacognition proposes three levels of functioning of metacognition: the nonconscious, the personal awareness, and the social level. In the nonconscious level, monitoring and control function out of the person's awareness but may inform the personal level awareness in the form of metacognitive experiences (e.g., metacognitive feelings and judgments). The personal awareness level of metacognition refers to the person becoming aware of his/her own thinking and learning and the subjective experiences (i.e., metacognitive experiences and metacognitive knowledge) that go with cognitive processing. Control is exercised by the individual on her/his thinking based on these subjective experiences. The third is the social level of metacognitive functioning, which is based on reflection on one's own vis-à-vis other people's metacognitive experiences, metacognitive knowledge, and metacognitive skills. This allows communication between individuals at a meta level, reflection and analysis of metacognitive products, and exercising of control in a co- or shared regulation manner. This level of functioning of metacognition is present in the interactions between parents and children, teachers and students, and peers, as well as between researchers of metacognitive phenomena and the development of the science of metacognition.

The MASRL model, on the other hand, expands the conceptualization of personal awareness as a level that comprises not only metacognitive experiences but also motivational and affective experiences (emotions, moods, motivational feelings, e.g., effort exertion) (Efklides 2011, 2016, 2018). Although metacognition is involved in the regulation of cognition, and affective regulation in the regulation of affect and effort, there are interactions between the two regulatory systems based on the awareness of subjective states during task processing. For example, feeling of difficulty during task processing may inform metacognitive control for strategy use but also motivational control based on the perceived cost that the needed effort may confer. Furthermore, being in positive or negative mood modulates feeling of difficulty and, hence, the perceived cost and subsequent decision on the kind of regulation (metacognitive, motivational, or affective) needed. However, subjective experiences are not conceived of as sole products of cognitive and affective processing. They are also influenced by personal characteristics (cognitive, metacognitive, motivational, and affective) as traits. Self-regulation, from this point of view, is task-specific but also a manifestation of stability and continuity of the self as the organizing principle that integrates the past, the present, and the future.

In this context, the chapters in this volume are representative of research that argues for a more comprehensive conception of the person as a social being that builds on own and others' metacognitive, motivational, and emotional experiences to self-, co-, or shared regulation in learning situations or challenges faced in the lifespan development. The volume has been organized along three parts: (I) the mechanism underlying the relations between metacognition and affect, (II) metacognition and affect in self- and co-regulation, and (III) metacognition and affect in the lifespan development.

Part I: The Mechanism Underlying the Relations Between Metacognition and Affect

This part of the volume starts with the chapter by Witherby, Tauber, and Dunlosky titled "*Why do Emotional Stimuli Influence Judgments of Learning? Theory, Evidence, and Future Directions.*" Starting from Efklides' contribution on the role of affect and emotions in self-monitoring processes, the authors try to uncover the mechanism that underlies the influence of emotion on individuals' monitoring judgments. They first review and discuss evidence for the emotional salience effect on the magnitude of judgments of learning (JOLs) and, then, introduce a theoretical model for explaining the above effect. They start from the main theoretical assumption of JOL theories that JOLs are largely inferential and they are influenced by a number of available cues via two mechanisms: (a) people's beliefs about their own and others' learning and (b) experiences or feelings that are triggered during online processing of the learning material. They present evidence which shows that, even though people's beliefs and experiences (either fluency or arousal) during processing can explain at least a portion of emotional salience effects on JOLs, the existing evidence does not clearly establish the proposed theoretical pathways, leaving ample space for future research in the area. The authors emphasize the need to investigate the influence of stimulus valence or/and mood on other metacognitive judgments, such as the feeling of knowing and confidence judgments, as well as the need to use multiple measures in order to evaluate the combined influence of processing fluency and physiological arousal during the processing of emotional stimuli. Further, they argue that an individual differences perspective should be included in future empirical attempts to evaluate the magnitude of contribution of each of the above mechanisms to people's monitoring judgments.

In the next chapter titled "*The role of fluency and dysfluency in metacognitive experience*," Schwartz and Jemstedt continue the discussion on the role of perceptual and retrieval fluency as primary sources of accurate and inaccurate metacognitive judgments. They acknowledge, as Witherby, Tauber, and Dunlosky did in the previous chapter, the discrete influence of both processing fluency and beliefs on the learning judgments as well as a fluency x beliefs interaction effect, despite this still being hard to pinpoint. The authors review evidence that supports the impact of processing fluency on metacognition, indicating either its adaptive or its distorting function for self-regulated learning. In particular, they show how processing fluency may lead us to inaccurate control decisions via increases in the metacognitive feeling of confidence. They stress, thus, the need for studying metacognitive illusions, namely situations in which our metacognitive judgments do not accurately monitor our learning process and performance, in order to uncover the mechanisms underlying metacognitive monitoring and control decisions.

Whereas the focus of the two previous chapters was on the experiences or feelings that are triggered during processing of the material to be learnt, Vogl, Pekrun, and Loderer in the next chapter titled "*Epistemic emotions and metacognitive feelings*" discuss similarities, differences, and links between epistemic emotions and metacognitive feelings. They argue that, while both share common features, such as an affective core experience and their effects on cognitive processing, they differ in terms of their functions and their constituents. They acknowledge, though, that there are not established yet clear-cut boundaries between them, which could direct future research in the area. They present empirical evidence that supports the critical role of metacognitive feelings, especially that of feeling of confidence, in the formation and experience of epistemic states that are affectively charged, such as surprise, curiosity, and confusion. At the end of the chapter, the authors argue that studying the links between metacognitive feelings and epistemic emotions is a very promising research area and draw our attention to many open questions for future study, concerning the function and constituents of less studied epistemic states, such as doubt, the relations of epistemic emotions with other metacognitive feelings, such as the feeling of knowing, as well as their distinct influences on cognitive processing, motivation, and behavior.

In the last chapter of Part I titled "*Metacognitive experience across the creative process*," Antonietti, Cancer, Colombo, and Iannello discuss the role of metacognition in the less studied and challenging domain of creativity. They start by identifying the specific cognitive mechanisms that are involved in creative thinking and present their WCR model, which involves three major mental operations in creative thinking, namely, widening, connection, and reorganization of the mental field. Having this model as a basis for inquiry, they review and discuss evidence about the possible role of different facets of metacognition, that is, knowledge, experiences, and control in fostering creativity. In the last part of the chapter, they try to answer the question if metacognitive awareness is beneficial in increasing the level of creativity by presenting evidence from a creative thinking training program that uses metacognitive prompts in a sample of primary school children. The results showed that training in activating the above three basic mental creative operations increased children's creative skills. Further, the group that was prompted to reflect on the way they worked in various activities, i.e., reflecting on their ability, effort, and liking the task before and after their involvement, outperformed the control group only in one aspect of creativity: that of widening their mental field. At the same time, the above metacognitive prompts were found to hinder reorganization. The authors highlight the need for further research in the field, in order to delimit the beneficial or detrimental influences different facets of metacognition and different levels of metacognitive functioning may have on creative processes according to Efklides' model.

Part II: Metacognition and Affect in Self- and Co-regulation

The chapters in this part of the volume focus on the functioning of metacognition in the social level and provide evidence for the dynamic interplay of metacognition and affect in educational settings. Vauras, Volet, and Iiskala in the chapter titled "*Socially-shared metacognitive regulation in collaborative science learning*" build on Efklides' initial idea that metacognition and metacognitive regulation is not a purely individual phenomenon but has a strong social nature. They discuss conceptualization issues of social regulation of cognition and, then, they select the challenging area of science learning and present evidence on the role of socially shared metacognitive regulation (SSMR) in different collaborative science learning environments. They provide a detailed review of the empirical data from their own and others' work in the last fifteen years for the most critical elements of the SSMR, such as the focus, the functions and the triggering factors of SSMR, as well as the relationship of SSMR and desired learning outcomes. Specifically, they point out the complexity of the relations between SSMR and learning outcomes, due to possible mediating factors related to the type of the task and the focus and functions of SSMR. Further, they argue that conceptual understanding is evidenced as the most important focus of SSMR for quality learning outcomes with the metacognitive experiences as one of the most crucial triggers for this kind of SSRM. Facing (socio)cognitive conflicts and receiving error feedback from others in collaborative learning contexts are acknowledged as the other two critical triggers of SSMR. They highlight the need for evidence on the role of affective reactions as part of the SSMR process and the role of feedback as a trigger factor for accurate monitoring and control decisions in SSMR.

The following two chapters provide evidence for the role of affect in self- and co-regulation of learning in the domain of math problem solving, while the last two chapters of Part II discuss evidence for the role of feedback from teachers and parents in fostering children's SRL skills in school and home. Specifically, the chapter by Singh and Muis, titled "*The role of social emotions and co-regulation of learning during complex math problem solving*," provides empirical evidence regarding the role of affect in monitoring and control decisions in collaborative learning contexts. The authors discuss the antecedents and consequences of social emotions in collaborative learning, in the area of complex math problem solving. Using a triangulated multi-method approach of self-reports, discourse analysis, and individual interviews, they provide evidence for the role of social emotion in co-regulatory processes in a group of elementary students. The results of their study indicate the significant role of task value and perceived control beliefs as antecedents of social emotions. They seem to serve as buffers against disengagement from the learning activity. Further, social emotions are preceded by social appraisals, such as being competent, autonomous, and related to the social context. These appraisals, in turn, affect co-regulatory processes and the social emotions function as mediators of the feelings of relatedness and the use of functional co-regulatory strategies. The authors discuss the educational implications of the findings and point out the important role of teachers in communicating to their students (either explicitly or by modeling) all the necessary information as regards the functions, the processes, and the benefits of SRL and CoRL.

Kramarski, Tzohar-Rozen, and Gadasi in their chapter titled "*Metacognition and meta-Emotion in kindergarten: Is the combination necessary for self-regulation in mathematical problem solving?*" provide empirical evidence from an intervention study that does not only engage children in interactive learning environments with the emphasis on content-related learning, but, instead, it explicitly teaches them how to regulate their cognitive, metacognitive, and emotional aspects of learning, especially when they have to deal with complex problem-solving tasks. Specifically, they discuss the necessity of applying interventions that simultaneously support the metacognitive and the affective aspects of SRL even from kindergarten. They provide empirical evidence of the effectiveness of a combined metacognitive and emotional support (MES) program in the domain of mathematics as compared to only a metacognitive support (MS) and a control (no SRL support) program. While both intervention programs increased children's performance and verbal metacognitive statements along the three phases of SRL (planning, monitoring and control, and evaluation), the combined MES group showed the greatest lasting gains two months after the intervention, especially in the complex tasks. Further, the combined MES group showed the greatest immediate as well as lasting gains in emotional regulation as compared to both MS and control programs. They also discuss the need to give time to the system to assimilate the metacognitive and emotional regulation strategies in order to use them in future learning experiences. They highlight that SRL skills need time to develop and improve, especially in young children.

The next two chapters review evidence on the role of teachers' and parents' practices to foster children's SRL skills in different learning contexts. Specifically, van Loon and Roebers in the chapter titled "*Using feedback to support children when monitoring and controlling their learning*" present an overview of research on the effects of different kinds of feedback on kindergarten and elementary school children's monitoring and control decisions in learning contexts. They focus on Efklides' (2008) social level of metacognition and discuss the effects of feedback on metacognition and learning in the task x person level of interaction, as this is conceptualized in Efklides' (2011) MASRL model. Namely, they examine the effects of teacher, internal task, and peer feedback on monitoring and control decisions while the child is working on a learning task. They provide well-established evidence that feedback could be helpful when it is developmentally appropriate and takes into consideration children's individual differences in their learning skills. They argue that children can benefit the most from informative feedback regarding the progress of processing, that is, to give children information about the actual level of their performance. Further, they highlight the need to investigate motivational and affective factors (e.g., personal goal orientations, feelings of competence) as moderators of the feedback influences on metacognition and learning.

Dermitzaki and Kallia continue the above discussion in their chapter titled "*The role of parents and teachers in fostering children's self-regulated learning skills*" and review current evidence that highlights the contribution of parents and teachers in the development of children's SRL skills. Specifically, in the first part of their chapter they discuss the contribution of different aspects of parental support, such as cognitive, metacognitive, and emotional in children's academic and SRL skills. Given that early parent–child interactions can function as the initiators of the development of various self-monitoring and regulating skills, the authors indicate the need to better understand the (individual and child-related or contextual) factors that contribute to the adoption of specific parental support practices. In the second part of their chapter, they discuss evidence regarding the role of teachers in fostering children's SRL skills. The authors argue that explicit instruction of SRL skills in real classrooms is not frequently observed. Given the well-evidenced cognitive and motivational gains for students whenever explicit instruction of learning strategies takes place in classroom, they indicate the need to intervene and strengthen teachers' beliefs, knowledge, and practices of SRL via well-designed professional development programs.

Part III: Metacognition and Affect in the Lifespan Development

In the last part of the volume, there are four chapters that discuss the development of metacognition and self-regulatory skills as well as changes in the interaction of metacognition with motivation and affect during the lifespan. The first two chapters focus on social influences that support the development of metacognition and regulatory skills in young children, while the next two chapters provide evidence for metacognitive functioning in older adults.

Misailidi in her chapter titled "*Understanding cognitive mental states and emotions in early childhood: Dissociation and interconnectedness*" discusses, within the framework of the theory of mind (ToM), evidence from recent developmental and neuropsychological studies for the development of abilities to understand cognitive mental states and emotions in early childhood. She argues that, even though the above two abilities follow distinct developmental trajectories early in life, they are at the same time interconnected components of a complex system that is developing dynamically in early childhood. They seem to function independently at the beginning of life, while later on they form interdependent dynamic interaction networks, which provide coherence to the system. She also argues that a great challenge for future research is to investigate the distinct role of young children's abilities to understand cognitive and emotional mental states as possible precursors of different components of metacognitive development. These attempts could shed light as well on the debate regarding the unitary vs. the componential nature of ToM.

Whitebread in the next chapter entitled "*Influences on the emergence and development of cognitive and emotional regulation in early childhood*" provides an overview of his and others' work in the last two decades on the development of metacognitive and self-regulatory abilities in young children. Recognizing that much of the relevant research has been guided or inspired by Efklides' work, he uses her multifaceted and multilevel model of metacognition as the basis for discussing evidence regarding the development of metacognitive and regulatory processes from the nonconscious level to the emerging personal awareness level and the influences of social environment on this development. In the first part of the chapter, he presents well-established evidence indicating that there are nonconscious as well as conscious processes of metacognition. The transition, though, from nonconscious to conscious awareness in young children is influenced considerably by contextual factors and social experiences. The evidence clearly indicates that children by the age they enter preschool or kindergarten education show profound individual differences in their metacognitive and self-regulatory abilities, which continue to grow after entering primary school. In the second part of the chapter, he reviews research regarding the social factors that support the emergence and development of metacognition and self-regulation. He argues that early parenting and educational practices are critical features of the early child's social environment since they have been systematically found to be associated with the emergence and development of individual differences in children's metacognitive and self-regulation abilities. At the end of the chapter, he reviews and discusses evidence from intervention studies designed to support children's cognitive and emotional regulation by addressing significant aspects of home and school environment. Given the success of these programs, especially for children who are at risk to develop weak regulatory abilities, he once again points out the importance of taking into consideration the social level of metacognition in Efklides' model, especially when we are to understand the processes that support the early development of cognitive and emotional regulation.

In relation to the developmental trajectory from the inverse side, that is, older adulthood and the declines in cognitive functioning that have been well documented in aging literature, McGillivray discusses intrinsic and extrinsic motivational influences in older adults' metacognitive monitoring and control. In the chapter entitled *"Strategic, emotional, and motivational influences on metacognition in older adulthood,"* McGillivray reviews evidence which suggests that metamemory judgments and control decisions are affected by motivational and emotional factors, such as interest, the value and importance of to-be-remembered information, or its emotional content. She claims that, in general, older adults strategically select to focus on valuable information. At times, they demonstrate more selectivity in their metacognitive control behaviors, compared to younger adults, and this could be at the expense of less important information. Besides objective value of information, she claims that often one's own interest or goals determine the overall "worth" of information. She suggests that with advancing age, subjective interest or curiosity could have an even larger effect on memory. As regards the effects of emotional information on metacognitive monitoring, she points out that, contrary to a wealth of literature on affective effects on memory, there are fewer studies on emotions' effects on metacognitive judgments of older adults. Further, given that research evidence for the well-known "positivity effect" is inconclusive, she argues that if it exists, it may at times operate on an implicit level that does not affect metacognitive judgments in older adults. Hence, according to McGillivray, more research is needed to explore the impact of various memory-moderating factors on metamemory monitoring and control decisions, in order to further inform theories of cognitive aging and improve quality of life of older adults.

The improvement of quality of life of adults could be achieved via metacognitive training programs, that is, cognitive training programs which incorporate metacognitive components. In the last chapter entitled "*Metacognition in cognitive rehabilitation in adults: a literature review*," Bampa, Moraitou, and Metallidou discuss the benefits of metacognitive training programs in older and younger adults with cognitive deficits. They review nine randomized controlled trial training studies that targeted to promote both metacognitive knowledge (e.g., through awareness regarding their condition and its consequences on several domains in everyday life, and declarative, procedural, and conditional metacognitive knowledge about various coping strategies) and metacognitive regulation through feedback and discussion upon exercises and homework assignments. In the first part of the chapter, they present and discuss findings of five studies examining the efficacy of metacognitive training programs in older adults and in the second part the findings of four studies examining the efficacy of metacognitive training programs in younger adults confronting cognitive difficulties due to underlying neurological conditions. The findings showed that metacognitive training is beneficial for both adult populations not only in respect of their metacognitive functioning but also in respect of their subjective well-being. Besides the limitations, the authors argue the interventions presented clearly suggest that future attempts should combine training that aims to enhance metacognitive knowledge as regards memory and flexible use of cognitive strategies with training to improve self-efficacy about cognitive functioning and promote well-being. Further, future research should address methodological limitations in order to gain a better understanding of the beneficial effects of incorporating metacognition in cognitive training programs.

New Insights and Challenges in Metacognition Research

After more than 40 years of research in metacognition (Flavell 1976), it is now well recognized that metacognitive phenomena are far more complex than initially perceived. Moreover, metacognition is present in every aspect of human behavior, despite our will or desire to enable or ignore it. It is an integral part of our cognitive system, a constant source of inner feedback and control, via feedback loops between monitoring and control processes, which makes it a key component in self-regulation of cognition and behavior. It is more than evidenced, though, that metacognition does not mirror our cognitive functioning. Instead, it is a product of inferential processes, which leaves space for inaccurate monitoring and unsuccessful control decisions in everyday functioning. Also, metacognition, as an integral part of self-regulation, does not act independently from affect and motivation, and is not a purely individual phenomenon but has a strong social nature. Ten years after the first book on *Trends and Prospects in Metacognition Research* (Efklides and Misailidi 2010), the authors of this book, inspired by Efklides' work in the area, provide new insights into metacognition research and point out promising avenues of future investigation and effective interventions in various contexts and populations. They present and discuss their own or others' current evidence that underscores the social nature of metacognitive monitoring and metacognitive control and provide new insights for the mechanism underlying the relations between metacognition and affect in learning situations or challenges faced in the lifespan development.

Starting from the mechanism underlying the interaction between metacognition and affect, there is accumulated evidence that our beliefs about learning and cognitive functioning as well as subjective experiences of processing fluency lead us to either accurate or inaccurate control decisions via their influence on metacognitive feelings (e.g., feeling of confidence), even though the mechanism of their interaction is still an open question (Schwartz and Jemstedt, this volume). Further, the emotional salience effect on our JOLs is evidenced in various experimental settings, even though we are far from knowing how various affective factors (either personal or stimulus-related) interact with metacognitive experiences (Witherby, Tauber, and Dunlosky, this volume). The study of our metacognitive illusions, that is, how monitoring, especially the misleading one, "translated" to ineffective control decisions and the moderated or mediated role of various affective factors, is indicated as a prominent goal in future studies. The influences of emotionally charged stimuli/tasks or one's emotional and motivational state seem to play a critical role in understanding the interplay of monitoring and control decisions, not only during cognitive processing in an experimental environment, but, most importantly, in everyday functioning in various settings (e.g., educational, professional) or while we try to accomplish different personal and/or developmental goals (McGillivray, this volume). Monitoring and control have been found to interact with affective factors, such as motivation and emotions, to determine the person's decision making and action.

This line of thinking is now becoming part of theorizing and research in various contexts, including self-regulated learning (e.g., Efklides et al. 2018), decision making (Finn 2010), mindfulness as a booster of well-being (Jankowski and Holas 2014), and development of metacognition in young children (Efklides and Misailidi 2019; Whitebread, this volume). However, there is still much to be learnt about the mechanism underlying the interactions of metacognition with affect and its effects on self-regulation. A key construct in understanding the metacognition x affect interaction, which should be underscored in future attempts, is metacognitive experiences, especially those that are affectively charged. It is clear by now that calibrated metacognitive experiences lead to successful control decisions. Moreover, recent evidence showed that they exert significant influences on the formation and experience of epistemic states that are affectively charged and, via those, on cognitive processing, motivation, and behavior (Vogl, Pekrun, and Loderer, this volume). This line of research is at its first steps and clearly calls for further evidence. Finally, metacognitive experiences may either facilitate or hinder creative operations when they are used as prompts (Antonietti, Cancer, Colombo, and Iannello, this volume). The role of metacognitive processes in different stages of creative thinking is a very promising and fascinating area with relatively less and inconsistent evidence (see review by Jia et al. 2019), which definitely will "widen our mental field."

A second critical factor that impacts metacognition is social interaction in the context of collaborative learning or co-regulation of learning. Social interaction may involve parents, teachers, or peers as sources of feedback and may take place at informal or formal learning contexts. Research evidence on the socially shared metacognitive regulation (SSMR) in educational contexts clearly points out the complexity of relations between different functions of SSMR and learning outcomes (Vauras, Volet, and Iiskala, this volume). The mediated role of social emotions in monitoring and control decisions in self- and co-regulation in collaborative learning environments may explain part of the above complexity (Singh and Muis, this volume). Future studies should focus on the role of various affective reactions as part of the SSMR process, especially those following feedback from peers and teachers. Feedback triggers monitoring and control decisions and could be helpful, according to evidence, provided that it is developmentally appropriate (van Loon and Roebers, this volume). Given that feedback triggers affective reactions as well, future attempts should investigate the moderating role of those reactions. Motivation and affect could shed light on the way students interpret, value, and use feedback to direct their learning efforts. Kramarski, Tzohar-Rozen, and Gadasi (this volume) present evidence for the greatest cognitive gains of a combined metacognitive and emotional support intervention, as compared to a metacognitive support, in young children's problem-solving skills. It is a great challenge for future interventions to address both aspects of self- and co-regulation.

The above results, also, suggest that the role of teachers in fostering self- and co-regulation is critical not only for teaching cognitive and metacognitive strategies and skills but also for helping students to become aware of and regulate their emotions, especially the negative ones. It is more than evidenced in the chapters of the volume that teachers' beliefs, attitudes, and feedback practices do matter. At the same time, recent evidence suggests that teachers lack deeper knowledge regarding the role of metacognition in fostering SRL (Dignath and Büttner 2018). Given that evidence from intervention studies indicates that school-aged students substantially benefit with regard to their achievement from direct metacognitive instruction (see meta-analyses by de Boer et al. 2018 and Donker et al. 2014), future studies should focus on training teachers how to teach and which kind of skills is most critical to teach. Transferring knowledge from research evidence on metacognition and SRL into teaching practice is not an easy task. We have to take into consideration (a) the complexity of the above constructs, (b) the kinds of skills that should be trained, to which students and when, in order to be developmentally appropriate, and (c) how to prepare teachers to implement SRL-related interventions in the classroom (Efklides and Metallidou 2020).

The third critical factor that may interfere with metacognitive monitoring and control is development. Development of metacognition and interactions with affect in the lifespan has not received much attention in the past. However, this trend is changing in an effort to decipher the effects of cognitive and affective theory of mind on self-regulation in young children and older adults. For older adults, metacognition and affect may also be critical for interventions aiming to enhance cognitive functioning. The social roots in the development of metacognition and its interaction with affect and motivation are evidenced from early childhood perception of others' cognitive and affective reactions and children's theory of mind (Misailidi, this volume) to their early social and learning experiences within the family and the school context (Dermitzaki and Kallia, this volume; see also Pino-Pasternak et al. 2019). In fact, as Whitebread argues (this volume), contextual factors and social experiences, such as early parenting and educational practices, play a critical role in the transition from nonconscious metacognitive processes to conscious personal cognitive and emotional awareness. Further, intervention studies for supporting young children's cognitive and emotional regulation through their social networks have been proved very successful, especially for children who are at risk to develop weak regulatory abilities. We need to keep in mind, though, that metacognitive and emotion regulation takes time to develop. It seems that the system needs to assimilate the new knowledge and skills in order to apply and transfer them successfully (Kramarski et al. this volume). Most of the authors of the volume emphasize the need to have an individual differences perspective as well when we try to understand the interplay of metacognition and affect in children. Future studies should also incorporate in their theoretical framework individual differences in cognitive and metacognitive skills, motivation and affect as significant moderators in any attempt to understand or foster monitoring and control processes in children.

The role of self and personal goals is even more critical when we try to understand the interplay of metacognition and affect in adults, especially in older adults and in clinical populations. Recent research evidence suggests that at least some aspects of metacognitive monitoring and control in memory tasks remain intact in older adults, despite certain impairments in their actual memory functioning, and this cannot be explained by their age-related cognitive declines due to neurobiological aging (for reviews, see Castel et al. 2016; Hertzog 2016). Metamemory judgments and control decisions in older adults are clearly affected by motivational and emotional factors, such as interest, the value and importance of to-be-remembered information, or its emotional content (McGillivray, this volume). Older adults are "strategic regulators" even at the expense of their actual performance. Identifying the impact of motivational and affective moderating factors on monitoring and control decisions, not only in experimental memory tasks but in their everyday learning and acting challenges, should direct future research in the area. This would allow us to further inform theories of cognitive aging and to improve the quality of life of older adults through "meaningful" interventions that permit the optimal employment of monitoring and control processes. Metacognitive training in older and younger adults with cognitive deficits is beneficial for both populations not only for their metacognitive functioning but also for their subjective well-being (Bampa et al., this volume). The question, then, for future attempts is under which conditions we could ensure the optimal benefit for the quality of life of older or younger adults with cognitive deficits. At the same time, methodological limitations related to ecological validity of tasks and measures we use in investigating those populations should be acknowledged.

To sum up, the mentioned areas in metacognition research and theory are gaining prominence and have major implications for understanding self- and co-regulation of learning and successful cognitive and social functioning. However, there are also major challenges both methodological and theoretical, particularly with respect to bridging the basic experimental research on metacognition with educational research and research in developmental contexts and vice versa. These challenges will create the prospects for significant breakthroughs in integrated theory in metacognition in the years to come.

References

Castel, A. D., Middlebrooks, C. D., & McGillivray, S. (2016). Monitoring memory in old age: Impaired, spared, and aware. In J. Dunlosky & S. K. Tauber (Eds.), *Oxford handbook of metacognition* (pp. 519–535). New York: Oxford University Press.

De Boer, H., Donker, A. S., Kostons, D. D. N. M., & van der Werf, G. P. C. (2018). Long-term effects of metacognitive strategy instruction on student academic performance: A meta-analysis. *Educational Research Review, 24*, 98–115.

Dignath, C., & Büttner, G. (2018). Teachers' direct and indirect promotion of self-regulated learning in primary and secondary school mathematics classes: Insights from video-based classroom observations and teacher interviews. *Metacognition and Learning, 13*, 127–157.

Donker, A. S., de Boer, H., Kostons, D., Dignath-van Ewijk, C. C., & van der Werf, M. P. C. (2014). Effectiveness of learning strategy instruction on academic performance: A meta-analysis. *Educational Research Review, 11*, 1–26.

Efklides, A. (2006). Metacognition and affect: What can metacognitive experiences tell us about the learning process? *Educational Research Review, 1*, 3–14.

Efklides, A. (2008). Metacognition: Defining its facets and levels of functioning in relation to self-regulation and co-regulation. *European Psychologist, 13*, 277–287.

Efklides, A. (2011). Interactions of metacognition with motivation and affect in self-regulated learning: The MASRL model. *Educational Psychologist, 46*, 6–25.

Efklides, A. (2016). Metamemory and affect. In J. Dunlosky & S. K. Tauber (Eds.), *Oxford handbook of metacognitio*n (pp. 245–267). New York: Oxford University Press.

Efklides, A. (2018). Gifted students and self-regulated learning: The MASRL model and its implications for SRL. *High Abilities Studies*. https://doi.org/10.1080/13598139.2018.1556069

Efklides, A. & Metallidou, P. (2020). Applying metacognition and self-regulated learning in the classroom. In L.-f. Zhang (Ed.), *Oxford research encyclopedia of education*. New York: Oxford University Press. https://doi.org/10.1093/acrefore/9780190264093.013.961

Efklides, A. & Misailidi, P. (2010). (Eds.), *Trends and prospects in metacognition research*. New York: Springer.

Efklides, A., & Misailidi, P. (2019). Emotional self-regulation in the early years: The role of cognition, metacognition and social interaction. In D. Whitebread, V. Grau, K. Kumpulainen, M. McClelland, N. Perry & D. Pino-Pasternak (Eds.), *The Sage handbook of developmental psychology and early childhood education* (pp. 502–516). London: Sage Publications.

Efklides, A., Schwartz, B., & Brown, V. (2018). Motivation and affect in SRL: Does metacognition play a role? In D. Schunk & J. Greene (Eds.), *Handbook of self-regulation of learning and performance* (2nd ed., pp. 64–82). New York: Routledge.

Finn, B. (2010). Ending on a high note: Adding a better end to effortful study. *Journal of Experimental Psychology: Learning, Memory, and Cognition, 36*, 1548–1553.

Flavell, J.H. (1979). Metacognition and cognitive monitoring–A new era of cognitive-developmental inquiry. *American Psychologist, 34*, 906–911.

Hertzog, C. (2016). Aging and metacognitive control. In J. Dunlosky & S.K. Tauber (Eds.), *Oxford handbook of metacognitio*n (pp. 537–558). New York: Oxford University Press.

Jankowski, T., & Holas, P. (2014). Metacognitive model of mindfulness. *Consciousness and Cognition, 28*, 64–80.

Jia, X., Li, W., & Cao, L. (2019). The role of metacognitive components in creative thinking. *Frontiers in Psychology, 10*, 1–11 (2019). https://doi.org/10.3389/fpsyg.2019.02404

Nelson, T. O. (1996). Consciousness and metacognition. *American Psychologist, 51*, 102–116.

Pino-Pasternak, D., Valcan, D., & Malpique, A. (2019). Associations between the home environment, parenting and self-regulation in early childhood. In D. Whitebread, V. Grau, K. Kumpulainen, M. McClelland, N. Perry, & D. Pino-Pasternak (Eds.), *The Sage handbook of developmental psychology and early childhood education* (pp. 487–501). London: Sage Publications.

School of Psychology, Aristotle University of Thessaloniki, Thessaloniki, Greece

Panayiota Metallidou
Despina Moraitou

Contents

Part I
The Mechanism Underlying the Relations Between Metacognition and Affect

Chapter 1
Why Do Emotional Stimuli Influence Judgments of Learning? Theory, Evidence, and Future Directions

Amber E. Witherby, Sarah K. Tauber, and John Dunlosky

Abstract When people monitor their memory, their judgments of how much they have learned are influenced by the emotional valence of the to-be-learned material. A challenge is to discover why emotion influences people's monitoring judgments. Toward meeting this challenge, we discuss theory about how emotions may impact memory monitoring (through beliefs or experiences) and the prevailing evidence relevant to evaluating these theories. To foreshadow, our critical review of the evidence (a) suggests that people's beliefs about the relation between emotion and memory partly explain the effect of emotion on monitoring and (b) reveals avenues for future research to more fully understand the role of emotion in memory monitoring.

Keywords Emotion · Metacognition · Judgments of learning · Emotional-salience effect · Monitoring

1.1 Introduction

Emotion is a vital cue because it can have pervasive influences on people's cognitive processes and behaviors. The impact of emotion on memory in particular has been extensively investigated (for reviews, see Kensinger 2009a, b). In general, people remember emotional information better compared to non-emotional (i.e., neutral) information (for a meta-analysis, see Murphy and Isaacowitz 2008). In contrast to

A. E. Witherby (✉)
Department of Psychology, Iowa State University, Ames, IA, USA
e-mail: witherby@iastate.edu

S. K. Tauber
Department of Psychology, Texas Christian University, Fort Worth, TX, USA
e-mail: uma.tauber@tcu.edu

J. Dunlosky
Department of Psychological Sciences, Kent State University, Kent, OH, USA
e-mail: jdunlosk@kent.edu

D. Moraitou, P. Metallidou (eds.), *Trends and Prospects in Metacognition Research across the Life Span*, https://doi.org/10.1007/978-3-030-51673-4_1

the voluminous literature on emotion and memory, since 1979 when John Flavell's article in the *American Psychologist* (Flavell 1979) ignited interest in people's beliefs, monitoring, and control of their memory (i.e., *metamemory*), limited systematic research has been conducted on the contribution of human emotion to metamemory processes (for a notable exception, emotional responses have been considered a defining feature of tip-of-the-tongue state, Schwartz 2002).

As a major contributor to research on metamemory over the past few decades, Anastasia Efklides reminded us that metamemory researchers should not only consider people's minds and memories but also their emotions. She emphasized the core role that affect and emotions play in people's self-monitoring and self-regulation (e.g., Efklides 2006, 2011, 2016; Efklides and Petkaki 2005), and by doing so, she drew attention to the importance of emotions to our metacognitive experiences and self-regulatory processes. Inspired by her efforts, researchers have recently begun to investigate the relation between emotion and people's judgments of their memory during episodic memory tasks. Accordingly, in the present chapter, our goals are to review the existing literature on how emotion impacts people's memory judgments as well as to provide a theoretical framework for exploring why emotion impacts these judgments. We begin with a brief overview of emotion and metacognitive monitoring and then we review the literature of the impact of emotion on monitoring, followed by a discussion of the theoretical mechanisms that may explain how emotion influences monitoring judgments. We conclude by providing some suggestions for future research that are aimed at further understanding how emotion influences monitoring.

1.2 Overview of Emotion and Metacognitive Monitoring

When investigating memory and metacognition, researchers often ask participants to study items that vary on a single dimension. For instance, participants might study related and unrelated word pairs (e.g., Mueller et al. 2013), concrete and abstract words (e.g., Witherby and Tauber 2017), or words presented in a large or small font (e.g., Rhodes and Castel 2008). By contrast, emotion is a multifaceted construct, and emotional stimuli can vary on the dimensions of valence and arousal (e.g., Bradley et al. 1992; Kensinger and Corkin 2004; Kuppens et al. 2013; Posner et al. 2005). *Valence* refers to a person's subjective emotional evaluation of a given stimulus (e.g., Fairfield et al. 2015). For instance, when viewing a picture of a wedding, a person may feel happy and evaluate it as a positive experience. By contrast, when viewing a picture of a spider, a person may feel afraid and evaluate it as a negative experience. Thus, ratings of valence can range from extremely negative to extremely positive, with mid-levels representing neutral information. *Arousal* refers to an objective measure of a person's level of sympathetic nervous system activation (e.g., Fairfield et al. 2015). That is, arousal represents a person's physiological response to a stimulus. Levels of arousal can range from low (i.e., not arousing) to high (i.e., very arousing). Moreover, these dimensions can interact to create nuanced emotional categories. For instance, a picture of people while water rafting could be considered positive and high on arousal, whereas a picture of a baby kitten could be considered positive and low on arousal.

Metacognitive monitoring refers to people's assessments of their cognitive processes (for a review, see Dunlosky and Metcalfe 2009). Within the domain of memory, monitoring refers to people's evaluations of their own learning and memory. To investigate memory monitoring, participants are presented with information to learn for a later test and make evaluative judgments about their memory. One commonly used judgment, which is the focus of the present chapter, is a *judgment of learning* (JOL). JOLs are prospective memory assessments with which people predict how likely they will be to remember a given item on a future test (for a review, see Rhodes 2016). JOLs have received a great deal of research scrutiny, in part because people use them to make decisions during learning, which can influence later memory (e.g., Dunlosky and Hertzog 1997; Metcalfe and Finn 2008; Thiede 1999; for reviews, see Dunlosky and Ariel 2011; Rhodes 2016). For example, if a person gives an item a high JOL (i.e., indicating that the item has been well learned), she will be unlikely to invest additional resources into learning it. By contrast, if a person gives an item a low JOL (i.e., indicating that the item has been poorly learned), she may devote more study time to it to increase the likelihood that she will remember it later. Given that JOLs play an important role in self-regulated study, much research has been aimed at revealing how people make JOLs, which is the focus of the remainder of this chapter.

To illustrate a typical method used to explore how people make JOLs, consider an experiment in which participants are tasked with learning a list of words that vary in valence. Some of the words are positive (e.g., *money*), some of the words are negative (e.g., *coffin*), and some of the words are neutral (e.g., *chair*). During an initial learning phase, participants study the words and estimate the likelihood that they will remember them on a later test. After studying and judging all words, participants complete a memory test. Using this method, researchers interested in impact of emotion on monitoring have primarily focused on answering two key questions. Does the valence of the to-be-learned information influence people's JOLs? And, if so, how—that is, what is the mechanism that links emotional stimuli to people's JOLs? We discuss the answers to each of these questions in the following sections.

1.3 Impact of Emotion on Judgments of Learning

Does the valence of the to-be learned information influence JOLs? To answer this question, Zimmerman and Kelley (2010, Experiment 2) had participants study and make JOLs for a list of words that were negative and neutral. JOLs were made on a scale from 0 (certain will not recall the word) to 100 (certain will recall the word).

Table 1.1 Review of the literature on the impact of emotion on judgments of learning

Stimuli	Example or explanation	Sources
Single words	Positive: cake, diamond Negative: rat, mold Neutral: office, basket	Hourihan et al. (2017), Tauber and Dunlosky (2012), Tauber et al. (2019), Undorf and Bröder (2020), Undorf et al. (2018), Zimmerman and Kelley (2010)
Word pairs	Positive: circus—treasure Negative: prison—cancer Neutral: violin—avenue	Undorf and Bröder (2020), Zimmerman and Kelley (2010)
Pictures of scenes	Positive: picture of a wedding Negative: picture of a cemetery Neutral: picture of a highway	Hourihan (2019), Hourihan and Bursey (2017), Otani et al. (2014), Tauber et al. (2017)
Pictures of facial expressions	Positive: happy expression Negative: fearful expression Neutral: neutral expression	Nomi et al. (2013), Witherby and Tauber (2018)

After studying and judging all words, participants' memory for the items was tested.[1] JOLs were significantly higher for negative relative to neutral words. In follow-up experiments, Zimmerman and Kelley replicated this outcome and extended it by demonstrating that participants also gave higher JOLs to positive words relative to neutral words. The finding that participants' JOLs are higher for emotional (both positive and negative) relative to neutral words has been termed the *emotional salience effect on JOLs* (Tauber et al. 2017). As reviewed in Table 1.1, this effect has been replicated with several different kinds of stimuli, including single words, word pairs, pictures of emotional and neutral scenes, and pictures of emotional and neutral facial expressions (for similar outcomes with decisions about memorability, see Tomaszczyk and Fernandes 2013).

[1]A test is typically used to evaluate the accuracy of JOLs. Although accuracy has driven many research programs, our interest in the current chapter is on the degree to which differences in emotional stimuli impact JOL magnitude, and why such effects arise. For interested readers, our assessment of the preliminary outcomes (from papers cited in the present chapter) is that JOL accuracy does not consistently differ as a functional of item valence. Given that our current focus is on the JOLs themselves, we will not consider judgment accuracy (or test outcomes) further in this chapter.

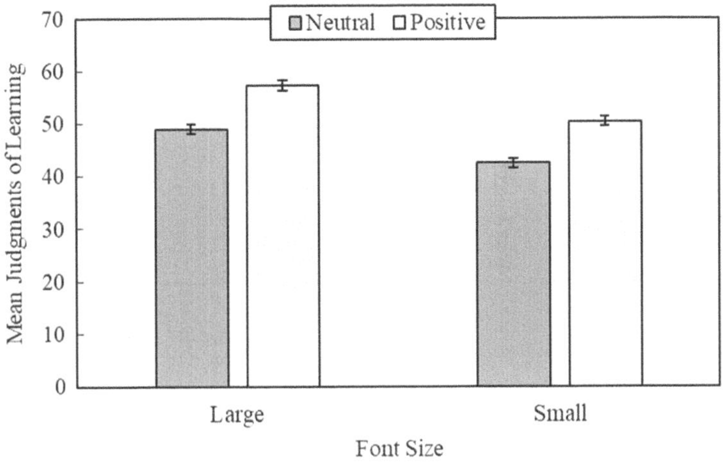

Fig. 1.1 Mean judgments of learning as a function of valence (positive and neutral) and font size (large and small), Witherby and Tauber (unpublished data). Error bars represent within-participant standard error (Loftus and Masson 1994)

When investigating the emotional salience effect on JOLs, researchers have primarily isolated valence as the only stimulus-relevant cue. This procedure is useful for understanding the independent impact of valence on JOLs. It is also important to understand how people integrate cues when making JOLs (cf. Undorf and Bröder 2020; Undorf et al. 2018). Witherby and Tauber (unpublished data) investigated the impact of valence on JOLs when font size also varied.[2] Font size was manipulated because it typically has an impact on JOLs (for a review, see Mueller et al. 2014), and hence we could explore whether one cue—valence or font size—overshadowed the other or whether they have a combined impact on the magnitude of JOLs. Participants studied and made JOLs for a list of words that were positive or neutral. Half of the words were presented in a large font (48 pt) and half of the words were presented in a smaller font (18 pt). As evident in Fig. 1.1, participants gave higher JOLs to positive relative to neutral words, $F(1, 79) = 48.15, p < .001, \eta_p^2 = .38$, and for words presented in a large font relative to words presented in a small font, $F(1, 79) = 36.26, p < .001, \eta_p^2 = .32$. The interaction was not significant, $F < 1$. Thus, participants' JOLs were influenced by both cues, and the effect sizes were large both for the emotional salience effect and the font size effect on JOLs. Most relevant, valence had a strong effect on JOLs even when it was not isolated as the only stimulus-relevant cue.

Nomi et al. (2013) were the first to investigate participants' JOLs for emotional and neutral facial expressions. They presented participants with faces that displayed

[2]For unpublished data discussed in this chapter, we report descriptive and inferential statistics for the raw data, which have been uploaded to the Open Science Framework and can be accessed at https://osf.io/uazkx/

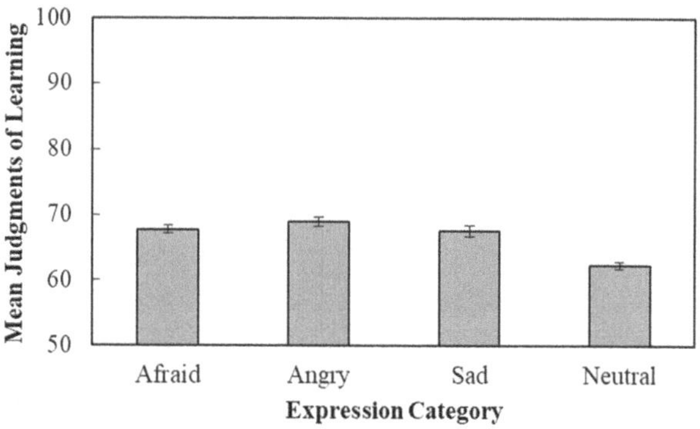

Fig. 1.2 Mean judgments of learning for each expression category. Error bars represent within-participant standard error (Loftus and Masson 1994). Reprinted by permission of Taylor & Francis LTD, http://www.tandfonline.com. (Adapted from Witherby and Tauber 2018)

angry, happy, or neutral expressions. After studying each face, participants identified the emotion that was expressed by selecting "happy", "angry", or "neutral" and made a JOL. Participants demonstrated an emotional salience effect on JOLs, but their JOLs did not differ between the happy and angry expressions. Consistent with Nomi et al. (2013), most of the research presented in Table 1.1 has shown that participants' JOLs do not differ between items of positive and negative valence. Participants typically judge negative information (e.g., a picture of a robbery) and positive information (e.g., a picture of a birthday party) to be equally memorable.

Pictures of facial expressions can provide a more fine-grained evaluation of how different categories of emotion impact participants' JOLs beyond verbal materials. That is, because emotional stimuli are multifaceted, within each level of valence different categories of emotion exist. For instance, negative items could evoke fear, sadness, or anger, and positive items could evoke happiness, love, or satisfaction. Critically, these distinct categories of emotion may uniquely impact JOLs. Witherby and Tauber (2018) investigated the degree to which participants' JOLs discriminate between categories of negative emotion. Participants studied faces that displayed an angry, sad, fearful, or neutral expression. After studying each, participants identified the emotion that was expressed and made a JOL on a scale from 50% to 100%. This scale was used because participants completed a recognition test on which chance performance was at 50%. Although an emotional salience effect was evident, participants' JOLs did not discriminate between angry, sad, and fearful expressions (see Fig. 1.2). That is, participants provided higher JOLs for emotional relative to neutral items, but their JOLs were insensitive to categories of negative emotion.

Although college students' JOLs (who are the majority of participants in JOL studies about emotion) appear to be insensitive to different categories of emotion, older adults may be more sensitive. In particular, according to socioemotional selectivity theory, encoding processes for emotional and neutral stimuli may differ between older and younger adults because older adults are motivated to remember different kinds of emotional information (e.g., Charles et al. 2003; Mather and Carstensen 2005). Younger adults may place equal emphasis on remembering positive and negative experiences (which may explain why their JOLs do not differ for these items) or they may place a greater emphasis on remembering negative relative to positive experiences. By contrast, according to socioemotional selectivity theory, older adults place more emphasis on remembering positive relative to negative experiences. Thus, from this perspective, older adults' JOLs would be expected to discriminate between positive and negative items with JOLs being higher for positive than for negative items. Note, however, that older adults do not always emphasize positive experiences over negative ones (e.g., Denburg et al. 2003; Kensinger et al. 2002; Murphy and Isaacowitz 2008), so their JOLs may not distinguish between categories of emotion (i.e., positive and negative items).

To test these predictions, Tauber and Dunlosky (2012) had older and younger adults study a series of positive, negative, and neutral words and make a JOL for each. Consistent with the previously reviewed research, younger adults provided higher JOLs for positive and negative words compared to neutral words, but their JOLs for positive and negative words did not differ. By contrast, older adults' JOLs were slightly higher for negative words relative to neutral words but were insensitive to positive words. That is, JOLs for positive words were numerically in between their JOLs for negative and neutral words, and they did not significantly differ from either. This outcome is inconsistent with the idea that older adults are biased to focus on positive experiences (as per socioemotional selectivity theory). In follow-up work, Tauber et al. (2017) investigated older and younger adults' JOLs for pictures of positive and neutral scenes. Pictures are more complex than are single words (e.g., Schlochtermeier et al. 2013; Tempel et al. 2013) and often elicit larger emotional effects relative to single words (e.g., De Houwer and Hermans 1994; Kensinger and Schacter 2006). In this case, both older and younger adults gave higher JOLs to positive pictures than to neutral pictures. These outcomes highlight an important consideration for evaluating the impact of emotion on JOLs. Namely, the strength of the emotion manipulation is likely to vary depending on the type of stimuli that are used, which in turn could influence the extent to which participants' JOLs are sensitive to emotion.

1.4 Why Does Emotion Influence Judgments of Learning?

As reviewed above (and in Table 1.1), preliminary research on emotion and JOLs has established two outcomes that require explanation: (a) JOLs are higher for emotional relative to neutral information, and (b) JOLs do not discriminate between categories of emotion. As for explaining these outcomes, current theory indicates that JOLs do not directly tap memory strength but instead are largely inferential; that is, people base their JOLs on any number of cues that are available when the judgment is made (i.e., Koriat 1997). A common assumption of JOL theories is that any cue can influence JOLs via two mechanisms: (a) beliefs about one's learning or (b) experiences or feelings that are triggered while processing the to-be-judged content (Koriat 1997; Mueller and Dunlosky 2017). Regarding beliefs, people have a lifetime of experience learning and remembering information, and thus, they have lay theories about how their memory functions. To illustrate, consider a person who

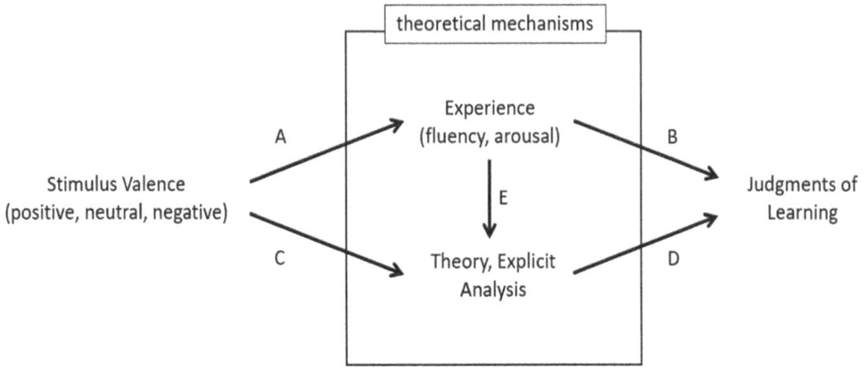

Fig. 1.3 Framework for exploring theoretical explanations for the emotional salience effect wherein stimulus valence influences people's judgments of learning

believes that she is more likely to remember positive information relative to neutral information. She may use her belief to make informed memory predictions by giving higher JOLs to positive items than to neutral items. Concerning experiences or feelings, people's judgments about their learning may also be influenced by feelings that arise while they process the to-be-judged content. For instance, when learning new information, a person may process some items more fluently relative to others. If so, the experience of fluent processing may have a direct impact on her judgments and would result in higher JOLs to items that were processed fluently relative to those that were processed less fluently.

These two factors—beliefs and experiences—are theorized to represent *distinct* contributions to people's judgments. In particular, the contribution of beliefs comprises an explicit, conscious—or analytic—influence on people's judgments. For instance, from the analytic-processing theory (Mueller and Dunlosky 2017), people presumably search for cues about the to-be-judged items that they believe will be relevant to subsequently remembering the items, and then they use those cues to adjust their judgments so as to improve judgment accuracy. By contrast, experiential factors influence judgments in an unconscious, non-analytic manner. This difference in how the two factors impact JOLs is essential, because if experiences also impact judgments via analytic processes then the two factors would not be distinct. That is, if a person experiences that processing a particular item is relatively fluent and then gives that item a higher JOL because she believes fluent processing is associated with better memory, then the experience of fluency itself is simply another cue (one of many) that can impact judgments through beliefs (cf. Dunlosky et al. 2015). In this case, fluency is not special at all and a model of JOLs would include only a single, belief-based mechanism.

Our focus is on explaining the emotional salience effect on the magnitude of JOLs. And, in the model presented in Fig. 1.3, the potential impact of stimulus valence on JOLs is illustrated with respect to the two-factor theory of JOLs described above, in which beliefs and experiences are represented as distinct contributions to people's JOLs. One way in which valence can impact JOLs is by producing different kinds of experiences when processing a to-be-judged item, such as fluent processing of an item or the arousal that could be evoked by an emotionally-laden item. This possible influence of stimulus valence on people's experiences while processing an item is illustrated by Path A. Note, however, that we are not suggesting that valence and these experiences (and in particular, arousal) are perfectly correlated or dependent, because the two can be dissociated and are theoretically and psychologically distinct (as noted above). For instance, a variable other than stimulus valence may be manipulated that is unrelated to valence yet produces emotional arousal, and it would be interesting to evaluate whether it would also impact JOLs. Given that the focus of this review is on the relation between stimulus valence and JOLs, the model illustrates the possible relation between valence and experience as a theoretical pathway that requires empirical investigation to confirm its contribution to emotional salience effects on JOLs.

Most important, the paths in Fig. 1.3 from stimulus valence through *Experience* directly to JOLs (Paths A and B) represent the contribution of experience, whereas the paths through *Theory, Explicit Analysis* (Paths C and D) represent the contribution of beliefs. Path E represents the possibility that experience may impact JOLs through beliefs (as demonstrated by Mueller and Dunlosky 2017). If Path E contributes to JOL effects and Path B does not, then the theory devolves into a single-factor (belief-based) model.[3] Importantly, the contribution of these pathways to how emotion impacts JOLs can be evaluated empirically. In the next sections, we review the available evidence in the context of this model, so as to provide preliminary conclusions on how emotional stimuli impact JOLs and to highlight where further research is needed to fully evaluate predictions from the model.

1.4.1 The Possible Contribution of People's Beliefs

To measure beliefs, researchers commonly construct a vignette of a hypothetical experiment and ask participants to respond to it (cf. Koriat et al. 2004). As a recent example, Jia et al. (2016, Experiment 3a) presented participants with a description of an experiment in which students studied 32 written Chinese words. Half of the words (i.e., 16) were high frequency and half were low frequency. Participants were informed that high frequency words are common because they appear often in

[3]The model in Figure 1.3 highlights pathways that have been commonly investigated in the JOL research, but other perspectives may also be considered. In particular, a reviewer suggested that theory may influence people's experience (a bi-directional arrow on Path E), and others have argued that an unconscious heuristic may mediate the relation between an experience (e.g., fluency) and JOLs. The former idea is intriguing, and other pathways not considered here may also exist. Our discussion will pertain to the pathways represented in Figure 1.3, which provide a useful framework for considering prior research on emotion and JOLs and a great deal of testable hypotheses to drive future research.

both written and spoken form, whereas low frequency words are less common because they appear rarely in either form. Participants estimated that students in the hypothetical experiment would have recalled significantly more high frequency words relative to low frequency words. These outcomes suggest that people believe that high frequency words are easier to learn and remember than are low frequency words. Similarly, researchers have established that people have beliefs about the impact of many other cues on their learning (for a review, see Tauber et al. 2019). Even so, little is known about the contribution of beliefs to the emotional salience effect on JOLs.

To directly probe participants about their beliefs about the impact of emotion on learning, Witherby and Tauber (2018) gave participants a belief survey which described a hypothetical experiment. In the experiment, students studied faces that displayed angry, sad, or afraid expressions. Participants estimated how many of each expression students would have remembered. Most participants (58%) estimated that students would have remembered more faces displaying one emotional expression than the other two. Relative to the other emotional expressions, 53% of these participants gave the highest estimates to angry faces, 33% gave the highest estimates to sad faces, and 14% gave the highest estimates to afraid faces. An additional 34% percent of participants estimated that memory performance would be the same regardless of emotion. The remaining 8% gave the highest estimates to two emotional expressions (e.g., angry and afraid) relative to the other emotion (e.g., sad). Thus, participants had diverse beliefs about the impact of emotion on learning, which supports Path C of the model in Fig. 1.3. Nonetheless, these outcomes do not provide evidence about people's beliefs concerning the memorability of emotional information compared to neutral information. Moreover, although people have beliefs about emotion, these outcomes do not demonstrate the extent to which those beliefs contribute to JOLs.

Other evidence supports the suggestion that people have beliefs about the impact of emotional, relative to neutral, stimuli on their learning and extends it to propose that they may use such beliefs as a basis for their JOLs. This research capitalizes on the fact that emotional stimuli can vary on valence and physiological arousal. Using a clever design, Hourihan et al. (2017, Experiment 2) explored the degree to which valence impacted participants' JOLs. To do so, they used normative ratings of valence and arousal for words. They created word lists for which words differed in valence (neutral versus negative), but not arousal. By doing so, they were able to view the independent contribution of valence to participants' JOLs while holding ratings of arousal constant. JOLs were significantly higher for negative words than for neutral words. From the belief perspective, valence is the cue of most interest because it is likely to contribute to participants' JOLs through beliefs about the impact of emotion on learning. This is because valence is a categorical descriptor (e.g., negative, positive, or neutral), so determining the valence of a to-be-learned item is dependent upon a subjective interpretation of each item. Thus, this outcome suggests that valence contributes to the emotional salience effect on JOLs (i.e., Paths C and D of Fig. 1.3), which is consistent with the belief account of JOLs (cf. Tauber et al. 2017).

The contribution of beliefs to JOLs can also be evaluated using prestudy JOLs (cf. Castel 2008). Prestudy JOLs are given before an item is presented for study, which prevents participants from gaining experience with processing the to-be-judged item. Thus, beliefs will largely contribute to participants' prestudy JOLs, especially for the first items presented for study because participants have limited experience with the items (Mueller et al. 2013). Undorf and Bröder (2020) investigated the impact of valence on JOLs by presenting participants with word pairs that were normatively rated as high on emotion (i.e., emotional word pairs) or low on emotion (i.e., neutral word pairs). Of less interest, they also manipulated the concreteness of the word pairs. Participants either made JOLs immediately after studying the word pairs (i.e., immediate JOLs), or made prestudy JOLs before studying the word pairs. To make prestudy JOLs, participants were told, "you are about to study a word pair with a concreteness of X and an emotionality of Y, please estimate your chance of free recall." The "Y" was replaced with the normative value of the word pair, which ranged from 1 to 7, and participants were told that "words high in emotionality evoke pleasant or unpleasant feelings (e.g., love, poison), whereas words low in emotionality evoke no feelings (e.g., percentage)." Consistent with prior research, immediate JOLs were higher for emotional relative to neutral word pairs. Prestudy JOLs were also higher for emotional than for neutral word pairs. These outcomes are consistent with the hypothesis that people's beliefs contributed to their prestudy JOLs, and likewise, may also contribute to their immediate JOLs.

Taken together, these outcomes are consistent with the hypothesis that beliefs explain at least a portion of the emotional salience effects on JOLs. Even so (and as previously noted), the paucity of research on people's beliefs about how emotion influences their learning warrants a call for more research. First, simply because beliefs on one measure are consistent with the effect of a cue on JOLs does not necessitate the conclusion that beliefs drive the effect of that cue on JOLs. That is, even if participants have a belief that is consistent with their JOLs, the extent to which this belief is used to inform their JOLs is unclear (i.e., evidence for Path C in Fig. 1.3 does not necessitate Path D). To address this issue, experiments need to be designed so that an independent measure of beliefs could be obtained (e.g., global estimates of performance) and used to evaluate whether participants' beliefs mediate the relationship between valence and JOLs (cf. Ariel et al. 2014; Frank and Kuhlmann 2017). Second, participants' beliefs about other cues are not always consistent with the impact of that cue on their JOLs (Frank and Kuhlmann 2017). For instance, younger adults believe that memory declines with aging. However, younger adults' JOLs are not lower when they make them on behalf of an average older adult (vs. an average younger adult), suggesting that younger adults' belief about cognitive aging does not inform their JOLs (Tauber et al. 2019).

Other methodologies have been used to measure participants' beliefs, and they may prove useful in estimating the contribution of beliefs to the emotional salience effects on JOLs. For instance, the learner-observer paradigm is an effective way to measure participants' beliefs (Undorf et al. 2017) and the degree to which both beliefs and experiences (as per Fig. 1.1) contribute to JOL effects (Matvey et al. 2001). With this paradigm, participants view to-be-learned items and make JOLs predicting future memory performance. By contrast, observers view a participant's experience during learning without being instructed to learn and remember any items. Then, they make JOLs predicting recall for that participant, rather than for themselves. Observers arguably rely on their beliefs about cue effects on learning, whereas participants can use both their beliefs and experiences when actually studying the given information (for details on the subtleties of using the learner-observer method, see Matvey et al. 2001).

1.4.2 The Possible Contribution of Experiences During Learning

Although valenced stimuli may be arousing, most often, experiences during learning have been conceptualized in terms of processing fluency, which refers to the ease with which items are processed during learning. Thus, to explore the possibility that the experience of fluent processing while studying contributes to emotion effects on JOLs, a critical question that must be answered first is, are emotional stimuli processed more fluently relative to neutral stimuli? This is represented by Path A in Fig. 1.3.

Some evidence suggests that emotional stimuli can be processed more fluently relative to neutral stimuli. For instance, one way that processing fluency has been investigated is with a lexical decision task (e.g., Mueller et al. 2013; Witherby and Tauber 2017; for limits of using a single measure of fluency, see Yang et al. 2018). Participants are presented with a list of words and non-words (e.g., vaded) and must decide as quickly as possible whether each is a word or not. Shorter response times on this task indicate increased processing fluency. Kuchinke et al. (2007) had participants complete a lexical decision task for which they were presented with non-words and words that were positive, negative, and neutral. In addition, half of the words were high-frequency and half were low-frequency. Of most interest, response times were shorter for positive and negative words relative to neutral words (cf., Challis and Krane 1998; Kuchinke et al. 2005; Kousta et al. 2009; Williamson et al. 1991; for evidence that lexical decision response times do not differ based on valence, see Imbir et al. 2016). Thus, emotional information may be processed more fluently than neutral information (supporting Path A in Fig. 1.3). Given support for Path A of the model (Fig. 1.3), a key issue is whether processing fluency contributes to the emotional salience effect on JOLs (Paths B, D, or E in the model).

Ample evidence suggests that fluency can contribute to other cue effects on JOLs (Besken 2016; Besken and Mulligan 2014; Susser and Mulligan 2015; Susser et al. 2017; Undorf and Erdfelder 2015). As one example, Susser and Mulligan (2015) evaluated the influence of a motoric cue (in this case, handwriting) on participants' JOLs. To do so, participants copied words with their dominant or non-dominant hand and the amount of time to write each was recorded. Writing time provides an

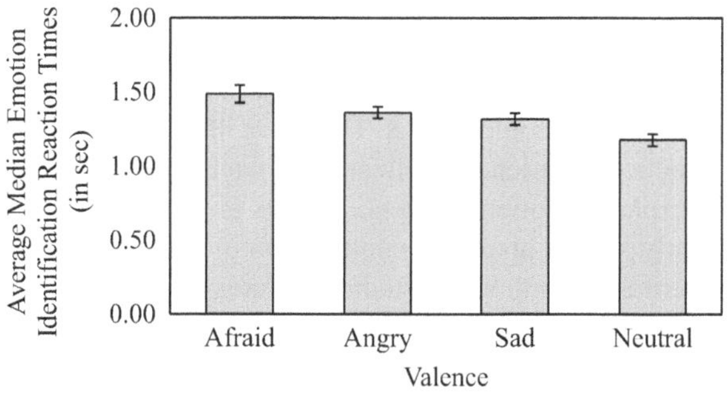

Fig. 1.4 Median response times in an emotion identification task for angry, afraid, sad, and neutral facial expressions (previously unpublished data from Witherby and Tauber 2018). Response times were only included for expressions that were correctly identified. Error bars represent within-participant standard error (Loftus and Masson 1994)

index of fluency, and participants were faster at writing words with their dominant hand than with their non-dominant hand. As important, JOLs were significantly higher for words written by the dominant hand relative to the non-dominant hand, although recall performance did not differ.

Preliminary evidence suggests that processing fluency may not contribute to the emotional salience effect on JOLs. Witherby and Tauber (2018) had participants study a series of afraid, angry, sad, and neutral facial expressions. Participants identified the emotion that was expressed and make a JOL for each. Although participants demonstrated an emotional salience effect on JOLs, response times for the emotion identification task were in the opposite direction of what would be expected if emotional faces were processed more fluently relative to neutral faces. As shown in Fig. 1.4, response times were shorter for neutral faces relative to emotional faces (afraid, $t(45) = 4.35$, $p < .001$, $d = .71$; angry, $t(45) = 3.96$, $p < .001$, $d = .59$; sad, $t(45) = 4.54$, $p < .001$, $d = .69$), and response times did not differ for the three categories of emotional expressions, $ts < 1$[4]. It should be noted that measuring processing fluency was *not* the goal of this research, and as such, design features of the experiment limit the conclusions that should be drawn about the degree to which emotional information is processed more fluently than is neutral information. Thus, additional research is needed to directly evaluate the extent to which processing fluency contributes to the emotional salience effect on JOLs.

The contributions of fluency to cue effects on JOLs are typically small, and in some cases nonexistent. For instance, measures of processing fluency do not always mediate the relationship between a cue and JOLs (e.g., Mueller et al. 2013, 2016; Susser et al. 2016; Witherby and Tauber 2017). And, even when measures of fluency do contribute to cue effects on JOLs, beliefs may still play an important role (e.g.,

[4]The reaction time data were not presented in the original paper. Therefore, the raw data for this experiment has been uploaded to the Open Science Framework and can be accessed at https://osf.io/jra3v/

Frank and Kuhlmann 2017; Mueller et al. 2013; Susser et al. 2017). In addition to the experience of fluent processing, emotional stimuli may produce differences in physiological arousal (another kind of experience in Fig. 1.3) which maybe a central experience that influences people's JOLs. That is, as illustrated in Fig. 1.3, emotional materials may produce experiences of fluency as well as physiological arousal, and both may partly explain emotional salience effects on JOLs.

Little is currently known about the contribution of arousal to emotion effects on JOLs. In one experiment, participants studied pictures of scenes and made a JOL for each (Tauber et al. 2017). The pictures varied in normative ratings of arousal and valence with the variables fully crossed. In other words, the pictures were high-arousal and positive (e.g., loving embrace), low-arousal and positive (e.g., a person fishing), high-arousal and neutral (e.g., pilot in a cockpit), or low-arousal and neutral (e.g., farmer in a field). Participants' JOLs did not differ based on normative ratings of arousal, but they were significantly higher for positive relative to neutral pictures. Thus, an emotional salience effect was evident even when normative ratings of arousal were held constant. This does not support the experience-based account of JOLs (i.e., Path B of Fig. 1.3). Even so, arousal is likely idiosyncratic, so normative ratings of arousal may poorly inform how each individual person will respond (physiologically) to an item and how that physiological response contributes to their JOLs. Thus, a stronger evaluation of arousal to JOLs would require an independent measure of the arousal each participant experienced when learning the words.

In sum, participants' experiences—either fluency or arousal—during learning may play a role in the emotional salience effect on JOLs. However, researchers have yet to systematically explore this possibility. One way to explore it would be to have participants learn emotional materials, measure their experiences during learning, and have them make JOLs for the items. Participants' experiences could be measured using multiple measures of processing fluency (e.g., self-paced study time, lexical decision times, number of trials to acquisition) or multiple measures of physiological arousal (e.g., pupil reactivity, galvanic skin response, respiratory sinus arrhythmia). Moreover, a strong approach to this work would be to conduct mediation analyses to determine if these measures mediate the relationship between valence and JOLs. By doing so, the measures of experiences could be used to simultaneously estimate the degree to which both fluency and arousal could statistically account for the emotional salience effect on JOLs.

1.5 Other Directions for Future Research

The research reviewed in this chapter has advanced our knowledge of the impact of emotion on JOLs. Even so, several issues deserve further attention. The preliminary evidence does not definitively establish any of the complete pathways in the model presented in Fig. 1.3. Thus, as outlined in the prior sections, more research is needed to inform the degree to which participants' beliefs and experiences explain the emotional salience effect on JOLs. In the following sections, we provide additional directions for future research that are necessary for developing a clearer understanding of when and why emotion influences JOLs.

1.5.1 How Does Emotion Influence Monitoring?

One intriguing avenue for future research is to investigate the possible indirect effect of people's experiences during learning on JOLs through their beliefs (i.e., Path E in Fig. 1.3). That is, people may have the belief that emotional items that are processed more easily will be better remembered relative to neutral items that are processed with more difficulty. Similarly, given that emotional items tend to increase physiological arousal, people may believe that emotional items that elicit high arousal are more likely to be remembered than are neutral items that elicit low arousal. Critically, they may use these beliefs about their experiences during learning to make JOLs (cf. Dunlosky et al. 2015; Mueller et al. 2016).

Recent evidence is consistent with this prediction. Mueller and Dunlosky (2017, Experiment 1) had participants learn words that varied in font color—half of the words were presented in blue font and half were presented in green font. Critically, half of the participants were given false information that blue words would be easier to process compared to green words, whereas the remaining participants were not given any instructions regarding how font color influences processing speed. After studying each word, participants made a JOL. Participants who were not given instructions about processing speed gave similar JOLs to blue and green items. By contrast, participants who were told that blue words were easier to process gave higher JOLs to blue words relative to green words. This effect was replicated when participants were told that green words were easier to process compared to blue words (i.e., JOLs were higher for green relative to blue words). Moreover, in two experiments, Mueller and Dunlosky (2017) demonstrated that font color did not influence processing speed as measured with a lexical decision task (Experiment 6) and with self-paced study time (Experiment 7). Thus, participants used inaccurate beliefs about processing fluency to make JOLs.

One test of whether a mechanism contributes to the emotional salience effect on JOLs requires evidence that the variance in the measure of a given mechanism (e.g., beliefs and/or experiences) mediates the relationship between stimulus valence and participants' JOLs. Thus, experimental designs measuring (a) participants' beliefs about emotion, (b) participants' experiences when learning emotional and neutral information, and (c) participants' beliefs about those experiences would provide informative evidence both for the direct roles of beliefs (i.e., Path B) and experiences (i.e., Path D) in the emotional salience effect on JOLs, as well as the indirect role of experiences through participants' beliefs (i.e., Path E).

Another important goal for research will be to evaluate how, and why, valence influences other metacognitive judgments (e.g., feeling of knowing judgments, confidence judgments, ease of learning judgments). The influence of valence on remember/know judgments has received some empirical attention (e.g., Ochsner 2000; Phelps and Sharot 2008; Sharot et al. 2004). In the remember/know paradigm, participants are presented with a list of items to learn followed by a recognition test. On the recognition test, participants judge whether they remember the item (i.e., they can recollect specific details about the item), know the item (i.e., it feels familiar, but they cannot recollect specific details), or if it is new (i.e., it was not presented during study). In general, people are more likely to "remember" negative information compared to positive or neutral information, and they are more likely to "know" positive and neutral information compared to negative information (e.g., Mickley and Kensinger 2008; Ochsner 2000). In addition, some researchers have investigated how valence influences tip-of-the-tongue (TOT) states. Currently, evidence is mixed with some evidence that TOT states are more likely for emotional compared to non-emotional information (e.g., Schwartz 2010) and some evidence that TOT states are uninfluenced by valence (e.g., D'Angelo and Humphreys 2012).

In this chapter, we have been interested almost exclusively in how stimulus valence impacts JOLs. But, JOLs may also be influenced by a person's current emotional state (i.e., mood), which is another aspect of emotion that we briefly consider here. For instance, when people are in a negative mood, they may feel pessimistic about their learning and predict that they will not remember much of the information. By contrast, when people are in a positive mood, they may feel optimistic and predict that they will remember a lot of the information. Initial work has established that positive mood, relative to negative or neutral moods, tends to lead to increased retrospective confidence judgments, whereas mood typically has little effect on performance (e.g., Ifcher and Zarghamee 2014; Sidi et al. 2018; Prinz et al. 2019). Thus, positive mood appears to result in overconfidence when compared with negative and neutral moods. Future work exploring how mood influences other judgments (e.g., JOLs) will be important for developing a more complete understanding of the role of emotion on metacognitive monitoring. Like valence of the to-be-learned information, mood could influence people's judgments through their beliefs about mood or through their experiences during learning (cf. Figure 1.3). Moreover, mood could interact with the valence of the to-be-learned information to influence judgments. For instance, an interesting empirical question is whether people will show mood-congruent judgments (e.g., higher JOLs for negative items when the person is in a negative mood). If so, is this driven by beliefs (e.g., a person has the belief that they will remember negative information better relative to positive or neutral information when in a negative mood) or experiences (e.g., negative items are processed more fluently than are positive or neutral items when a person is in a negative mood)?

1.5.2 Individual Differences

Most of the current research has explored the extent to which emotion influences JOLs for college-aged participants. Thus, an important goal will be to evaluate the generalizability of the emotional salience effect on JOLs with other populations. The strength of each path in the model presented in Fig. 1.3 may vary for different groups of people because the mechanisms that contribute to emotion effects on JOLs may differ.

Evidence from two publications have shown that older adults use emotion to inform their JOLs in a similar fashion as do younger adults (Tauber and Dunlosky 2012; Tauber et al. 2017). However, this effect appears to be attenuated when older adults make JOLs for positive and neutral words (Tauber and Dunlosky 2012). Additional work is necessary to (a) replicate the effects and (b) evaluate how emotion impacts JOLs when older adults learn other kinds of materials (e.g., emotional and neutral facial expressions). It will also be important to explore the mechanisms that contribute to older adults' JOLs, because researchers have yet to evaluate the extent to which fluency and beliefs contribute to any cue effect on JOLs for older adults. Moreover, exploring the contribution of fluency and beliefs to their JOLs for emotional information in particular will be necessary for increasing understanding the emotional salience effect on JOLs.

In addition, researchers have recently begun exploring how non-typically developing individuals monitor their learning. For instance, in only two studies have researchers investigated how individuals with Autism Spectrum Disorder (ASD) monitor their learning with JOLs, and in both cases, participants learned neutral information (Grainger et al. 2016; Wojcik et al. 2014). The conclusion from these studies is that monitoring abilities appear to be spared in individuals with ASD. That is, their JOLs are similar to, and as accurate as, typically developing individuals. Nonetheless, individuals with ASD have deficits that are specific to processing and responding to emotional information (e.g., Mazefsky et al. 2013). Thus, valence may impact JOLs differently for individuals with ASD compared to typically developing individuals. Given that individuals with ASD may have different beliefs about learning emotional information (e.g., they may be aware that emotional information is challenging for them) or they may have different experiences when learning emotional and neutral information (e.g., they may process neutral information more fluently relative to emotional information), they may not show an emotional salience effect on JOLs and may even show the opposite effect and provide higher JOLs for neutral information relative to emotional information. Exploring how valence influences JOL magnitude for individuals with ASD, relative to typically developing individuals, will be important for understanding whether they have deficits when monitoring their learning of emotional information. If individuals with ASD do have impairments when monitoring their learning of emotional information, this may contribute to their more general deficits with responding appropriately to emotional information. Exploring this issue is critical so that, if need be, interventions can be developed to attenuate any impairments.

1.6 Concluding Remarks

In the past decade, increased emphasis has been placed on understanding how people monitor their learning of emotional information. And, since Anastasia Efklides' pioneering work on the role of affect in metacognition, robust emotional salience effects on JOLs have been demonstrated. Specifically, people predict that emotional information is more likely to be remembered than is neutral information. Even so, many unanswered questions remain. How do people's beliefs about emotion and experiences when learning emotional information impact their JOLs? Does processing fluency differ for emotional and neutral information, and if so, does this contribute to people's JOLs? Does physiological arousal contribute to JOLs? And, can the role of fluency and arousal in people's JOLs be accounted for by their beliefs? Do individual differences moderate the emotional salience effect on JOLs? If so, why? Answering these questions (as well as others) will be important for moving forward JOL theory.

Acknowledgments The writing of this chapter was supported by the James S. McDonnell Foundation 21st Century Science Initiative in Understanding Human Cognition Collaborative Activity Grant under grant number 220020483.

References

Ariel, R., Hines, J. C., & Hertzog, H. (2014). Test framing generates a stability bias for predictions of learning by causing people to discount their learning beliefs. *Journal of Memory and Language, 75*, 181–198.

Besken, M. (2016). Picture-perfect is not perfect for metamemory: Testing the perceptual fluency hypothesis with degraded images. *Journal of Experimental Psychology: Learning, Memory, and Cognition, 42*, 1417–1433.

Besken, M., & Mulligan, N. W. (2014). Perceptual fluency, auditory generation, and metamemory: Analyzing the perceptual fluency hypothesis in the auditory modality. *Journal of Experimental Psychology: Learning, Memory, and Cognition, 40*, 429–440.

Bradley, M. M., Greenwald, M. K., Petry, M. C., & Lang, P. J. (1992). Remembering pictures: Pleasure and arousal in memory. *Journal of Experimental Psychology: Learning, Memory, and Cognition, 18*, 379–390.

Castel, A. D. (2008). Metacognition and learning about primacy and recency effects in free recall: The utilization of intrinsic and extrinsic cues when making judgments of learning. *Memory & Cognition, 36*, 429–437.

Challis, B. H., & Krane, R. V. (1998). Mood induction and the priming of semantic memory in a lexical decision task: Asymmetric effects of elation and depression. *Bulletin of the Psychonomic Society, 26*, 309–312.

Charles, S. T., Mather, M., & Carstensen, L. L. (2003). Aging and emotional memory: The forgettable nature of negative images for older adults. *Journal of Experimental Psychology: General, 132*, 310–324.

D'Angelo, M. C., & Humphreys, K. R. (2012). Emotional cues do not increase the likelihood of tip-of-the-tongue states. *Memory & Cognition, 40*, 1331–1338.

De Houwer, J., & Hermans, D. (1994). Differences in the affective processing of words and pictures. *Cognition and Emotion, 8*, 1–20.

Denburg, N. L., Buchanan, T. W., Tranel, D., & Adolphs, R. (2003). Evidence for preserved emotional memory in normal older persons. *Emotion, 3*, 239–253.
Dunlosky, J., & Ariel, R. (2011). Self-regulated learning and the allocation of study time. In B. H. Ross (Ed.), *The psychology of learning and motivation: Advances in research and theory* (Vol. 54, pp. 103–140). San Diego: Elsevier Academic Press.
Dunlosky, J., & Hertzog, C. (1997). Older and younger adults use a functionally identical algorithm to select items for restudy during multitrial learning. *The Journals of Gerontology: Series B: Psychological Sciences and Social Sciences, 52*, 178–186.
Dunlosky, J., & Metcalfe, J. (2009). *Metacognition*. Thousand Oaks: Sage.
Dunlosky, J., Mueller, M. L., & Tauber, S. K. (2015). The contribution of processing fluency (and beliefs) to people's judgments of learning. In D. S. Lindsay, A. P. Yonelinas, & H. L. Roediger (Eds.), *Remembering: Attributions, processes, and control in human memory: Essays in honor of Larry Jacoby* (pp. 46–64). New York: Psychology Press.
Efklides, A. (2006). Metacognitive experiences: The missing link in the self-regulated learning process. *Educational Psychology Review, 18*, 287–291.
Efklides, A. (2011). Interactions of metacognition with motivation and affect in self-regulated learning: The MASRL model. *Educational Psychologist, 46*, 6–25.
Efklides, A. (2016). Metamemory and affect). In J. Dunlosky & S. K. Tauber (Eds.), *The Oxford handbook of metamemory* (pp. 245–267). New York: Oxford University Press.
Efklides, A., & Petkaki, C. (2005). Effects of mood on students' metacognitive experiences. *Learning and Instruction, 15*, 415–431.
Fairfield, B., Mammarella, N., Palumbo, R., & Di Domenico, A. (2015). Emotional metamemories: A review. *Brain Sciences, 5*, 509–520.
Flavell, J. H. (1979). Metacognition and cognitive monitoring: A new area of cognitive developmental inquiry. *American Psychologist, 34*, 906–911.
Frank, D. J., & Kuhlmann, B. G. (2017). More than just beliefs: Experience and beliefs jointly contribute to volume effects on metacognitive judgments. *Journal of Experimental Psychology: Learning, Memory, and Cognition, 43*, 680–693.
Grainger, C., Williams, D. M., & Lind, S. E. (2016). Judgment of learning accuracy in high-functioning adolescents and adults with autism spectrum disorder. *Journal of Autism and Developmental Disorders, 46*, 3570–3582.
Hourihan, K. L. (2019). Misleading emotions: Judgments of learning overestimate recognition of negative and positive emotional images. *Cognition and Emotion, 34*, 1–12.
Hourihan, K. L., & Bursey, E. (2017). A misleading feeling of happiness: Metamemory for positive emotional and neutral pictures. *Memory, 25*, 35–43.
Hourihan, K. L., Fraundorf, S. H., & Benjamin, A. S. (2017). The influences of valence and arousal on judgments of learning and on recall. *Memory and Cognition, 45*, 121–136.
Ifcher, J., & Zarghamee, H. (2014). Affect and overconfidence: A laboratory investigation. *Journal of Neuroscience, Psychology, and Economics, 7*, 125–150.
Imbir, K. K., Spustek, T., & Żygierewicz, J. (2016). Effects of valence and origin of emotions in word processing evidenced by event related potential correlates in a lexical decision task. *Frontiers in Psychology, 7*, 1–14.
Jia, X., Li, P., Li, X., Zhang, Y., Cao, W., Cao, L., & Li, W. (2016). The effect of word frequency on judgments of learning: Contributions of beliefs and processing fluency. *Frontiers in Psychology, 6*, 1–10.
Kensinger, E. A. (2009a). *Emotional memory across the adult lifespan*. New York: Psychology Press.
Kensinger, E. A. (2009b). Remembering the details: Effects of emotion. *Emotion Review, 1*, 99–113.
Kensinger, E. A., & Corkin, S. (2004). The effects of emotional content and aging on false memories. *Cognitive, Affective, & Behavioral Neuroscience, 4*, 1–9.
Kensinger, E. A., & Schacter, D. L. (2006). Processing emotional pictures and words: Effects of valence and arousal. *Cognitive, Affective, & Behavioral Neuroscience, 6*, 110–126.

Kensinger, E. A., Brierley, B., Medford, N., Growdon, J. H., & Corkin, S. (2002). Effects of normal aging and Alzheimer's disease on emotional memory. *Emotion, 2*, 118–134.
Koriat, A. (1997). Monitoring one's own knowledge during study: A cue-utilization approach to judgments of learning. *Journal of Experimental Psychology: General, 126*, 349–370.
Koriat, A., Bjork, R. A., Sheffer, L., & Bar, S. K. (2004). Predicting one's own forgetting: The role of experience-based and theory-based processes. *Journal of Experimental Psychology: General, 133*, 643–656.
Kousta, S.-T., Vinson, D. P., & Vigliocco, G. (2009). Emotion words, regardless of polarity, have a processing advantage over neutral words. *Cognition, 112*, 473–481.
Kuchinke, L., Jacobs, A. M., Grubich, C., Võ, M. L.-H., Conrad, M., & Herrmann, M. (2005). Incidental effects of emotional valence in single word processing: An fMRI study. *NeuroImage, 28*, 1022–1032.
Kuchinke, L., Võ, M. L.-H., Hofmann, M., & Jacobs, A. M. (2007). Pupillary responses during lexical decisions vary with word frequency but not emotional valence. *International Journal of Psychophysiology, 65*, 132–140.
Kuppens, P., Tuerlinckx, F., Russell, J. A., & Barrett, L. F. (2013). The relation between valence and arousal in subjective experience. *Psychological Bulletin, 139*, 917–940.
Loftus, G. R., & Masson, M. E. J. (1994). Using confidence intervals in within-subject designs. *Psychonomic Bulletin and Review, 1*, 476–490.
Mather, M., & Carstensen, L. L. (2005). Aging and motivated cognition: The positivity effect in attention and memory. *Trends in Cognitive Sciences, 9*, 496–502.
Matvey, G., Dunlosky, J., & Guttentag, R. (2001). Fluency of retrieval at study affects judgments of learning (JOLs): An analytic or nonanalytic basis for JOLs? *Memory and Cognition, 29*, 222–233.
Mazefsky, C. A., Herrington, J., Siegel, M., Scarpa, A., Maddox, B. B., Scahill, L., & White, S. W. (2013). The role of emotion regulation in autism spectrum disorder. *Journal of the American Academy of Child and Adolescent Psychiatry, 52*, 679–688.
Metcalfe, J., & Finn, B. (2008). Evidence that judgments of learning are causally related to study choice. *Psychonomic Bulletin and Review, 15*, 174–179.
Mickley, K. R., & Kensinger, E. A. (2008). Emotional valence influences the neural correlates associated with remembering and knowing. *Cognitive, Affective, & Behavioral Neuroscience, 8*, 143–152.
Mueller, M. L., & Dunlosky, J. (2017). How beliefs can impact judgments of learning: Evaluating analytic processing theory with beliefs about fluency. *Journal of Memory and Language, 93*, 245–258.
Mueller, M. L., Tauber, S. K., & Dunlosky, J. (2013). Contributions of beliefs and processing fluency to the effect of relatedness on judgments of learning. *Psychonomic Bulletin and Review, 20*, 378–384.
Mueller, M. L., Dunlosky, J., Tauber, S. K., & Rhodes, M. G. (2014). The font-size effect on judgments of learning: Does it exemplify fluency effects or reflect people's beliefs about memory? *Journal of Memory and Language, 70*, 1–12.
Mueller, M. L., Dunlosky, J., & Tauber, S. K. (2016). The effect of identical word pairs on people's metamemory judgments: What are the contributions of processing fluency and beliefs about memory? *The Quarterly Journal of Experimental Psychology, 69*, 781–799.
Murphy, N. A., & Isaacowitz, D. M. (2008). Preferences for emotional information in older and younger adults: A meta-analysis of memory and attention tasks. *Psychology and Aging, 23*, 263–286.
Nomi, J. S., Rhodes, M. G., & Cleary, A. M. (2013). Emotional facial expressions differentially influence predictions and performance for face recognition. *Cognition and Emotion, 27*, 141–149.
Ochsner, K. N. (2000). Are affective events richly recollected or simply familiar? The experience and process of recognizing feelings past. *Journal of Experimental Psychology: General, 129*, 242–261.

Otani, H., Von Glahn, N. R., Libkuman, T. M., Goernert, P. N., & Kato, K. (2014). Emotional salience and the isolation effect. *Journal of General Psychology, 141*, 35–46.

Phelps, E. A., & Sharot, T. (2008). How (and why) emotion enhances the subjective sense of recollection. *Current Directions in Psychological Science, 17*, 147–152.

Posner, J., Russell, J. A., & Peterson, B. S. (2005). The circumplex model of affect: An integrative approach to affective neuroscience, cognitive development, and psychopathology. *Development and Psychopathology, 17*, 715–734.

Prinz, A., Bergmann, V., & Wittwer, J. (2019). Happy but overconfident: Positive affect leads to inaccurate metacomprehension. *Cognition and Emotion, 33*, 606–615.

Rhodes, M. G. (2016). Judgments of learning: Methods, data, and theory. In J. Dunlosky & S. K. Tauber (Eds.), *The Oxford handbook of metamemory* (p. 6580). New York: Oxford University Press.

Rhodes, M. G., & Castel, A. D. (2008). Memory predictions are influenced by perceptual information: Evidence for metacognitive illusions. *Journal of Experimental Psychology: General, 137*, 615–625.

Schlochtermeier, L. H., Kuchinke, L., Pehrs, C., Urton, K., Kappelhoff, H., & Jacobs, A. M. (2013). Emotional picture and word processing: An fMRI study on effects of stimulus complexity. *PLoS One, 8*, e55619.

Schwartz, B. L. (2002). *Tip-of-the-tongue states: Phenomenology, mechanism, and lexical retrieval*. Mahwah: Lawrence Erlbaum Associates Publishers.

Schwartz, B. L. (2010). The effects of emotion on tip-of-the-tongue states. *Psychonomic Bulletin and Review, 17*, 82–87.

Sharot, T., Delgado, M. R., & Phelps, E. A. (2004). How emotion enhances the feeling of remembering. *Nature Neuroscience, 7*, 1376–1380.

Sidi, Y., Ackerman, R., & Erez, A. (2018). Feeling happy and (over)confident: The role of positive affect in metacognitive processes. *Cognition and Emotion, 32*, 876–884.

Susser, J. A., & Mulligan, N. W. (2015). The effect of motoric fluency on metamemory. *Psychonomic Bulletin and Review, 22*, 1014–1019.

Susser, J. A., Jin, A., & Mulligan, N. W. (2016). Identity priming consistently affects perceptual fluency but only affects metamemory when primes are obvious. *Journal of Experimental Psychology: Learning, Memory, and Cognition, 42*, 657–662.

Susser, J. A., Panitz, J., Buchin, Z., & Mulligan, N. W. (2017). The motoric fluency effect on metamemory. *Journal of Memory and Language, 95*, 116–123.

Tauber, S. K., & Dunlosky, J. (2012). Can older adults accurately judge their learning of emotional information? *Psychology and Aging, 27*, 924–933.

Tauber, S. K., Dunlosky, J., Urry, H. L., & Opitz, P. C. (2017). The effects of emotion on younger and older adults' monitoring of learning. *Aging, Neuropsychology, and Cognition, 24*, 555–574.

Tauber, S. K., Witherby, A. E., & Dunlosky, J. (2019). Beliefs about memory decline in aging do not impact judgments of learning (JOLs): A challenge for belief-based explanations of JOLs. *Memory and Cognition, 47*, 1102–1119.

Tempel, K., Kuchinke, L., Urton, K., Schlochtermeier, L. H., Kappelhoff, H., & Jacobs, A. M. (2013). Effects of positive pictograms and words: An emotional word superiority effect? *Journal of Neurolinguistics, 26*, 637–648.

Thiede, K. W. (1999). The importance of monitoring and self-regulation during multitrial learning. *Psychonomic Bulletin and Review, 6*, 662–667.

Tomaszczyk, J. C., & Fernandes, M. A. (2013). A positivity effect in older adults' memorability judgments of pictures. *Experimental Aging Research, 39*, 254–274.

Undorf, M., & Bröder, A. (2020). Cue integration in metamemory judgments is strategic. *Quarterly Journal of Experimental Psychology, 73*, 629–642.

Undorf, M., & Erdfelder, E. (2015). The relatedness effect on judgments of learning: A closer look at the contribution of processing fluency. *Memory & Cognition, 43*, 647–658.

Undorf, M., Zimdahl, M. F., & Bernstein, D. M. (2017). Perceptual fluency contributes to effects of stimulus size on judgments of learning. *Journal of Memory and Language, 92*, 293–304.

Undorf, M., Söllner, A., & Bröder, A. (2018). Simultaneous utilization of multiple cues in judgments of learning. *Memory and Cognition, 46*, 507–519.

Williamson, S., Harpur, T. J., & Hare, R. D. (1991). Abnormal processing of affective words by psychopaths. *Psychophysiology, 28*, 260–273.

Witherby, A. E., & Tauber, S. K. (2017). The concreteness effect on judgments of learning: Evaluating the contribution of fluency and beliefs. *Memory and Cognition, 45*, 639–650.

Witherby, A. E., & Tauber, S. K. (2018). Monitoring of learning for emotional faces: How do fine-grained categories of emotion influence participants' judgments of learning and beliefs about memory? *Cognition and Emotion, 32*, 860–866.

Wojcik, D. Z., Waterman, A. H., Lestié, C., Moulin, C. J., & Souchay, C. (2014). Metacognitive judgments-of-learning in adolescents with autism spectrum disorder. *Autism, 18*, 393–408.

Yang, C., Huang, T. S.-T., & Shanks, D. R. (2018). Perceptual fluency affects judgments of learning: The font size effect. *Journal of Memory and Language, 99*, 99–110.

Zimmerman, C. A., & Kelley, C. M. (2010). "I'll remember this!". Effects of emotionality on memory predictions versus memory performance. *Journal of Memory and Language, 62*, 240–253.

Chapter 2
The Role of Fluency and Dysfluency in Metacognitive Experiences

Bennett L. Schwartz and Andreas Jemstedt

Abstract Metacognition is a broad term that means different things to researchers in different sub-areas. A major contribution of Anastastia Efklides is to bring together disparate approaches in metacognition under one theoretical perspective. In this paper, we examine the concept of fluency and how it has been employed in metacognition research. Fluency-based judgments are generally considered to be the primary source of inaccuracy of metacognitive judgments as well as the primary reason why metacognitive control goes astray in self-regulated learning. We discuss how and when fluent processing influences metacognition, when fluency leads to accurate judgments and when it leads to illusions.

Keywords Metacognition · Fluency · Judgments of learning · Self-regulated learning · Illusions

2.1 Introduction

Metacognition is a broad term that means many different things to researchers in different sub-areas of Psychology (Metcalfe and Son 2012; Proust 2015; Wells and Colbear 2012). In general, it means cognition about cognition, but this definition is so vague as to be useless. In some cases, metacognition may refer to the cognitive processes that underlie our thinking, whereas in other cases, metacognition may refer to the thoughts themselves, if those thoughts' content is our own thinking. Thus, the process by which we assess whether we have learned a new word is metacognition, but so too is the conscious thought that the item has been learned. Thus, any

B. L. Schwartz (✉)
Florida International University, Miami, FL, USA
e-mail: schwartb@fiu.edu

A. Jemstedt
Stockholm University, Stockholm, Sweden
e-mail: andreas.jemstedt@psychology.su.se

D. Moraitou, P. Metallidou (eds.), *Trends and Prospects in Metacognition Research across the Life Span*, https://doi.org/10.1007/978-3-030-51673-4_2

discussion of metacognition requires some defining of the approach one is taking to the topic. One of the major contributions of Anastastia Efklides is to bring together disparate approaches in metacognition under one theoretical perspective (Efklides 2008, 2011, 2016, 2018; Efklides et al. 2018). Indeed, her work on metacognition, more than anyone's, has brought the theoretical and applied perspectives of Educational psychology and Cognitive psychology together.

At the risk of simplifying her theory, Efklides divides metacognition into two interdependent domains. First, there is metacognitive knowledge, which refers to explicit verbalizable beliefs that we have about how our minds work (Efklides 2011; also see Flavell 1979). Thus, I may know that I am poor at recognizing faces, I may think that further study in preparation of a test is unnecessary as I have learned everything, and I may believe that, at my age, I will not be able to learn to speak Greek. Knowledge has the property of being right or wrong. For example, on standardized tests, despite my belief about my sub-par face recognition ability, I may actually score better than the median (that is, I am above average) on face recognition. Second, there are metacognitive experiences which refers to the feelings that we experience as we learn, remember, and think about our own learning. For example, I may feel that I have studied this translation pair sufficiently to remember it on a test or I may feel like I can remember a word, even though at the moment I cannot recall it (e.g., Schwartz and Cleary 2016). Metacognitive experiences are inherently subjective—they may be correlated with later memory performance, but the inability to later recall a word does not mean that the tip-of-the-tongue state was not experienced genuinely (Arango-Muñoz 2019). That is, our metacognitive experiences occur regardless of whether they are accurate or not. Our research has focused on metacognitive experience, and we will explore this aspect of metacognition throughout this chapter.

Another important aspect of Efklides' contribution to the field of metacognition has been her attention to self-regulated learning (2011, 2018). Self-regulated learning refers to how people channel their cognitive resources, time, and effort in order to master new learning. For example, a student may have to choose what topic to study, when to study it, and what study strategy to adopt. Efklides has been one of the leaders of the optimist approach to self-regulated learning, arguing that when left to themselves, most people engage in relatively efficient means of directing their own learning (Efklides et al. 2018). Others are more pessimistic and point out all the errors, illusions, and misconceptions that can derail a person's efficient studying (Bjork et al. 2013). In this paper, we will discuss when fluency is adaptive and leads people to study the right way as well as when it leads them astray, creating illusions. Resolving the conflict between the optimists and the pessimists in the role of metacognition in self-regulated learning is yet another important contribution of Efklides' work.

Almost from the beginning of research on metacognition, researchers have conducted studies that concern how fluency (the ease of processing stimuli) or familiarity (whether stimuli have been encountered recently) affects judgments (Begg et al. 1989; Nelson and Narens 1990; Reder 1987). Early in the study of metacognition it became apparent that mechanisms that underlie metacognition often did not directly measure the strength of memory storage (or retrieval strength) but relied on heuristic information which in many cases were correlated with memory strength (Koriat 1993; Metcalfe 1993). Among these heuristics are the ease of which an item was studied, retrieved, or even perceived. In other words, processing fluency influences our metacognitive judgments. The idea is that processing fluency can be potentially misleading because an item that is perceived or processed fluently will be judged as likely to be remembered, even when fluency does not correlate with better performance. Thus, fluency may cause us to underestimate the difficulty we will have learning the item or remembering it later (Undorf et al. 2017). As such, we suspect that fluency-based judgments are considered to be a source of inaccuracy of metacognitive judgments as well as the primary reason why metacognitive control goes astray in self-regulated learning. In this chapter, we explore situations in which fluency is predictive of later performance, and we will also consider if fluency can be used to help with self-regulated learning. We will also consider many of the situations in which fluency does indeed produce illusory confidence. But to start, we give a general review on what processing fluency is and how it affects metamemory (see Reber and Greifeneder 2017 for a review).

2.2 Processing Fluency

Processing fluency refers to the ease of perceiving a particular stimulus or the ease of retrieving a particular item from memory (see Alter and Oppenheimer 2009; Jemstedt et al. 2018; Undorf et al. 2018). Fluency itself may be considered experiential in nature, that is, it is the feeling of how a cognitive process is operating (Oppenheimer 2008). Indeed, Oppenheimer (2008) defines fluency as "Fluency—the subjective experience of ease or difficulty with which we are able to process information—is one of the most prominent metacognitive cues used in reasoning." (p. 237). Processing fluency is divided into several distinct sub-categories (Reber and Greifeneder 2017). Reber and Greifeneder define four categories of fluency during cognitive processing. Perceptual fluency is the ease by which information is processed during perception or during its first encounter. Encoding fluency is the ease by which new information can be assimilated into memory. Conceptual fluency is the ease by which we can understand new information. Lastly, retrieval fluency is the ease by which information is retrieved from memory. For our purposes here, we focus on two of those categories—perceptual fluency and retrieval fluency. Perceptual fluency is how fluently people can perceive a stimulus. Researchers have manipulated perceptual fluency by changing perceptual aspects of a given stimulus to make them easier or more difficult to perceive. Thus, a bright stimulus has higher perceptual fluency than a much dimmer stimulus. In experiments, perceptual fluency has been manipulated in a number of ways. For example, perceptual fluency has been manipulated by presenting words in alternating upper- and lower-case letters (low fluency) compared to only upper-case letters (high fluency) (e.g., Jemstedt et al. 2018), by presenting words in large fonts compared to small fonts (e.g., Rhodes and

Castel 2008), and by presenting words in a clear font compared to an unclear font (e.g., Simmons and Nelson 2006).

Retrieval fluency refers to how easily or quickly information is retrieved from memory (e.g., Benjamin et al. 1998). For example, when asked the capital of France, Paris comes to mind quickly, demonstrating high retrieval fluency. However, it may take longer to retrieve that Dushanbe is the capital of Tajikistan, meaning lower retrieval fluency. Similarly, a recently presented item on a serial list will be more easily retrieved than one from the pre-recency part of the list. Benjamin et al. showed that in both of these situations people rely on retrieval fluency to make judgments of learning (JOLs), that is, predictions of future recall based on current learning, even though such retrieval fluency does not predict later free recall. For instance, in Experiment 1, when participants were given general-information questions, such as "What is the capital of Jamaica?". Retrieval fluency of the answers ("Kingston") predicted the JOLs participants made for later free recall. However, later when the free recall test was given, low-fluency answers were more likely to be recalled than high-fluency answers. Benjamin et al. demonstrates that retrieval fluency is important in making JOLs, but also shows that it is misapplied to the free recall test because participants used the ease of retrieval during cued recall and applied it to free recall, for which earlier retrieval fluency does not predict success. Similarly, Koriat and Ma'ayan (2005) showed that people respond with higher JOLs to answers that are quickly retrieved from memory than answers that take longer to retrieve from memory. Because perceptual fluency and retrieval fluency have much in common, when we speak of them together, we will use the term processing fluency unless distinguishing between perceptual and retrieval fluency is relevant to the study in question.

Considerable research in the field of metacognition demonstrates that processing fluency affects many different metacognitive judgments (see Besken and Mulligan 2014; Jemstedt et al. 2018; Rhodes 2016; Thomas et al. 2016; Undorf et al. 2018). The typical judgments used by metacognition researchers include ease-of-learning judgments (EOLs), judgments of learning (JOLs), feeling-of-knowing judgments, and post-answer confidence. Processing fluency influences the magnitude of all these judgments (Kornell et al. 2011; Metcalfe et al. 1993). For instance, repeating the cue word in a word pair results in higher feeling-of-knowing judgments and increases the number of reported tip-of-the-tongue states (Metcalfe et al. 1993). That familiar cues garner higher feeling-of-knowing judgments has been observed many times (e.g., Thomas et al. 2016). With respect to JOLs, in a now classic study, Rhodes and Castel (2008) found that words written in larger font sizes were more fluently processed and resulted in larger JOLs than words written in smaller font sizes (also see Blake and Castel 2018). With respect to ease-of-learning, we recently showed that words written in all-caps (SUNSET) were processed more fluently and given higher EOLs than words written in alternating caps and lower-case letters (sUnSeT) (Jemstedt et al. 2018). This follows from an earlier study in which Begg et al. (1989) asked participants to judge how easy words were to study or how easy they were to memorize. In the Begg et al. study, participants made judgments on words that varied in how easy they were to imagine and how frequently they were used in the English language, two factors correlating with processing fluency. Words were judged as more easy to memorize and to study if they had higher imaginability and higher word frequency (Begg et al. 1989). To summarize, processing fluency impacts metacognition and does so across metacognitive judgments at each stage in the learning and retrieval process.

Consider another study specifically designed to demonstrate how fluency distorts the accuracy of our metamemory. Toftness et al. (2018) had participants watch a lecture given by an actor. In one version, the actor delivered the material smoothly, with appropriate pauses, with appropriate gestures and mannerisms. In the other version, the actor delivered the same material, but hunched over the podium, reading from his notes, and without looking at the camera. In keeping with Toftness et al.'s hypotheses, students rated that they had learned more from the fluent presentation, but actually learned no more from the fluent than from the dysfluent presentation. Toftness et al. claim this pattern to be counter-intuitive, which it may be indeed for people not familiar with the research presented here, but it conforms to the idea that fluency can produce an illusion of learning. In another interesting study on fluency and metamemory with real-world stimuli, Ball et al. (2014) showed that perceptual fluency (as marked by font size) influenced JOLs made about psychological concepts and definitions.

2.3 Fluency Versus Belief in JOLs and EOLs

There has been a view which is seen as opposed to the view that fluency influences metacognitive judgments. In particular, it may be that it is people's beliefs about what influences their learning rather than fluency itself that causes metacognitive judgments to increase (e.g., Mueller and Dunlosky 2017). In this view, people form expectations about what will make an item more memorable. This belief or expectation then causes people to make higher judgments rather for those items for which they believe is more memorable. Mueller and his colleagues (e.g., Mueller and Dunlosky 2017; Mueller et al. 2014) have claimed that some effects of fluency actually reflect belief. There is a considerable literature that supports the idea that beliefs influence metacognitive judgments, but whether or not beliefs can explain fluency effects has been the focus of an important debate within the field of metacognition (see Blake and Castel 2018; Mueller et al. 2014; Undorf and Zimdahl 2018; Yang et al. 2018). For example, if I believe that bigger fonts should be more memorable, then I am likely to give a higher JOL to a word in a larger font than one in a smaller font. The belief view and the fluency view are not mutually exclusive. In fact, both beliefs and fluency can affect metacognitive judgments, but they have often been placed in contrast with one another (Mueller et al. 2014). Although the debate as to how much beliefs can explain fluency effects is beyond the scope of this paper, we briefly consider our current work that shows that both processing fluency and beliefs independently influence ease-of-learning judgments (also see Yang et al.

2018). In addition, we briefly discuss two possible ways beliefs and fluency may influence judgments.

We recently examined processing fluency and beliefs with regards to ease-of-learning judgments (Jemstedt et al. 2018). In our study, we were able to look for independent contributions from processing fluency and beliefs in order to determine if both contribute to the magnitude of ease-of-learning judgments. Participants made ease-of-learning judgments either on words written in all-caps (SUNSET) or in alternating caps and lower-case letters (sUnSeT). The alternating letters were designed to induce dysfluency during processing, leading to lower ease-of-learning judgments, which is exactly what we found. However, at the end of each experiment, we asked participants about their beliefs with regards to which type of stimuli would be more memorable. We found an interaction between the presentation conditions and beliefs. When people believed that all-caps would result in better memory, there was a bigger difference between the ease-of-learning judgments made on all-caps and those made on alternating letters. When people believed that alternating letters would be more memorable, however, there was still higher mean ease-of-learning judgments for the all-caps in one of the experiments. That is, their global belief was that alternating letters would help learning, but their individual ease-of-learning judgments were still affected by fluency. Thus, this interaction suggests that beliefs alter to what degree processing fluency influences their EOL judgments, but it does not mean that processing fluency does not have a role.

In another paper, Blake and Castel (2018) directly manipulated beliefs about the effect of font size on JOLs. In some conditions, participants were told that larger font size resulted in excellent memory relative to smaller font sizes. In other conditions, participants were told that smaller font size resulted in excellent memory relative to larger font sizes. When people were encouraged to believe that larger font sizes were good for memory, their JOLs were higher for large fonts than for smaller fonts. However, when participants were encouraged to believe that smaller fonts were good for memory, the JOLs were about the same for both large and small fonts. Thus, like Jemstedt et al. (2018), this study supports a role for beliefs, but does not rule out the importance for processing fluency in creating the font-size effect. In both studies, participants adjusted their judgments based on their beliefs. Thus, Blake and Castel's results support a role for beliefs, but do not rule out the importance for processing fluency in creating the font-size effect.

Undorf et al. (2017) addressed the issue of fluency in font size with a creative way of demonstrating that fluency is essential in the font-size effect independent of beliefs. In Undorf et al., participants were presented with stimuli that were initially so small as to be unrecognizable. Then the researchers increased the size of the stimuli either gradually or more rapidly. Participants made JOLs when they could identify the stimuli. Because JOLs did not occur until stimuli were recognized, prior beliefs about the effects of font size could be minimized. Undorf et al. used pictures of common objects, faces, and words as stimuli in their different experiments. In keeping with the perceptual-fluency view, Undorf et al. found that the faster participants identified the stimuli, the higher their JOLs were. Moreover, JOLs were higher when the stimuli were revealed more quickly. Thus, experience created by the faster transition to conscious recognition led to an increase in the JOL, consistent with the fluency view, but not the belief view. In a final experiment, they compared participants who were provided with beliefs that faster revelation increases recall but did not actually see the stimuli and participants who were provided with beliefs about this revelation effect and saw the stimuli. Only the latter group that actually saw the revelation of stimuli gave higher JOLs to stimuli that were revealed more quickly. Thus, both in the procedure and with an explicit manipulation, Undorf et al. were able to rule out belief effects in this paradigm. Therefore, although beliefs do effect JOLs, perceptual fluency is also a factor.

Although people are often asked to learn single-words (as in a grocery list) or paired-associates, as in learning language vocabulary, a question remains if the font size effect would persist in metacognition about learning larger sections of material. Recently, Luna et al. (2018) examined the font-size effect with respect to complete sentences. With short sentences, a font-size effect remains, but with longer-sentences the font-size effect was greatly reduced, presumably as more informative sources of information become available such as whether the sentence is understandable, relatable to self, or other factors that influence JOLs. Nonetheless, Luna et al. showed that font-size effects are possible for sentence stimuli.

Given that there is now evidence to support the view that both beliefs and processing fluency affect JOLs, a question arises to the nature of how beliefs and fluency interact. More specifically, it is still unknown to what degree beliefs are involved in the effect that fluency has on metacognition. That is to say, fluency may have a direct effect on metacognition or it may be that people need to interpret fluency via their beliefs in order for it to have an effect. One of many possibilities is that people interpret fluency differently depending on how they expect fluency to influence their learning and memory, and there is some evidence that people do have beliefs about fluency. For example, when Mueller and Dunlosky (2017) informed participants that the color of words affected how easily the words were processed by their brain, participants' JOLs followed the manipulated beliefs. This indicates that people can have beliefs about fluency, and they alter their JOLs based on these beliefs. Indeed, beliefs just induced by experimenters have immediate influence on people's JOLs. Thus, one potential reason why fluency affect metacognitive judgments is because people hold beliefs related to fluent or disfluent processing of information and simply make metacognitive judgments based on these beliefs. Another possibility is that fluency and beliefs work in parallel to construct judgments. It may be that people experience fluency, and this experience affects their metacognitive judgment without the involvement of beliefs. At the same time, people are more actively adjusting their judgments based on explicit beliefs. In this view, fluency could have a direct effect on judgments even when fluency and beliefs about fluency have opposite effects on judgments. It is also possible that the opposite expectations based on belief and the effects of fluency might simply cancel each other. We wonder if people may be able to adjust for the effect of fluency on their judgments if they believe that they should not trust fluency in a specific task (see Oppenheimer 2004).

If fluency and beliefs affect metacognitive judgments, it may be possible to find different effects of fluency when judgments are speeded and unspeeded. There are a number of studies which have showed that the feeling of familiarity (often related to fluency) affect metacognitive judgments even when participants have to make speeded judgments (e.g., Metcalfe and Finn 2008). At the same time, it seems reasonable to assume that applying one's beliefs about a property of a learning situation requires some time. If we imagine that an item is effortful to process (low fluency) but an individual believes this low fluency should improve memory of that item, we may get different judgments from this individual depending on whether the judgment is speeded or unspeeded. Consequently, if fluency can have a direct effect, it means that a property of a learning situation (e.g., word is presented in alternating letters or all caps), could both affect metacognition through its effect on fluency and because people have beliefs about how the property should affect memory or learning. Understanding the interaction of fluency and beliefs and how they affect metacognition will be central for developing theories of how metacognitive judgments are formed.

2.4 Fluency or Familiarity in Feeling-of-Knowing Judgments and Tip-of-the-Tongue States

The literature on feeling of knowing and tip-of-the-tongue states usually takes a different tack. Because these judgments tap into retrieval of learned information rather than learning, the concept of fluency is usually thought of in terms of the familiarity of the cue—which is the only stimuli present when feeling-of-knowing judgments or tip-of-the-tongue states are asked for. Thus, because of the way that feeling-of-knowing judgments and tip-of-the-tongue states are elicited, it is easier to assess if the magnitude of the metamemory judgments is affected by the fluency of the cue rather than the target (Schwartz and Cleary 2016; Schwartz and Metcalfe 2011, 2014). A typical feeling-of-knowing paradigm involves having someone study word-pairs for later retrieval. After study, people are given a recall test. If the target cannot be recalled in response to the cue, a feeling-of-knowing judgment is called for. A later recognition test occurs allowing the judgments to be correlated with recognition. Tip-of-the-tongue states are usually tested on already learned knowledge (such as word definitions, general-knowledge, or by showing faces of famous people). An inability to recall is followed by a tip-of-the-tongue query. Usually, a recognition test follows to allow assessment of accuracy (Schwartz and Metcalfe 2011). The first author of this paper has written extensively about this topic in the past, so will not dwell on it here. But the upshot of this research is that when making either feeling-of-knowing judgments or tip-of-the-tongue states, making the cue more familiar (or fluent) increases the magnitude of feeling-of-knowing judgments or the likelihood of a tip-of-the-tongue state (Schwartz and Cleary 2016; Thomas et al. 2016). Thus, these findings are analogous to what is found with JOLs and EOLs.

2.5 Fluency in Domains Other than Metamemory

In cognitive domains other than metamemory, processing fluency can either increase or decrease the magnitude of the particular judgments being examined. One of the domains in which processing fluency has been applied to is judgments of whether a statement is true or not. Research shows that increasing the fluency of a statement increases the perceived truthfulness of that statement. Thus, for example, repeating a statement causes that statement to be judged as more likely to be true than if repeated fewer times (Begg et al. 1992; Hasher et al. 1977; see Goldinger and Hansen 2005). In another study, Reber and Schwarz (1999) showed that presenting a statement in a clearer color causes that statement to be judged as more likely to be true than if seen in a less clear color. Unkelbach (2006) showed that recognition judgments decreased when participants were explicitly instructed that easier to see stimuli would be more likely to be stimuli they had not seen earlier. Other research shows that constructing lies takes more time and is basically harder than telling the truth (Verschuere et al. 2011). This suggests that lying can serve as a proxy for fluency in studies examining the effects of fluency on memory and metamemory. Moreover, Besken (2018) had participants answer general-information questions with either truthful or dishonest answers. After generating an answer, participants made JOLs as to the likelihood that they would remember that answer later in a free recall test. She found that people recalled more of their own lies than their truthful statements during the recall test, but that they predicted they would remember more of the truths during the JOL phase. Besken, therefore, generated a double dissociation—dysfluency produced better memory for lies, but fluency increased JOLs for truth. To summarize, fluency is associated with truth-telling and creates an illusion of better memory, even though we remember our lies better.

Song and Schwarz (2008) looked at fluency with regards to the Moses illusion. In the Moses illusion, people do not notice the falsehood implicit in the question, "how many animals did Moses bring on the arc?" (and other similar questions). Because the question calls upon a biblical context, people do not notice that it was Noah, not Moses, who built the arc in the Bible, whereas Moses parted the Red Sea. Song and Schwarz presented Moses-illusion questions in either an easy-to-read font (fluent condition) or a difficult-to-read font (disfluent condition). When the font was easy, participants were less likely to notice the errors in the sentences than when the font was more difficult. That is, fluency of reading the sentences was mistaken for truth. Alternatively, one can think of this result in terms of the difficult font/low fluency fonts. That is, the difficult-to-read font helped people detect errors in the question. Thus, it is possible to interpret this result as dysfluency makes people more careful or analytic.

Processing fluency is also associated with a number of other metacognitive or evaluative judgments (Reber and Greifeneder 2017). These include judgments of beauty, frequency, and clarity. Items that are processed more fluently are thought to be more beautiful than items processed less fluently (Schwarz 2018). Perceptually clear faces are more likely to be judged as previously viewed than perceptually distorted faces (Kleider and Goldinger 2004). When people read texts written in complex or simple language, people judge the authors of the texts with the simple language (i.e., more fluent language) as more intelligent (Oppenheimer 2008).

In a fascinating study, Goldinger and Hansen (2005) designed an unusual means of varying processing fluency and how people interpret their own experience of fluency. In this study, people's subjective experience was altered by externally creating a vibration, which was incorporated into people's subjective experience. In the study, Goldinger and Hansen required participants to study words for a later recognition test, but the participants sat in a chair that buzzed. The buzz was actually a vibration administered underneath the seat. In one condition, the buzzing occurred below the threshold of awareness, whereas in a second condition people could consciously feel the buzzing of the chair. Thus, there were two conditions—above and below threshold buzzing. The hypothesis was that when buzzing was above threshold, people would discount the experience of buzzing, knowing that it came from the odd chair that they were sitting in. But when the buzzing was below threshold, it might change their experience—but they would not know why. Indeed, they suspected that people would experience the unrecognized tingling as having to do with the test words that they were looking at. Thus, when the buzz was below threshold, people were not able to attribute the change in their excited subjective state caused by the buzz to its proper source, and thus may have mislabeled it as caused by familiarity with the target. Under these conditions, the buzz led to more "old" decisions, increasing both the hit and the false alarm rate. When the buzz was obvious (above threshold), people could easily discount any feeling of familiarity caused by the buzz. Thus, when the buzz was above threshold, it had no effect on "old" decisions. Thus, the same boost in fluency caused by the buzz led to different behaviors when people were aware of the source of that processing. However, such an analysis has yet to be applied to processing fluency with respect to metacognition.

2.6 Why Does Processing Fluency Increase but Never Decrease Metacognitive Confidence?

Earlier in this chapter, we reviewed the evidence that shows that processing fluency increases metacognitive confidence across a range of judgments. The question we ask here is why processing fluency only increases metacognitive confidence. Unkelbach (2006) showed that it was possible to get people to notice a negative correlation between fluency and old judgments in an old/new recognition task. Might there be some situations in which an increase in processing fluency is associated with a decrease in confidence? Certainly, there are situations in which the fluent processing of items leads to worse retrieval for those items later (Benjamin et al. 1998; Weissgerber and Reinhard 2017). For example, Benjamin et al. found that low-fluency answers to general-information questions were better free-recalled than high-frequency answers. To date, however, there are no situations in which metacognitive judgments decrease as processing fluency increases. Why is this when processing fluency is clearly associated with poor recall in some situations (e.g., Weissgerber and Reinhard 2017)? If a lack of fluent processing (i.e., dysfluency) can produce desirable difficulty, and desirable difficulty can result in better memory performance, why is it that our metacognitive systems cannot detect it, learn it, or respond to it?

We make two claims here that are rare in the literature on metacognition, one of which we can support with data, the other of which is currently speculation. The first is that, under normal circumstances (such as a student studying for an exam), fluency within a set of items correlates with memory performance, and therefore using fluency as a proxy for later memory is adaptive. Second, under the right circumstances, it ought to be possible to show that metacognitive confidence increases with dysfluency and decreases with fluency. As of yet, we are unaware of any studies showing that metacognitive confidence increases with dysfluency, but there are at least two studies that show that memory performance increases for more fluent stimuli (Mueller et al. 2013; Schwartz et al. in progress). For example, in Mueller et al. (2013), participants studied related and unrelated word pairs. For example, an unrelated pair could be "cat-fork," whereas a related pair could be "hat-check." At test, participants were given both a lexical decision task to assess fluency as well as a recall test. In this straightforward design, fluency and retrieval should be linked, which indeed they were. Target words in the pairs were recognized faster as real words on a lexical decision task (fluency) when pairs were related compared to unrelated. Furthermore, related pairs were associated with higher recall. That is, fluency was likely positively related to recall (although Mueller et al. did not directly examine this effect).

In our study, we looked at situations in which fluency predicts recall more directly (Schwartz et al. in progress). In this study, people who were musically literate were chosen as participants. All participants had to pass a music-reading test in order for participation to count. Once musical literacy was confirmed, participants were asked to learn small sequences of music (two bars). For some sequences, the music was presented in a familiar key signature (the number of sharps and flats), such as the key of C. This was considered the fluent condition. For other sequences, the same musical sequence was presented in an unfamiliar key signature, such as the key of F sharp. The music in an unfamiliar key signature was considered the dysfluent condition. Thus, for any participant, half of the items were in the fluent condition, and half were in the dysfluent condition. We found that participants gave higher JOLs to the fluent items, consistent with a large body of work on JOLs (Rhodes and Tauber 2011). However, the fluent items were also recognized better as well, documenting a situation in which fluency and retrieval are congruent.

We return to the Toftness et al. (2018) study. They found that students expected to learn more from a fluent speaker than a non-fluent speaker, when, in fact, there were no differences. We wonder if in the real world, people present information more fluently when they are more knowledgeable about a topic and are more likely to read from notes or show other signs of dysfluency when they are less knowledgeable about the topic. Thus, in the real world, the fluent speaker might indeed indicate a better source of learning than the dysfluent speaker. Indeed, we suspect that there would be an interesting interaction if the fluent/dysfluent speaker manipulation was crossed with a knowledgeable/unknowledgeable manipulation. In the fluent/unknowledgeable condition, we suspect that participants might pick up on the fact that their teacher may be funny and a good speaker, but he does not know the material. This might be one of those situations in which fluency should result in a lower estimation of learning than the dysfluent but knowledgeable speaker. To summarize, because fluency is used as a surrogate for confidence in learning and retrieving, it is logical to expect that under many circumstances, fluency should be positively correlated with learning and retrieving. However, most of the situations studied by metacognition researchers focus on those situations in which fluency and memory performance are inversely related. Thus, a goal for research in this area, going forward, is to identify those situations in which fluency and performance go hand in hand.

In general, researchers interested in metamemory have approached learning as if learning was a single process that gradually accumulates. However, many models of memory are more complex. For example, Bjork and Bjork (1992) conceptualized learning in terms of two strengths, retrieval strength and storage strength. Retrieval strength is equivalent to accessibility and reflects the ease with which information can be retrieved, whereas storage strength is equivalent to availability and reflects the permanence of the memory (see Tulving and Pearlstone 1966). Bjork and Bjork then demonstrated that many learning phenomena can be explained by postulating that retrieval strength and storage strength reflect different underlying processes of learning and do not always correlate with each other. We wonder if metacognitive judgments might actually be able to tap into these different systems. If so, perceptual fluency might be a good guide for retrieval strength. That which is easy to perceive might be easy to retrieve under short-term conditions. However, perhaps people are aware that perceptual fluency might not reflect the processes that are necessary for solid long-term learning. Thus, if it is made clear to participants that they are making judgments about what they will remember a year from now rather than 10 min from now, perhaps they will show a negative correlation between perceptual fluency and metacognitive judgments.

2.7 Conclusions

In this chapter, we have reviewed the evidence that shows that processing fluency has an important relation to metacognition. In the metacognitive judgments reviewed here, processing fluency is one source of information of metacognition from tip-of-the-tongue states to JOLs. In addition to processing fluency, the beliefs we have about how memory processes work is also important in making judgments (Efklides 2018). In particular, we reviewed the literature on JOLs which shows that processing fluency and beliefs independently contribute to making the judgment. That judgements are based on processing fluency even when processing fluency does not predict performance on the ongoing task is critical to future understanding of these issues.

As cognitive scientists, we wish to explore the mechanisms underlying metacognition. As scientists interested in both application and theory, we also want to understand the relation of those mechanisms to ordinary learning. Thus, we want to know when metacognition is adaptive for improving learning and when it actually gets in the way. Studying illusions or failures of cognition has been a traditional method of ferreting out the processes and mechanisms underlying our cognition (Bjork et al. 2013). Thus, it has long been understood that visual illusions help us understand the major processes involved in visual perception, but that generally our visual systems are quite good at allowing us to negotiate the actual world. We argue for a similar situation with respect to metacognitive illusions, that is, those situations in which our metacognitive judgments do not reflect our performance. Metacognitive illusions are important to study because they tell us about the process of how metacognition comes about. In this chapter, we focus on how fluency can distort metamemory. But beyond that, we must seek to understand them in terms of how we use metacognition in everyday life. When we do so, we may see that many of the factors that seem irrational at first are actually useful to prepare people to learn more and more efficiently (Efklides 2011). Thus, even though this chapter has focused much on the reasons why metacognition may be inaccurate, in the end, we endorse Efklides' positive view—that metacognition is beneficial for learning (Efklides 2016, 2018).

References

Alter, A. L., & Oppenheimer, D. M. (2009). Uniting the tribes of fluency to form a metacognitive nation. *Personality and Social Psychology Review, 13*, 219–235. https://doi.org/10.1177/1088868309341564.

Arango-Muñoz, S. (2019). Cognitive phenomenology and metacognitive feelings. *Mind and Language, 34*, 247–262. https://doi.org/10.1111/mila.12215.

Ball, B. H., Klein, K. N., & Brewer, G. A. (2014). Processing fluency mediates the influence of perceptual information on monitoring learning of educationally relevant materials. *Journal of Experimental Psychology: Applied, 20*, 336–348.

Begg, I., Duft, S., Lalonde, P., Melnick, R., & Sanvito, J. (1989). Memory predictions are based on ease of processing. *Journal of Memory and Language, 28*, 610–632.

Begg, I. M., Anas, A., & Farinacci, S. (1992). Dissociation of processes in belief: Source recollection, statement familiarity, and the illusion of truth. *Journal of Experimental Psychology: General, 121*, 446–458. https://doi.org/10.1037//0096-3445.121.4.446.

Benjamin, A. S., Bjork, R. A., & Schwartz, B. L. (1998). The mismeasure of memory: When retrieval fluency is misleading as a metamnemonic index. *Journal of Experimental Psychology: General, 127*, 55–68. https://doi.org/10.1037/0096-3445.127.1.55.

Besken, M. (2018). Generating lies produces lower memory predictions and higher memory performance than telling the truth: Evidence for a metacognitive illusion. *Journal of Experimental Psychology: Learning, Memory, and Cognition, 44*, 465–484.

Besken, M., & Mulligan, N. W. (2014). Perceptual fluency, auditory generation, and metamemory: Analyzing the perceptual fluency hypothesis in the auditory modality. *Journal of Experimental Psychology: Learning, Memory, and Cognition, 40*, 429–440. https://doi.org/10.1037/a0034407.

Bjork, R. A., & Bjork, E. L. (1992). A new theory of disuse and an old theory of stimulus fluctuation. In A. F. Healy, S. M. Kosslyn, & R. M. Shiffrin (Eds.), *From learning processes to cognitive processes: Essays in honor of William K. Estes* (Vol. 2, pp. 35–67). Hillsdale: Lawrence Erlbaum.

Bjork, R. A., Dunlosky, J., & Kornell, N. (2013). Self-regulated learning: Beliefs, techniques, and illusions. *Annual Review of Psychology, 64*, 417–444.

Blake, A. B., & Castel, A. D. (2018). On belief and fluency in the construction of judgments of learning: Assessing and altering the direct effects of belief. *Acta Psychologica, 186*, 27–38.

Efklides, A. (2008). Metacognition: Defining its facets and levels of functioning in relation to self- and co-regulation. *European Psychologist, 13*, 277–287. https://doi.org/10.1027/1016-9040.13.4.277.

Efklides, A. (2011). Interactions of metacognition with motivation and affect in self-regulated learning: The MASRL model. *Educational Psychologist, 46*, 6–25. https://doi.org/10.1080/00461520.2011.538645.

Efklides, A. (2016). Metamemory and affect. In J. Dunlosky & S. Tauber (Eds.), *The Oxford handbook of metamemory* (pp. 245–268). New York: Oxford University Press.

Efklides, A. (2018). Gifted students and self-regulated learning: The MASRL model and its implications for SRL. *High Abilities Studies, 30*, 79–102. https://doi.org/10.1080/13598139.2018.1556069.

Efklides, A., Schwartz, B. L., & Brown, V. (2018). Motivation and affect in self-regulated learning: Does metacognition play a role? In D. H. Schunk & J. A. Greene (Eds.), *Handbook of self-regulation of learning and performance* (pp. 64–82). New York: Routledge.

Flavell, J. H. (1979). Metacognition and cognitive monitoring: A new era of cognitive- developmental inquiry. *American Psychologist, 34*, 906–911.

Goldinger, S. D., & Hansen, W. A. (2005). Remembering by the seat of your pants. *Psychological Science, 16*, 525–529.

Hasher, L., Goldstein, D., & Toppino, T. (1977). Frequency and the conference of referential validity. *Journal of Verbal Learning and Verbal Behavior, 16*, 107–112.

Jemstedt, A., Schwartz, B. L., & Jönsson, F. U. (2018). Ease-of-learning judgments are based on both processing fluency and beliefs. *Memory, 26*, 807–815. https://doi.org/10.1080/09658211.2017.1410849.

Kleider, H. M., & Goldinger, S. D. (2004). Illusions of face memory: Clarity breeds familiarity. *Journal of Memory and Language, 50*, 196–211.

Koriat, A. (1993). How do we know that we know? The accessibility account of the feeling of knowing. *Psychological Review, 100*, 609–639.

Koriat, A., & Ma'ayan, H. (2005). The effects of encoding fluency and retrieval fluency on judgments of learning. *Journal of Memory and Language, 52*, 478–492. https://doi.org/10.1016/j.jml.2005.01.001.

Kornell, N., Rhodes, M. G., Castel, A. D., & Tauber, S. K. (2011). The ease-of-processing heuristic and the stability bias: Dissociating memory, memory beliefs, and memory judgments. *Psychological Science, 22*, 787–794. https://doi.org/10.1177/0956797611407929.

Luna, K., Albuquerque, P. B., & Martín-Luengo, B. (2018). Cognitive load eliminates the effect of perceptual information on judgments of learning with sentences. *Memory & Cognition*. https://doi.org/10.3758/s13421-018-0853-1.

Metcalfe, J. (1993). Novelty monitoring, metacognition, and control in a composite holographic associative recall model: Interpretations for Korsakoff amnesia. *Psychological Review, 100*, 3–22.

Metcalfe, J., & Finn, B. (2008). Familiarity and retrieval processes in delayed judgments of learning. *Journal of Experimental Psychology: Learning, Memory, and Cognition, 34*, 1084–1097. https://doi.org/10.1037/a0012580.

Metcalfe, J., & Son, L. K. (2012). Anoetic, noetic, and autonoetic metacognition. In M. Beran, J. R. Brandl, J. Perner, & J. Proust (Eds.), *The foundations of metacognition* (pp. 289–301). New York: Oxford University Press.

Metcalfe, J., Schwartz, B. L., & Joaquim, S. G. (1993). The cue-familiarity heuristic in metacognition. *Journal of Experimental Psychology: Learning, Memory, and Cognition, 19*, 851–861. https://doi.org/10.1037/0278-7393.19.4.851.

Mueller, M., & Dunlosky, J. (2017). How beliefs can impact judgments of learning: Evaluating analytic processing theory with beliefs about fluency. *Journal of Memory and Language, 93*, 245–258.

Mueller, M. L., Tauber, S. K., & Dunlosky, J. (2013). Contributions of beliefs and processing fluency to the effect of relatedness on judgments of learning. *Psychonomic Bulletin & Review, 20*, 378–384.

Mueller, M. L., Dunlosky, J., Tauber, S. K., & Rhodes, M. (2014). The font size effect on judgments of learning: Does it exemplify fluency effects or reflect people's beliefs about memory? *Journal of Memory and Language, 70*, 1–12.

Nelson, T. O., & Narens, L. (1990). Metamemory: A theoretical framework and new findings. In G. H. Bower (Ed.), *The psychology of learning and motivation: Advances in research and theory* (pp. 125–173). San Diego: Academic Press.

Oppenheimer, D. M. (2004). Spontaneous discounting of availability in frequency judgment tasks. *Psychological Science, 15*, 100–105.

Oppenheimer, D. M. (2008). The secret life of fluency. *Trends in Cognitive Sciences, 12*, 237–241. https://doi.org/10.1016/j.tics.2008.02.014.

Proust, J. (2015). The representational structure of feelings. In T. Metzinger & J. M. Windt (Eds.), *Open MIND* (Vol. 31). Frankfurt am Main: Open MIND Group. https://doi.org/10.15502/9783958570047.

Reber, R., & Greifeneder, R. (2017). Processing fluency in education: How metacognitive feelings shape learning, belief formation, and affect. *Educational Psychologist, 52*, 84–103.

Reber, R., & Schwarz, N. (1999). Effects of perceptual fluency on judgments of truth. *Consciousness and Cognition, 8*, 338–342.

Reder, L. M. (1987). Strategy selection in question answering. *Cognitive Psychology, 19*, 90–138.

Rhodes, M. G. (2016). Judgments of learning: Methods, data, and theory. In J. Dunlosky & S. Tauber (Eds.), *The Oxford handbook of metamemory* (pp. 65–80). New York: Oxford University Press.

Rhodes, M. G., & Castel, A. D. (2008). Memory predictions are influenced by perceptual information: Evidence for metacognitive illusions. *Journal of Experimental Psychology: General, 137*, 615–625.

Rhodes, M. G., & Tauber, S. K. (2011). The influence of delaying judgements of learning (JOLs) on metacognitive accuracy: A meta-analytic review. *Psychological Bulletin, 137*, 131–148. https://doi.org/10.1037/a0021705.

Schwartz, B. L., & Cleary, A. M. (2016). Tip-of-the-tongue states, déjà vu and other metacognitive oddities. In J. Dunlosky & S. Tauber (Eds.), *Oxford handbook of metamemory* (pp. 95–108). New York: Oxford University Press.

Schwartz, B. L., & Metcalfe, J. (2011). Tip-of-the-tongue (TOT) states: Retrieval, behavior, and experience. *Memory & Cognition, 39*, 737–749.

Schwartz, B. L., & Metcalfe, J. (2014). Tip-of-the-tongue (TOT) states: Mechanisms and metacognitive control. In B. L. Schwartz & A. S. Brown (Eds.), *Tip-of-the-tongue states and related phenomena* (pp. 15–31). New York: Cambridge University Press.

Schwarz, N. (2018). Of fluency, beauty, and truth: Inferences from metacognitive experiences. In J. Proust & M. Fortier (Eds.), *Metacognitive diversity* (pp. 25–46). New York: Oxford University Press.

Simmons, J. P., & Nelson, L. D. (2006). Intuitive confidence: Choosing between intuitive and nonintuitive alternatives. *Journal of Experimental Psychology: General, 135*, 409–428.

Song, H., & Schwarz, N. (2008). Fluency and the detection of misleading questions: Low processing fluency attenuates the Moses illusion. *Social Cognition, 26*, 791–799.

Thomas, A. K., Lee, M., & Hughes, G. (2016). Introspecting on the elusive: The uncanny state of the feeling of knowing. In J. Dunlosky & S. Tauber (Eds.), *Oxford handbook of metamemory* (pp. 81–94). New York: Oxford University Press.

Toftness, A. R., Carpenter, S. K., Geller, J., Lauber, S., Johnson, M., & Armstrong, P. (2018). Instructor fluency leads to higher confidence in learning, but not better learning. *Metacognition and Learning, 13*, 1–14.

Tulving, E., & Pearlstone, Z. (1966). Availability versus accessibility of information in memory for words. *Journal of Verbal Learning and Verbal Behavior, 5*, 381–391.

Undorf, M., & Zimdahl, M. F. (2018). Metamemory and memory for a wide range of font sizes: What is the contribution of perceptual fluency? *Journal of Experimental Psychology: Learning, Memory, and Cognition, 45*, 97–109. https://doi.org/10.1037/xlm0000571.

Undorf, M., Zimdahl, M. F., & Bernstein, D. M. (2017). Perceptual fluency contributes to effects of stimulus size on judgments of learning. *Journal of Memory and Language, 92*, 293–304. https://doi.org/10.1016/j.jml.2016.07.003.

Undorf, M., Söllner, A., & Bröder, A. (2018). Simultaneous utilization of multiple cues in judgments of learning. *Memory & Cognition, 46*, 507–519. https://doi.org/10.3758/s13421-017-0780-6.

Unkelbach, C. (2006). The learned interpretation of cognitive fluency. *Psychological Science, 17*, 339–345.

Verschuere, B., Spruyt, A., Meijer, E. H., & Otgaar, H. (2011). The ease of lying. *Consciousness and Cognition, 20*, 908–911. https://doi.org/10.1016/j.concog.2010.10.023.

Weissgerber, S. C., & Reinhard, M.-A. (2017). Is disfluency desirable for learning? *Learning and Instruction, 49*, 199–217.

Wells, A., & Colbear, J. S. (2012). Treating posttraumatic stress disorder with metacognitive therapy: A preliminary controlled trial. *Journal of Clinical Psychology, 68*, 373–381.

Yang, C., Huang, T. S.-T., & Shanks, D. R. (2018). Perceptual fluency affects judgments of learning: The font size effect. *Journal of Memory and Language, 99*, 99–110.

Chapter 3
Epistemic Emotions and Metacognitive Feelings

Elisabeth Vogl, Reinhard Pekrun, and Kristina Loderer

Abstract Epistemic emotions such as surprise, curiosity, and confusion occur during epistemic cognitive activities. They result from cognitive appraisals about the (mis-)alignment between new information and existing knowledge or beliefs. More specifically, epistemic emotions can be triggered by discrepant or contradictory information that prompts cognitive incongruity, and they can influence cognitive information processing and the generation of knowledge. Metacognitive feelings, on the other hand, are affective experiences that inform individuals about the status of their cognitive processes. Metacognitive feelings are products of inferential processes that are often non-conscious and non-analytic, and they can influence the regulation of cognition. These definitions suggest that both epistemic emotions and metacognitive feelings are closely connected to cognitive processing, which raises the question whether, and how, they relate to each other. In this chapter, we introduce the concept of epistemic emotions and discuss similarities, differences, and links between epistemic emotions and metacognitive feelings.

Keywords Epistemic emotion · Metacognitive feeling · Cognitive incongruity · Knowledge exploration · Curiosity

---

E. Vogl (✉)
Department of Psychology, LMU Munich, Munich, Germany
e-mail: elisabeth.vogl@psy.lmu.de

R. Pekrun
Department of Psychology, LMU Munich, Munich, Germany

Department of Psychology, University of Essex, Colchester, UK

Institute for Positive Psychology, Australian Catholic University, Sydney, NSW, Australia

K. Loderer
Department of Psychology, University of Augsburg, Augsburg, Germany

D. Moraitou, P. Metallidou (eds.), *Trends and Prospects in Metacognition Research across the Life Span*, https://doi.org/10.1007/978-3-030-51673-4_3

3.1 Introduction

Research has started to acknowledge the importance of affective phenomena during cognitive and metacognitive processes (Efklides 2006; Pekrun and Linnenbrink-Garcia 2014). Affective phenomena and their role in epistemic (knowledge-generating) activities are focal constructs not only in psychology but also other disciplines such as philosophy. In this chapter, we will consider two particular groups of affective processes that have been examined in this context: epistemic emotions and metacognitive feelings. Following a brief introduction of both concepts, we will discuss the qualities of these experiences, their functional role during epistemic activities, and possible linkages between them, taking both philosophical and psychological considerations into account.

3.2 Epistemic Emotions

3.2.1 Definition of Epistemic Emotions

The term "epistemic emotions" was originally coined by philosophers referring to affective states that can motivate human inquiry and critical reflection (see Brun et al. 2008; Morton 2010). In philosophy, it has been proposed that there might be emotions that are epistemic by nature (e.g., Scheffler 1991), but some "non-epistemic" emotions and feelings may also be epistemically relevant (e.g., Morton 2010). Scheffler (1991), for example, identified joy of verification and surprise as epistemic emotions because they relate to the content of a person's cognition (e.g., beliefs and expectations), inform about the status of inquiry, and can be used to guide it. Besides these two emotions, Morton (2010) argued that various other positive and negative emotions might also be epistemic, such as curiosity, fascination, intellectual courage, love of truth, meticulousness, excitement, humility, interest, (dis)satisfaction, frustration, worry, concern, and intellectual disappointment. Additionally, he proposed that "non-epistemic" emotions, such as fear, anger or sadness, can have epistemic consequences.

In psychology, epistemic emotions have been defined as emotions that relate to knowledge and the generation of knowledge (Pekrun and Stephens 2012; Pekrun et al. 2017b). They result from cognitive appraisals about the (mis-)alignment between new information and existing knowledge or beliefs (Muis et al. 2018). Cognitive incongruity resulting from this misalignment can prototypically trigger the epistemic emotions surprise, curiosity, and confusion (D'Mello and Graesser 2012; Muis et al. 2015a; Vogl et al. 2019a, b). In addition, anxiety may be experienced in case of severe incongruity and information that deeply disturbs existing cognitive schemas or beliefs, or frustration and boredom if the resolution of incongruity seems impossible (Pekrun and Stephens 2012). In contrast, enjoyment may be experienced when cognitive incongruity is resolved (Pekrun and Stephens

2012), or when dealing with the new information is in line with personal epistemic beliefs (Muis et al. 2015a), resulting in cognitive congruity.

3.2.2 *Quality of Epistemic Emotions*

Some of the epistemic emotions discussed in philosophy have also been described as epistemic emotions in psychology (e.g., surprise, curiosity, frustration, enjoyment; e.g., D'Mello and Graesser 2012; Pekrun and Stephens 2012). The affective status of other subjective states considered in philosophy (e.g., intellectual courage, meticulousness) is up for discussion. Specifically, it is debatable whether they qualify as emotional states given contemporary multicomponent definitions of emotions (e.g., Scherer 2009). These approaches propose that emotions are systems of coordinated psychological processes including an emotion-specific affective experience (feeling), cognitive processes, and motivational tendencies, as well as physiological and expressive components. In line with this approach, affective epistemic states also need to comprise these five components to be classified as epistemic emotions.

Interestingly, two out of the three prototypical epistemic emotions, namely surprise, curiosity, and confusion, are not classified as emotions traditionally. Specifically, while surprise has been labeled as a basic or fundamental human emotion (e.g., Ekman 1982, 1999), curiosity has its roots in the broader motivation literature (e.g., Berlyne 1954, 1960; Deci 1975; Kagan 1972), whereas confusion is often described as a mere cognitive state (Clore and Huntsinger 2007). However, in line with multicomponent approaches to emotions (e.g., Scherer 2009), curiosity and confusion have been shown to involve affective feelings, physiological arousal, motivational impulses, as well as specific patterns of facial expression (e.g., Markey and Loewenstein 2014; Reeve 1993; Rozin and Cohen 2003).

Philosophical accounts hold that some emotions may be epistemic by nature (e.g., surprise, curiosity, and confusion), whereas others maybe members of various groups of emotion, depending on their object focus (Pekrun et al. 2017b; Vogl et al. 2019a). Examples include social, moral, and achievement emotions. As noted, knowledge and the generation of knowledge are the objects of epistemic emotions; in social, moral, and achievement emotions, the objects are other persons, moral norms, or success and failure, respectively. For example, during cognitive activities, some emotions can be experienced as epistemic emotions or as achievement emotions (Pekrun and Perry 2014): A student's frustration can be considered an epistemic emotion if the focus is on the cognitive incongruity resulting from an unsolved problem, or an achievement emotion if the focus is on personal failure and the inability to solve the problem. As such, it is important to acknowledge that epistemic emotions can share affective properties with other groups of emotions, but differ from them in terms of their object focus (Brun et al. 2008). In addition, epistemic emotions can also target knowledge and knowledge generation related to achievement and achievement outcomes (e.g., when a student is curious to find out her exam grade, or surprised about failing an exam).

3.2.3 Origins of Epistemic Emotions

As indicated above, cognitive appraisals about the (mis-)alignment between new information and existing knowledge or beliefs (Muis et al. 2018) are central triggers of epistemic emotions. Additional antecedents of epistemic emotions, such as proximal expectancies of success and value related to the epistemic activity (Muis et al. 2015b, 2018; Pekrun and Perry 2014; Pekrun 2020), as well as more distal antecedents such as personality traits that influence how individuals react to unexpected information (e.g., need for structure or openness to experience; Gocłowska et al. 2014, 2017; Vogl et al. 2019a), also need to be considered to explain the experience of different epistemic emotions. For example, curiosity may be experienced when being confronted with new information that contradicts one's personal beliefs, but only if the information is valued and seems to be controllable (i.e., the incongruity can be resolved). In contrast, confusion might be experienced if contradictory information is valued, but does not seem to be easily controllable (i.e., the incongruity cannot easily be resolved).

3.2.4 Functions of Epistemic Emotions

In so-called circumplex models, affective states are grouped according to (a) the relative degree of positive versus negative valence, and (b) activation versus deactivation in a two-dimensional space (e.g., Feldman Barrett and Russell 1999). Similarly, discrete emotions can be categorized in a 2×2 taxonomy including positive-activating emotions (e.g., enjoyment), positive-deactivating emotions (e.g., relief and relaxation), negative-activating emotions (e.g., frustration and anxiety), and negative-deactivating emotions (e.g., boredom and hopelessness; Pekrun 2006; Pekrun and Perry 2014). Different groups but also different emotions within each group can influence cognitive information processing and the generation of knowledge in different ways (Pekrun et al. 2017b; Vogl et al. 2019a).

Interestingly, for some epistemic emotions it is not yet quite clear to which group they belong (e.g., surprise, curiosity). Surprise can generally be experienced as pleasant or unpleasant (Ortony and Turner 1990), but, empirical evidence suggests that it may be positively valenced in epistemic contexts (e.g., learning about climate change; Pekrun et al. 2017a, b). Surprise has been found to promote recall of unexpected events (Parzuchowski and Szymkow-Sudziarska 2008), elicit interest (Renninger and Hidi 2016), and prompt curiosity (Berlyne 1954, 1960; Loewenstein 1994). Epistemic curiosity has been described as the "drive to know" (Berlyne 1954, p. 187) and is regarded as a means to support learning in educational contexts (von Stumm et al. 2011). It is complex in that its valence can involve positive feelings of interest in new learning material as well as unpleasant feelings of uncertainty and tension due to a lack of knowledge (Litman and Jimerson 2004). However, the process of satisfying curiosity is itself pleasurable. Overall, curiosity can be pleasant, or unpleasant, or both (see Murayama et al. 2019; Pekrun 2019). In terms of functional properties for human behavior, curiosity has been found to promote the exploration of new knowledge (Berlyne 1954, 1960; Litman et al. 2005; Vogl et al. 2019a) and to enhance memory for new information (Gruber et al. 2014; Kang et al. 2009; Marvin and Shohamy 2016; Middlebrooks et al. 2016). The positive-activating epistemic emotion enjoyment has been associated with deep learning strategies such as elaboration and critical thinking (Muis et al. 2015a).

For negative-activating epistemic emotions such as confusion, anxiety, and frustration, relationships with task engagement and performance have been found to be more complex. For example, confusion can relate positively to engagement (Bosch and D'Mello 2017; D'Mello and Graesser 2012) and learning outcomes (Craig et al. 2004; D'Mello and Graesser 2014; D'Mello et al. 2014), because impasses (and the associated state of confusion) require active engagement and effortful cognitive processing to be overcome (Brown and VanLehn 1980; Mandler 1990). However, for confusion to be productive it is crucial that incongruity is ultimately resolved (D'Mello and Graesser 2014; D'Mello et al. 2014). One possibility for resolving cognitive incongruity is the exploration of new knowledge. New knowledge can help to better understand conflicting information or to decide which information is correct (Berlyne 1954, 1960; Vogl et al. 2019a). Epistemic anxiety is experienced when information challenges strong cognitive schemas or existential beliefs (Muis et al. 2018; Pekrun and Stephens 2012). Interestingly, epistemic anxiety can also have positive effects. For example, anxiety can motivate knowledge-generating behavior that aims to reduce uncertainty and fulfill needs for epistemic control (Miceli and Castelfranchi 2005). Frustration has often been associated with detrimental effects on knowledge generation (D'Mello and Graesser 2012). However, research on the effects of frustration on cognitive processes is not as consistently negative as one might expect (Baker et al. 2010; Muis et al. 2015b; Wong 1979). Similarly, to confusion and anxiety, frustration as a negative-activating emotion may possibly promote learning if the frustrated person is able to use it in order to strengthen motivation, effort, and exploratory behavior by maintaining positive expectancies of success (Pekrun 2012). The negative-deactivating emotion epistemic boredom, in contrast, has been found to impair knowledge generating processes, such as the use of metacognitive self-regulation and deep processing strategies (Muis et al. 2015a; Muis et al. 2015b).

3.3 Metacognitive Feelings

3.3.1 Definition of Metacognitive Feelings

In philosophy, de Sousa (2008, 2009) argued that epistemic feelings such as the feeling of certainty, the feeling of knowing and the feeling of familiarity are part of the epistemic process as well, in addition to epistemic emotions such as those discussed in the previous section. In line with this idea, Arango-Muñoz (2013) categorizes positive and negative epistemic feelings according to the functional stage in which they occur during cognitive and metacognitive processing, and the types of motivation they afford. He argues that positive epistemic feelings motivate initiation or continued execution of cognitive processes, whereas negative epistemic feelings motivate the search for alternative ways to reach a goal or for revision of action patterns. The author suggests that prior to retrieval of information from memory, a feeling of knowing initiates mental action, while a feeling of uncertainty motivates the search for adequate strategies. During an intermediate assessment of the cognitive process, the feeling of fluency indicates that it is safe to continue with the action, whereas a feeling of difficulty suggests a switch of strategies. During final evaluation of the process, a feeling of rightness motivates a person to terminate the action, whereas the feeling of error or of forgetting signals the necessity to revise the command.

Psychologists have examined similar constructs, albeit under a different label: metacognitive feelings (Efklides 2016, 2017; Efklides et al. 2018). Metacognitive feelings are experiences that represent one facet of metacognition (Efklides 2006), a term that is used to denote cognition of cognition (Flavell 1979) or a model of cognition (Nelson 1996). Just like metacognitive knowledge (i.e., beliefs about the self, the task, strategies, goals, cognitive functions), metacognitive experiences (i.e., feelings, judgements/estimates, online task-specific knowledge; Efklides 2006; Flavell 1979) inform metacognition about cognitive processes. These can be modified by metacognition by applying metacognitive skills such as effort allocation and time allocation, planning, monitoring, and evaluation.

3.3.2 Origins and Functions of Metacognitive Feelings

Efklides (2006) defines metacognitive feelings as affective (i.e., pleasant or unpleasant) experiences that inform individuals about the status of features of cognitive processing in an experiential way. They are products of inferential processes that are often non-conscious and non-analytic, and they can influence the regulation of cognition by monitoring the progress being made towards one's goal. Based on work by Carver and Scheier (1998) and Carver (2003), Efklides (2006, 2008) proposed that metacognitive feelings can relate to a feedback loop that informs about the attainment of one's goal (e.g., feeling of confidence and feeling of satisfaction), or a metaloop that monitors the rate of progress toward one's goal. Goal attainment relates to positive affect (e.g., feeling of satisfaction), whereas the more distant the goal attainment is the more negative affect is experienced (Efklides and Petkaki 2005). If the rate of progress is slower than anticipated, negative feelings arise (e.g., feeling of difficulty). If the rate is faster than anticipated, positive feelings arise (e.g., feeling of familiarity). Negative feelings can inform the person that more effort is needed to attain the goal, or that the goal should be abandoned if the experienced difficulty cannot be overcome (Carver and Scheier 1998). Positive feelings, in contrast, can inform the person that progress toward one's goal is better than expected and that, therefore, effort can be reduced (Carver 2003). However, positive feelings can also motivate to continue one's ongoing activity, to process information more deeply, and to engage more deeply with it (Fredrickson 2001). Efklides and Dina (2004) proposed that both arguments may be valid. Essentially, initially reduced effort may be restored at subsequent confrontation with the same task triggering positive feelings signaling that processing is running smoothly, and that it may be favorable to immerse more deeply into task processing.

The effect of metacognitive feelings on motivation maybe mediated by causal attributions regarding the outcome of cognitive processing (Efklides 2011). Metallidou and Efklides (2001) found, for example, that the feeling of confidence leads to attribution of ability, whereas the feeling of difficulty leads to attribution of task difficult. These attributions, in turn, have implications for subjective appraisal of control over and the value of achievement activities or their outcomes and may lead to engagement or to disengagement with the task (see expectancy-value theory of achievement motivation; Wigfield and Eccles 2000; control-value theory of achievement emotions; Pekrun and Perry 2014). Clearly, more research is needed to understand the differential effects of positive and negative metacognitive feelings. The additional categorization into activating- and deactivating-positive and -negative feelings may help to explain the seemingly contradicting effects. For example, the positive feeling of familiarity, which accompanies fluency of progressing, may be a positive-activating feeling signaling smooth processing that can motivate further engagement with the task, whereas the positive feeling of satisfaction may be a positive-deactivating feeling signaling that a person's goal or standard is reached and that effort can be reduced.

3.3.3 The Feeling of Confidence

In what follows, we focus on one particular metacognitive feeling, i.e., the feeling of confidence, which has important implications for knowledge generation, and has also been associated with epistemic emotions (Nerantzaki and Efklides 2019; Vogl et al. 2019a, b). Metacognition research on the feeling of confidence has been focusing on online task processing that takes place at a task-specific micro-level of self-regulated learning (Efklides 2011). The feeling of confidence relates to the meta-level feedback loop that informs about the attainment of one's goal. It is particularly important for learning and knowledge generation because it can influence the motivation to engage in a task by influencing the types of strategies employed to solve it (Boekaerts and Rozendaal 2010; Stone 2000). A slightly optimistic but still realistic feeling of confidence is thought to be key for positive effects on learning. Over- and under-confidence, on the other hand, indicates poor metacognitive monitoring accuracy, and can be detrimental for learning (Dunlosky and Rawson 2012; Efklides 2006). Future research needs to analyze common and differential characteristics of the feeling of confidence with related concepts such as self-concept and self-efficacy beliefs, which are person characteristics that are researched on a macro-level, more closely to determine their common and differential effects (Efklides 2011).

Similar to epistemic emotions, metacognitive feelings comprise an affective component that closely relates to cognitive processes and motivational tendencies. However, to the extent that they lack specific physiological and expressive components, they do not qualify as emotions as defined by multicomponent approaches of emotions (e.g., Scherer 2009).

3.4 The Interplay of Epistemic Emotions and Metacognitive Feelings

Efklides (2014) argued that the outcome of monitoring of cognitive processes is experienced in form of metacognitive or affective feelings, such as the feeling of familiarity, the feeling of knowing, the feeling of confidence, satisfaction, pleasure, surprise, curiosity, or frustration (i.e., in form of metacognitive feelings or epistemic emotions). Empirical evidence supports this assumption and shows that the experience of epistemic emotions and metacognitive feelings are closely connected. For example, Touroutoglou and Efklides (2010) found that cognitive incongruity gives rise to metacognitive and affective reactions such as the feeling of difficulty and surprise (see also Metcalfe and Finn 2012).

3.4.1 The Interplay of Surprise, Curiosity, and Confusion with the Feeling of Confidence

We recently investigated the interplay of epistemic emotions (i.e., surprise, curiosity, and confusion) and individuals' feelings of confidence (Vogl et al. 2019a). In three independent experimental studies, we used within-person analysis to investigate cognitive incongruity prompted by high-confidence errors (i.e., participants' feeling of confidence in their answers that turned out to be incorrect) during a trivia task as an antecedent of surprise, curiosity, and confusion. Exploration of knowledge was assessed as a potential outcome of these three emotions. In addition, we compared the epistemic emotions with two achievement emotions, pride and shame, in terms of their antecedents and functions for knowledge exploration. The goal of this comparison was to shed light on the unique functional mechanisms underlying these different groups of emotions. In essence, we expected different patterns of antecedents and effects for epistemic emotions versus achievement emotions.

In more detail, the trivia task consisted of 20 single sentence statements compiled from various sources that tap into general knowledge in several domains (Ebert and Klotzek 2008, 2010; Nelson and Narens 1980; Pöppelmann 2009). The statements were designed to produce various degrees of cognitive (in-)congruity. We included statements that are likely to produce high-confidence errors because they target common misconceptions in general knowledge (e.g., "Chameleons match their color to their environment") as well as statements that were not expected to induce such errors (e.g., "Jupiter is the largest planet of our solar system"). Additionally, participants had to indicate how confident they were that their answer was correct. Next, participants received feedback about the accuracy (i.e., correctness) of their answer and were asked how surprised, curious, confused, proud, and ashamed they felt at that moment. Afterwards, they were presented with the opportunity to explore the correct solution, and to request up to two more pieces of information related to the trivia item.

Within this design, we hypothesized that success (correct answer) and failure (incorrect answer) would be core triggers of pride and shame (Pekrun 2006; Weiner 1985, 2010), respectively, whereas surprise, curiosity, and confusion would be triggered by high-confidence errors (i.e., interaction of accuracy and confidence in one's reply; e.g., D'Mello and Graesser 2012; Loewenstein 1994; Scherer 2009). In addition, we expected positive effects of epistemic emotions on knowledge generating behavior (Berlyne 1954, 1960; D'Mello et al. 2014; Litman et al. 2005; Loewenstein 1994). Considering prior findings on positive effects of pride on motivation and perseverance on pride-inducing tasks and domains (e.g., Carver and Johnson 2010; Pekrun et al. 2017a; Williams and DeSteno 2008), we expected positive effects of pride on knowledge-generating behavior in case of correct answers. Due to inconsistent findings on the effects of shame on knowledge exploration, we did not formulate a directional hypothesis. In addition, we assumed a temporal order or the epistemic emotions and hypothesized that the effect of high-confidence errors on knowledge exploration would be mediated by surprise in the first step and curiosity and confusion in the second step (Berlyne 1954, 1960; D'Mello and Graesser 2012; Loewenstein 1994).

Corroborating our assumptions, our results pointed to distinct patterns of antecedents for epistemic versus achievement emotions: Feedback on the trivia task induced both epistemic and achievement emotions, but under different circumstances. Specifically, as expected, pride was predicted by correct answers (i.e., success), and shame was predicted by incorrect answers (i.e., failure). The effects of correct versus incorrect answers on pride and shame were substantial and fully consistent across studies. Similar to shame, the epistemic emotions surprise, curiosity, and confusion were also triggered by inaccuracy. However, the effects of inaccuracy on these emotions were specified by an interaction with individuals' prior feelings of confidence in the accuracy of their answer. In other words, surprise, curiosity, and confusion were induced by high-confidence errors: the intensity of these emotions depended on participants' confidence in the answers that turned out to be incorrect, implying incongruity between prior beliefs and the correct answer. The link between high-confidence errors and epistemic emotions was also substantial, and it was fully robust across all three studies and all three epistemic emotions included in this research.

Interestingly, the effects of the accuracy x confidence interaction indicate that confidence in correct answers was positively linked to pride, whereas confidence in incorrect answers was positively linked to shame. Importantly, however, these relationships were relatively weak, and notably weaker than those observed for surprise, curiosity, and confusion, suggesting that the feeling of confidence in one's knowledge is less relevant for the arousal of achievement emotions as compared with epistemic emotions. These results were replicated in two subsequent studies by Vogl et al. (2019b). Study 3 by Vogl et al. (2019a), further shed light on the dynamic interplay of multiple epistemic emotions suggesting that surprise may precede curiosity (Loewenstein 1994) and confusion (D'Mello and Graesser 2012). In supplemental analyses, we competitively evaluated additional models depicting alternative sequences of epistemic emotions, but the proposed order (i.e., surprise preceding curiosity/confusion) showed the best fit to the data. This indicates that there might be a temporal order in the experience of epistemic emotions. Nevertheless, the data are of correlational nature and experimental studies are needed to further test causal ordering of emotions.

In line with hypotheses, the data demonstrated that both surprise and curiosity related positively to subsequent motivation to explore as well as actual exploratory behavior. These links were fully robust across all three studies and across correctly as well as incorrectly answered trivia questions. The findings further suggest that cognitive incongruity promotes exploration, and that surprise and curiosity are mediators in this relationship. For confusion, the findings were somewhat less consistent. Confusion did not relate to exploration after correct answers, which is well explained by floor effects in the occurrence of this emotion after correct answers. Confusion after incorrect answers positively predicted exploration, in line with prior evidence indicating that confusion can promote cognitive performance (D'Mello et al. 2014); however, these effects were relatively weak, and they were significant in Studies 1 and 3 but not in Study 2. The small effect sizes for confusion could be due to variable effects of negative activating emotions, such as confusion, on motivation and behavior (Pekrun and Stephens 2012). It is possible that confusion strengthens motivation to explore in individuals who expect to successfully resolve their confusion, but undermines motivation and knowledge exploration in persons who expect that the resolution of confusion is less likely. Low expectations could drive these individuals to withdraw from, rather than persist through, the task at hand. Meta-analytic integration of the findings of Study 3 by Vogl et al. (2019a) and the results of two replication studies reported in Vogl et al. (2019b) support positive effects of all three epistemic emotions.

As for achievement emotions, pride after correctly answered items had positive effects on knowledge exploration, in line with prior findings on positive relations between pride and cognitive performance (e.g., Pekrun et al. 2017a; Pekrun et al. 2019; Williams and DeSteno 2008). In contrast, there were null relations between shame and exploration. Similar to the variable effects of confusion, this finding is consistent with theoretical perspectives and prior evidence that the effects of activating negative emotions can be complex and result in zero correlations with overall measures of performance (Pekrun and Stephens 2012; Turner and Schallert 2001). Interestingly, the positive effect of pride could not be replicated by Vogl et al. (2019b). More research is needed to understand the inconsistent effects of pride on knowledge exploration. However, the null effect of shame could be replicated. In sum, the findings clearly connect the experience of the epistemic emotions surprise, curiosity, and confusion with the feeling of confidence.

3.4.2 *The Interplay of Surprise, Curiosity, Confusion, and Wonder with the Feeling of Confidence and the Feeling of Comprehension*

In line with our results, Nerantzaki and Efklides (2019) also found interrelations between epistemic emotions (surprise, curiosity, confusion, wonder, and interest) and metacognitive feelings (feeling of certainty and feeling of comprehension) using a between-subjects design. Participants watched three learning scenarios with varying difficulty presenting two students using different learning strategies to prepare for an exam. Participants were asked to decide which student would be more successful in the exam. They received immediate feedback about the accuracy of their reply and a scientific explanation of the correct response. After that, participants were asked about their personal learning strategy use given the three scenarios.

Epistemic emotions were measured (a) after participants received feedback about the accuracy of their reply, (b) after they received the explanation of the correct answer, and (c) after their personal use of learning strategies. Participants' feeling of confidence was measured directly after responding to each scenario. Feeling of comprehension was measured after the presentation of a scientific explanation of the correct response. The authors expected epistemic emotions to be triggered by negative feedback and to vary as a function of scenario difficulty. In addition, they expected interrelations between epistemic emotions and a negative relationship between epistemic emotions and both metacognitive feelings.

In line with their hypotheses, Nerantzaki and Efklides (2019) found that epistemic emotions were triggered by negative feedback and they were more intensely experienced in time 1 as compared to times 2 and 3 in all scenarios. In addition, they found that the intensity of epistemic emotions varied as a function of scenario difficulty, i.e., epistemic emotions were more intensely experienced in the difficult scenario as compared to the moderately difficult and easy scenarios. With the exception of interest, epistemic emotions correlated positively with each other in time 1 in all scenarios. Correlations were less strong and less consistent in times 2 and 3 as well as between the three times of measurement. In contrast to hypotheses, Nerantzaki and Efklides (2019) found a positive relationship between surprise, wonder, and confusion with the feeling of confidence only in time 1 of the difficult scenario. In the moderately difficult and difficult scenario, feeling of comprehension was negatively related to confusion and wonder.

The findings about the relationship between epistemic emotions and the feeling of confidence may be explained by taking into account the interactive effect of accuracy and confidence on epistemic emotions. In the difficult scenario most participants received negative feedback. An intense feeling of confidence paired with negative feedback may have possibly driven the positive relationship between epistemic emotions and the feeling of confidence, which would be in line with findings by Vogl and colleagues (Vogl et al. 2019a, b). However, Nerantzaki and Efklides (2019) did not find a relationship between high-confidence errors and curiosity. Differences in the results might be attributable to the different research designs (between- vs. within-person design) and the fact that Nerantzaki and Efklides (2019) did not take into account the interactive effect of the feeling of confidence and accuracy on epistemic emotions. In sum, the findings connect epistemic emotions with metacognitive feelings, i.e., the experience of surprise, curiosity, confusion, and wonder with the feeling of confidence and the feeling of comprehension.

3.5 Conclusion

In sum, the body of research on epistemic emotions and metacognitive feelings indicates similarities and linkages of epistemic emotions and metacognitive feelings, but also suggests that they differ in terms of their qualities and their effects on knowledge acquisition. Specifically, epistemic emotions and metacognitive feeling share common features such as the affective core experience as well as effects on cognitive processing. Epistemic emotions have been associated with cognitive and motivational outcomes, but also with the initiation of behaviors such as inquiry and exploration (Berlyne 1954, 1960; Litman et al. 2005; Loewenstein 1994; Wong 1979), suggesting that their functions include setting off regulatory efforts targeting cognitive as well as behavioral engagement. Metacognitive feelings, in contrast, seem to be more closely bound to the regulation of cognitive processing, and less to the regulation of non-cognitive behaviors (see also Efklides 2011). In addition, epistemic emotions and metacognitive feelings seem to differ in terms of their characteristic constituents. While epistemic emotions qualify as emotions as defined by multicomponent definitions (e.g., Scherer 2009), metacognitive feelings are less closely associated with physiological and expressive processes (see also Efklides 2016). Nevertheless, the boundaries between epistemic emotions and metacognitive feelings are fuzzy, in particular when considering cognitively-grounded emotions such as surprise or confusion.

As for the relations between epistemic emotions and metacognitive feelings, empirical evidence suggests that metacognitive processes play an important role in the occurrence of epistemic emotions (e.g., Metcalfe and Finn 2012; Nerantzaki and Efklides 2019; Touroutoglou and Efklides 2010; Vogl et al. 2019a, b). In particular, they highlight the critical role of the metacognitive feeling of confidence in the accuracy of one's knowledge for the experience of surprise, curiosity, and confusion. In sum, first empirical evidence suggests that metacognitive feelings can not only influence the regulation of cognition but also the experience of epistemic emotions.

3.6 Open Questions for Future Research

Our discussion about the similarities, differences, and relations between epistemic emotions and metacognitive feelings was not completely in line with your preexisting conceptualization of these constructs? Great! We hope it sparked your curiosity to explore these concepts in more detail. There are still many open questions for future research. For example, we discussed a select subset of affectively-connotated epistemic states and their qualification as epistemic emotions as defined by multicomponent approaches to emotions (e.g., Scherer 2009). However, what about other states that might qualify as epistemic emotions, such as doubt (e.g., de Sousa 2008, 2009; Wesson and Pulford 2009), or the experience of awe (e.g., Shiota et al. 2007)? Are there specific component processes differentiating epistemic emotions from metacognitive feelings (e.g., physiological processes)? How do epistemic emotions interact with metacognitive feelings other than the feeling of confidence? For example, how is the feeling of knowing related to (epistemic) enjoyment? And can epistemic emotions and metacognitive feelings in fact be differentiated by a set of unique outcomes? It has been proposed that metacognitive feelings exclusively impact cognitive processing, whereas epistemic emotions can influence cognition, motivation, and behaviors more broadly. More research is needed to address these open problems.

Last but not least, the ultimate goal of this research could be to use the cumulative knowledge about epistemic emotions and metacognitive feelings to create appropriate measures as well as tools that foster adaptive epistemic emotions and metacognitive feelings to promote knowledge generation. For example, how can we use surprise to spark curiosity? When does an individual's surprise in reaction to unexpected information give rise to curiosity versus confusion? When is confusion productive and beneficial for knowledge acquisition? How can we promote realistic feelings of confidence in learners, all the while leaving room for playing with common misconceptions and triggering motivating experiences of surprise and curiosity that drive knowledge generation and conceptual change? As reflected in the sheer number of questions posed above, the similarities, differences, and relations between epistemic emotions and metacognitive feelings are not yet fully understood and they will hopefully spark a lively collaborative debate between research on emotions and metacognition.

References

Arango-Muñoz, S. (2013). The nature of epistemic feelings. *Philosophical Psychology, 27*, 1–19. https://doi.org/10.1080/09515089.2012.732002.

Baker, R., D'Mello, S., Rodrigo, M., & Graesser, A. C. (2010). Better to be frustrated than bored: The incidence and persistence of affect during interactions with three different computer-based learning environments. *International Journal of Human-Computer Studies, 68*, 223–241. https://doi.org/10.1016/j.ijhcs.2009.12.003.

Berlyne, D. E. (1954). A theory of human curiosity. *British Journal of Psychology, 43*, 180–191.

Berlyne, D. E. (1960). Toward a theory of exploratory behavior: II. Arousal potential, perceptual curiosity, and learning. In D. E. Berlyne (Ed.), *Conflict, arousal, and curiosity* (pp. 193–227). New York: McGraw-Hill Book Company. https://doi.org/10.1037/11164-008.

Boekaerts, M., & Rozendaal, J. S. (2010). Using multiple calibration indices in order to capture the complex picture of what affects students' accuracy of feeling of confidence. *Learning and Instruction, 20*, 372–382. https://doi.org/10.1016/j.learninstruc.2009.03.002.

Bosch, N., & D'Mello, S. (2017). The affective experience of novice computer programmers. *International Journal of Artificial Intelligence in Education, 27*, 181–206. https://doi.org/10.1007/s40593-015-0069-5.

Brown, J., & VanLehn, K. (1980). Repair theory: A generative theory of bugs in procedural skills. *Cognitive Science, 4*, 379–426.

Brun, G., Doğuoğlu, U., & Kuenzle, D. (Eds.). (2008). *Epistemology and emotions*. Aldershot: Ashgate.

Carver, C. S. (2003). Pleasure as a sign you can attend to something else: Placing positive feelings within a general model of affect. *Cognition and Emotion, 17*, 241–261. https://doi.org/10.1080/02699930302294.

Carver, C. S., & Johnson, S. L. (2010). Authentic and hubristic pride: Differential relations to aspects of goal regulation, affect, and self-control. *Journal of Research in Personality, 44*, 698–703. https://doi.org/10.1016/j.jrp.2010.09.004.

Carver, C. S., & Scheier, M. F. (1998). *On the self-regulation of behavior*. Cambridge: Cambridge University Press.

Clore, G. L., & Huntsinger, J. R. (2007). How emotions inform judgment and regulate thought. *Trends in Cognitive Sciences, 11*, 393–399. https://doi.org/10.1016/j.tics.2007.08.005.

Craig, S., Graesser, A., Sullins, J., & Gholson, B. (2004). Affect and learning: An exploratory look into the role of affect in learning with AutoTutor. *Journal of Educational Media, 29*, 241–250. https://doi.org/10.1080/1358165042000283101.

D'Mello, S., & Graesser, A. (2012). Dynamics of affective states during complex learning. *Learning and Instruction, 22*, 145–157. https://doi.org/10.1016/j.learninstruc.2011.10.001.

D'Mello, S., & Graesser, A. (2014). Confusion and its dynamics during device comprehension with breakdown scenarios. *Acta Psychologica, 151*, 106–116. https://doi.org/10.1016/j.actpsy.2014.06.005.

D'Mello, S., Lehman, B., Pekrun, R., & Graesser, A. (2014). Confusion can be beneficial for learning. *Learning and Instruction, 29*, 153–170. https://doi.org/10.1016/j.learninstruc.2012.05.003.

de Sousa, R. (2008). Epistemic feelings. In G. Brun, U. Doğuoğlu, & D. Kuenzle (Eds.), *Epistemology and emotions* (pp. 185–204). Aldershot: Ashgate.

de Sousa, R. (2009). Epistemic feelings. *Mind and Matter, 7*, 139–161.

Deci, E. L. (1975). *Intrinsic motivation*. New York: Plenum Press.

Dunlosky, J., & Rawson, K. A. (2012). Overconfidence produces underachievement: Inaccurate self evaluations undermine students' learning and retention. *Learning and Instruction, 22*, 271–280. https://doi.org/10.1016/j.learninstruc.2011.08.003.

Ebert, M., & Klotzek, T. (2008). *Neon UnnützesWissen I [Neon useless knowledge I]*. Munich: Wilhelm Heyne.

Ebert, M., & Klotzek, T. (2010). *Neon UnnützesWissen II [Neon useless knowledge II]*. Munich: Wilhelm Heyne.

Efklides, A. (2006). Metacognition and affect: What can metacognitive experiences tell us about the learning process? *Educational Research Review, 1*, 3–14. https://doi.org/10.1016/j.edurev.2005.11.00.1.

Efklides, A. (2008). Metacognition: Defining its facets and levels of functioning in relation to self- and co-regulation. *European Psychologist, 13*, 277–287. https://doi.org/10.1027/1016-9040.13.4.277.

Efklides, A. (2011). Interactions of metacognition with motivation and affect in self-regulated learning: The MASRL model. *Educational Psychologist, 46*, 6–25. https://doi.org/10.1080/00461520.2011.538645.
Efklides, A. (2014). How does metacognition contribute to the regulation of learning? An integrative approach. *Psychological Topics, 1*, 1–30.
Efklides, A. (2016). Metamemory and affect. In J. Dunlosky & U. Tauber (Eds.), *Oxford handbook of metamemory* (pp. 245–268). New York: Oxford University Press.
Efklides, A. (2017). Affect, epistemic emotions, metacognition, and self-regulated learning. *Teachers College Record, 119*, 135–144.
Efklides, A., & Dina, F. (2004). Feedback from one's self and the others: Their effect on affect. *Hellenic Journal of Psychology, 1*, 179–202.
Efklides, A., & Petkaki, C. (2005). Effects of mood on students' metacognitive experiences. *Learning and Instruction, 15*, 415–431. https://doi.org/10.1016/j.learninstruc.2005.07.010.
Efklides, A., Schwartz, B., & Brown, V. (2018). Motivation and affect in SRL: Does metacognition play a role? In D. Schunk & J. Greene (Eds.), *Handbook of self-regulation of learning and performance* (pp. 64–82). New York: Routledge.
Ekman, P. (1982). *Emotion in the human face*. New York: Cambridge University Press.
Ekman, P. (1999). Basic emotions. In T. Dalgleish & M. Power (Eds.), *Handbook of cognition and emotion*. New York: Wiley.
Feldman Barrett, L., & Russell, J. A. (1999). The structure of current affect: Controversies and emerging consensus. *Current Directions in Psychological Science, 8*, 10–14. https://doi.org/10.1111/1467-8721.00003.
Flavell, J. H. (1979). Metacognition and cognitive monitoring: A new era of cognitive-developmental inquiry. *American Psychologist, 34*, 906–911. https://doi.org/10.1037/0003-066X.34.10.906.
Fredrickson, B. L. (2001). The role of positive emotions in positive psychology: The broaden-and-build theory of positive emotions. *American Psychologist, 56*, 218–226.
Gocłowska, M. A., Baas, M., Crisp, R. J., & De Dreu, C. K. W. (2014). Whether social schema violations help or hurt creativity depends on need for structure. *Personality and Social Psychology Bulletin, 40*, 959–971. https://doi.org/10.1177/0146167214533132.
Gocłowska, M. A., Baas, M., Elliot, A. J., & De Dreu, C. K. W. (2017). Why schema-violations are sometimes preferable to schema- consistencies: The role of interest and openness to experience. *Journal of Research in Personality, 66*, 54–69. https://doi.org/10.1016/j.jrp.2016.
Gruber, M. J., Gelman, B. D., & Ranganath, C. (2014). States of curiosity modulate hippocampus-dependent learning via the dopaminergic circuit. *Neuron, 84*, 486–496. https://doi.org/10.1016/j.neuron.2014.08.060.
Kagan, J. (1972). Motives and development. *Journal of Personality and Social Psychology, 22*, 51–66. https://doi.org/10.1037/h0032356.
Kang, M. J., Hsu, M., Kajbich, I. M., Loewenstein, G., McClure, S. M., Wang, J. T., & Camerer, C. F. (2009). The wick in the candle of learning: Epistemic curiosity activates reward circuitry and enhances memory. *Psychological Science, 20*, 963–973. https://doi.org/10.1111/j.1467-9280.2009.02402.x.
Litman, J. A., & Jimerson, T. L. (2004). The measurement of curiosity as a feeling of deprivation. *Journal of Personality Assessment, 82*, 147–157. https://doi.org/10.1207/s15327752jpa8202_3.
Litman, J., Hutchins, T., & Russon, R. (2005). Epistemic curiosity, feeling-of-knowing, and exploratory behaviour. *Cognition and Emotion, 19*, 559–582. https://doi.org/10.1080/02699930441000427.
Loewenstein, G. (1994). The psychology of curiosity: A review and reinterpretation. *Psychological Bulletin, 116*, 75–98. https://doi.org/10.1037/0033-2909.116.1.75.
Mandler, G. (1990). Interruption (discrepancy) theory: Review and extensions. In S. Fisher & L. Cooper (Eds.), *On the move: The psychology of change and transition* (pp. 13–32). Chichester: Wiley.

Markey, A., & Loewenstein, G. (2014). Curiosity. In R. Pekrun & L. Linnenbrink-Garcia (Eds.), *Educational psychology handbook series. International handbook of emotions in education* (pp. 228–245). New York: Routledge/Taylor & Francis Group. https://doi.org/10.1037/t12348-000.

Marvin, C. B., & Shohamy, D. (2016). Curiosity and reward: Valence predicts choice and information prediction errors enhance learning. *Journal of Experimental Psychology: General, 145*, 266–272. https://doi.org/10.1037/xge0000140.

Metallidou, P., & Efklides, A. (2001). The effects of general success-related beliefs and specific metacognitive experiences on causal attributions. In A. Efklides, J. Kuhl, & R. M. Sorrentino (Eds.), *Trends and prospects in motivation research* (pp. 325–347). Dordrecht: Kluwer.

Metcalfe, J., & Finn, B. (2012). Hypercorrection of high confidence errors in children. *Learning and Instruction, 22*, 253–261. https://doi.org/10.1016/j.learninstruc.2011.10.004.

Miceli, M., & Castelfranchi, C. (2005). Anxiety as an "epistemic" emotion: An uncertainty theory of anxiety. *Anxiety, Stress and Coping, 18*, 291–319. https://doi.org/10.1080/10615800500209324.

Middlebrooks, C. D., McGillivray, S., Murayama, K., & Castel, A. D. (2016). Memory for allergies and health foods: How younger and older adults strategically remember critical health information. *Psychological Sciences and Social Sciences, 71*, 389–399. https://doi.org/10.1093/geronb/gbv032.

Morton, A. (2010). Epistemic emotions. In P. Goldie (Ed.), *The Oxford handbook of philosophy of emotion* (pp. 385–399). Oxford: Oxford University Press.

Muis, K. R., Pekrun, R., Sinatra, G. M., Azevedo, R., Trevors, G., Meier, E., & Heddy, B. C. (2015a). The curious case of climate change: Testing a theoretical model of epistemic beliefs, epistemic emotions, and complex learning. *Learning and Instruction, 39*, 168–183. https://doi.org/10.1016/j.learninstruc.2015.06.003.

Muis, K. R., Psaradellis, C., Lajoie, S. P., Di Leo, I., & Chevrier, M. (2015b). The role of epistemic emotions in mathematics problem solving. *Contemporary Educational Psychology, 42*, 172–185. https://doi.org/10.1016/j.cedpsych.2015.06.003.

Muis, K. R., Chevrier, M., & Singh, C. A. (2018). The role of epistemic emotions in personal epistemology and self-regulated learning. *Educational Psychologist, 53*, 165–184. https://doi.org/10.1080/00461520.2017.1421465.

Murayama, K., FitzGibbon, L., & Sakaki, M. (2019). Process account of curiosity and interest: A reward learning perspective. *Educational Psychology Review, 31*, 875–895. https://doi.org/10.1007/s10648-019-09499-9.

Nelson, T. O. (1996). Consciousness and metacognition. *American Psychologist, 51*, 102–116. https://doi.org/10.1037/0003-066X.51.2.102.

Nelson, T. O., & Narens, L. (1980). Norms of 300 general-information questions: Accuracy of recall, latency of recall, and feeling-of-knowing ratings. *Journal of Verbal Learning and Verbal Behavior, 19*, 338–368. https://doi.org/10.1016/S0022-5371(80)90266-2.

Nerantzaki, K., & Efklides, A. (2019). Epistemic emotions: Interrelationships and changes during task processing. *Hellenic Journal of Psychology, 16*, 177–199.

Ortony, A., & Turner, T. (1990). What's basic about basic emotions? *Psychological Review, 97*, 315–331. https://doi.org/10.1037//0033-295X.97.3.315.

Parzuchowski, M., & Szymkow-Sudziarska, A. (2008). Well, slap my thigh: Expression of surprise facilitates memory of surprising material. *Emotion, 8*, 430–434. https://doi.org/10.1037/1528-3542.8.3.430.

Pekrun, R. (2006). The control-value theory of achievement emotions: Assumptions, corollaries, and implications for educational research and practice. *Educational Psychology Review, 18*, 315–341. https://doi.org/10.1007/s10648-006-9029-9.

Pekrun, R. (2012). Emotions as drivers of learning and cognitive development. In R. A. Calvo & S. K. D'Mello (Eds.), *New perspectives on affect and learning technologies* (pp. 23–39). New York: Springer.

Pekrun, R. (2019). The murky distinction between curiosity and interest: State of the art and future prospects. *Educational Psychology Review, 31*, 905–914. https://doi.org/10.1007/s10648-019-09512-1.

Pekrun, R. (2020). Self-appraisals and emotions: A generalized control-value approach. In T. Dicke, F. Guay, H. W. Marsh, R. G. Craven & D. M. McInerney (Eds.), *Self – a multidisciplinary concept*. Charlotte: Information Age Publishing.

Pekrun, R., & Linnenbrink-Garcia, L. (Eds.). (2014). *International handbook of emotions in education*. New York: Routledge.

Pekrun, R., & Perry, R. P. (2014). Control-value theory of achievement emotions. In R. Pekrun & L. Linnenbrink-Garcia (Eds.), *International handbook of emotions in education* (pp. 120–141). New York: Routledge.

Pekrun, R., & Stephens, E. J. (2012). Academic emotions. In K. R. Harris, S. Graham, T. Urdan, S. Graham, J. M. Royer, & M. Zeidner (Eds.), *APA handbooks in psychology. APA educational psychology handbook, Vol 2: Individual differences and cultural and contextual factors* (pp. 3–31). Washington: American Psychological Association. https://doi.org/10.1037/13274-001.

Pekrun, R., Lichtenfeld, S., Marsh, H. W., Murayama, K., & Goetz, T. (2017a). Achievement emotions and academic performance: Longitudinal models of reciprocal effects. *Child Development, 88*, 1653–1670. https://doi.org/10.1111/cdev.12704.

Pekrun, R., Murayama, K., Marsh, H. W., Goetz, T., & Frenzel, A. C. (2019). Happy fish in little ponds: Testing a reference group model of achievement and emotion. *Journal of Personality and Social Psychology, 117*, 166–185. https://doi.org/10.1037/pspp0000230.

Pekrun, R., Vogl, E., Muis, K. R., & Sinatra, G. M. (2017b). Measuring emotions during epistemic activities: The epistemically-related emotion scales. *Cognition and Emotion, 31*, 1268–1276. https://doi.org/10.1080/02699931.2016.1204989.

Pöppelmann, C. (2009). *1000 Irrtümer der Allgemeinbildung: Aufgedeckt und richtiggestellt [1,000 common misconceptions uncovered and rectified]*. Munich: Compact.

Reeve, J. (1993). The face of interest. *Motivation and Emotion, 17*, 353–375. https://doi.org/10.1007/BF00992325.

Renninger, K. A., & Hidi, S. (Eds.). (2016). *The power of interest for motivation and learning*. New York: Routledge.

Rozin, P., & Cohen, A. B. (2003). High frequency of facial expressions corresponding to confusion, concentration, and worry in an analysis of naturally occurring facial expressions of Americans. *Emotion, 3*, 68–75. https://doi.org/10.1037/1528-3542.3.1.68.

Scheffler, I. (Ed.). (1991). *In praise of the cognitive emotions and other essays in the philosophy of education*. New York: Routledge.

Scherer, K. R. (2009). The dynamic architecture of emotion: Evidence for the component process model. *Cognition and Emotion, 23*, 1307–1351. https://doi.org/10.1080/02699930902928969.

Shiota, M. N., Keltner, D., & Mossman, A. (2007). The nature of awe: Elicitors, appraisals, and effects on self-concept. *Cognition and Emotion, 21*, 944–963. https://doi.org/10.1080/02699930600923668.

Stone, N. J. (2000). Exploring the relationships between calibration and self-regulated learning. *Educational Psychology Review, 12*, 437–475. https://doi.org/10.1023/A:1009084430926.

Touroutoglou, A., & Efklides, A. (2010). Cognitive interruption as an object of metacognitive monitoring: Feeling of difficulty and surprise. In A. Efklides & P. Misailidi (Eds.), *Trends and prospects in metacognition research* (pp. 171–208). New York: Springer.

Turner, J., & Schallert, D. L. (2001). Expectancy-value relationships of shame reactions and shame resiliency. *Journal of Educational Psychology, 93*, 320–329. https://doi.org/10.1037//0022-0663.93.2.320.

Vogl, E., Pekrun, R., Murayama, K., & Loderer, K. (2019a). Surprised–curious–confused: Epistemic emotions and knowledge exploration. *Emotion*. https://doi.org/10.1037/emo0000578.

Vogl, E., Pekrun, R., Murayama, K., Loderer, K., & Schubert, S. (2019b). Surprise, curiosity, and confusion promote knowledge exploration: Evidence for robust effects of epistemic emotions. *Frontiers in Psychology, 10*, 2474. https://doi.org/10.3389/fpsyg.2019.02474.

von Stumm, S., Hell, B., & Chamorro-Premuzic, T. (2011). The hungry mind: Intellectual curiosity is the third pillar of academic performance. *Perspectives on Psychological Science, 6*, 574–588. https://doi.org/10.1177/1745691611421204.

Weiner, B. (1985). An attributional theory of achievement motivation and emotion. *Psychological Review, 92*, 548–573. https://doi.org/10.1037/0033-295X.92.4.548.

Weiner, B. (2010). The development of an attribution-based theory of motivation: A history of ideas. *Educational Psychologist, 45*, 28–36. https://doi.org/10.1080/00461520903433596.

Wesson, C. J., & Pulford, B. D. (2009). Verbal expressions of confidence and doubt. *Psychological Reports, 105*, 151–160. https://doi.org/10.2466/pr0.105.1.151-160.

Wigfield, A., & Eccles, J. S. (2000). Expectancy-value theory of achievement motivation. *Contemporary Educational Psychology, 25*, 68–81. https://doi.org/10.1006/ceps.1999.1015.

Williams, L. A., & DeSteno, D. (2008). Pride and perseverance: The motivational role of pride. *Journal of Personality and Social Psychology, 94*, 1007–1017. https://doi.org/10.1037/0022-3514.94.6.1007.

Wong, P. T. (1979). Frustration, exploration, and learning. *Canadian Psychological Review/ Psychologie canadienne, 20*, 133–144. https://doi.org/10.1037/h0081509.

Chapter 4
Metacognitive Experience Across the Creative Process

Alessandro Antonietti, Alice Cancer, Barbara Colombo, and Paola Iannello

Abstract In the first part of the chapter, recent literature is critically discussed to examine the relationships between creativity and metacognition–intended as metacognitive knowledge, metacognitive awareness, and metacognitive control. In the second part, we report an experimental study on primary school children. Participants were engaged in a creative thinking training programme with two conditions where they were either asked or not asked to rate the level of ability, effort, and liking perceived both before (prediction) and after (retrospection) carrying out the creative tasks. Creativity scores increased as a consequence of the training. The prediction/retrospection task enhanced only one aspect of creative thinking, namely, the ability to widen the mental field. Calibration—the match between the subjective prediction of the performance and the actual performance—improved across the training, as well as the quality of the retrospective judgments about the performance. Possible future directions of research about the role of metacognition in creativity and implications for education are highlighted.

Keywords Creativity · Metacognitive experience · Calibration

4.1 Introduction

Originally, metacognition had been extensively investigated in fields such as memory and learning. Thanks to the contribution of eminent researchers, such as Anastasia Efklides—the dedicatee of this Festschrift—the field of application of

A. Antonietti (✉) · A. Cancer · P. Iannello
Department of Psychology, Catholic University of the Sacred Heart, Milan, Italy
e-mail: alessandro.antonietti@unicatt.it; alice.cancer@unicatt.it; paola.iannello@unicatt.it

B. Colombo
Neuroscience Lab, Division of Education and Human Studies, Champlain College, Burlington, VT, USA
e-mail: bcolombo@champlain.edu

D. Moraitou, P. Metallidou (eds.), *Trends and Prospects in Metacognition Research across the Life Span*, https://doi.org/10.1007/978-3-030-51673-4_4

metacognition became broader, including for instance emotion and motivation (Efklides et al. 2001; Efklides and Misailidi 2010).

Among the topics that have not been researched yet is the analysis of the relationship between metacognition and creativity. Several aspects of this relationship have been investigated to some extent, reporting inconsistent findings (Jia et al. 2019). These topics include whether people are aware of the processes occurring when they are thinking in a creative way (metacognitive awareness) and whether they can control such processes (metacognitive control), as well as whether they share relevant beliefs about these processes (metacognitive knowledge). The inconsistent results may depend, on the one hand, on the complexity of the construct of "metacognition", which is a multi-facet term (Efklides 2011), and, on the other hand, on the fuzziness of the concept of "creativity", which still lacks a unanimous definition. In addition, limits of the instruments to assess both metacognition and creativity constitute a further obstacle. Metacognition is mainly measured through self-report tools, which are subjective by their own nature. Subjectivity often affects the systems used to score creativity as well (Batey 2012).

Indeed, creativity is often conceived as underlying mental processes that are completely unrelated to metacognition. Innovative ideas are usually interpreted as outcomes of unconscious processes, which cannot be predicted and/or controlled by the individual. In addition, creativity is commonly conceived as a spontaneous activity that relies on fast processes, which individuals are not aware of. Creativity is also believed not to follow regularities or rules, and hence cannot be controlled. In other words, it seems that creativity is based on sudden insights or associations of concepts, which cannot be prepared, prompted, programmed, and monitored.

Some studies seem to support a lack of relations between creativity and metacognition. For example, Hong et al. (2010) analysed the relationships between metacognition, intrinsic motivation, and creative performance in students and found that metacognition was not associated with more originality in homework assignments. Preiss et al. (2016) also failed to observe a relation between metacognitive knowledge and the ability to find unusual uses of common objects and to find uncommon associations among words. Only a moderate correlation between metacognitive knowledge and creativity in filling and titling drawings (Lizarraga and Baquedano 2013) and in mathematics (Erbas and Bas 2015) has been reported.

However, a variety of strategies aimed at facilitating or inducing the emergence of original ideas have been devised and are currently proposed as effective ways to foster creativity. Thus, it is assumed that creative outcomes can be achieved thanks to specific cognitive processes, which can be intentionally orientated according to precise mental plans and can be taught (De Stobbeleir et al. 2011). It has been reported that interventions aimed at teaching how relevant strategies can be monitored and controlled—with monitoring and control being two aspects of metacognition—improved scores in creativity tasks (Hargrove 2013; Hargrove and Nietfeld 2015). Yet, contrasting findings, suggesting the ineffectiveness of interventions based on nudging monitoring and planning thinking processes, have been reported as well (Hong et al. 2016).

Starting from this background, the goal of this chapter is to provide a contribution to the investigation of the relationships between metacognition and creativity by identifying which specific cognitive mechanisms are involved in creative thinking (Sect. 4.2) and organising them conceptually in a model (the WCR model, W = Widening, C = Connecting, R = Reorganising) which can take into account the different facets of creativity (Sect. 4.3). On the light of this model, previous studies about the possible role of metacognition in creativity are reviewed (Sect. 4.4). Subsequently, an experimental study testing the level of awareness of children engaged in creative tasks and the influence of metacognitive hints on creative ideas generation is reported (Sect. 4.5). In the final part of the chapter, findings are discussed by considering the possible ways the topic in question (i.e., the relations between metacognition and creativity) can be faced in the future. The need of innovative perspectives—as those Anastasia Efklides developed in addressing other domains of metacognition—is stressed (Sect. 4.6).

4.2 The Mechanisms Involved in Creative Thinking

When considering the cognitive mechanisms at the basis of creativity, quite different theoretical assumptions still coexist. The first, as yet commonly shared, perspective assumes that creativity has to do mainly with the abundant and diversified production of ideas. Within this perspective, the fluid, flexible, and original generation of ideas often derives from the variation of existing ideas (Perkins 1988; Simonton 1999; Weisberg 1993). The creative process becomes similar to the process of evolution, which is determined by the generation of variations in the characteristics of existing species and their selection, leading to the maintenance of those that guarantee a greater capacity for survival (Johnson-Laird 1988).

An associationist conception is also quite common, seeing creativity as the ability to bring together ideas which are distant from each other. For example, Rothenberg (1979) identified creativity with the Janic (from Janus, the double-faced Roman deity who looks in two opposite directions) thinking. This cognitive process makes it possible to combine the terms of an antithesis, i.e., to be able to keep two opposite elements in mind simultaneously, and try to integrate them.

Thirdly, Schank (1988) suggested that a restructuring process is at the basis of creativity. According to this author, individuals, in order to understand reality, need knowledge structures. A knowledge structure that is used several times to account for events constitutes a "pattern of explanation". When faced with a stimulus, the cheapest strategy is to treat it in the same way as a familiar stimulus, by trying to apply a pattern of explanation that is valid for other known situations. Creativity emerges when the situation an individual is facing is new. In this case individuals will apply an explanation pattern where they are not expected to apply it. The creative process derives from an intentional mis-application of an explanation pattern. When faced with an event, the creative person does not go back to the routine explanation, but ventures into the unexpected.

4.3 The WCR Model

Inspired by this varied range of theories, the WCR model has been proposed (Antonietti and Colombo 2013, 2016). This model tries to synthesize them to produce a complete and coherent picture of the creative mechanisms. If we do not focus specifically on the single aspects that characterise each theory, we can identify three major mental operations which underlie creativity.

The first operation is the *widening* of the mental field. If individuals are able to produce many different and unusual ideas, if they take something existing and try to vary it, if they generate different ideas in order to identify at least one that survives the evaluation phase, they have a wealth of mental elements that increases the probability of identifying among them one that leads to something new and valuable. Therefore, broadening the mental horizon through the discovery or invention of new elements contributes to creativity.

Connecting, namely, the bridging of mental fields usually considered distant or antithetical, is the second basic operation of creativity. It consists in establishing links between very different realities.

The third operation is *reorganising* the mental field, either through its internal restructuring or through the application of an apparently inappropriate interpretative scheme. This scheme would apply well to other situations but would be unconventional for the situation at hand, resulting in a new vision which highlights non-obvious and interesting meanings.

4.3.1 Supports from Neuroscience

Results from neuroscience research lend support to the idea that the mental operations discussed above are involved in creative thinking. In fact, today we can go beyond anecdotal evidence to support the link between creativity and the right hemisphere. This has been proven by the changes in blood flow in this part of the cerebral cortex in creative tasks, especially in individuals who provide original responses (Dacey and Lennon 1998; Martindale 1999). Going further, it is possible to correlate the *widening* of the mental field to the right prefrontal cortex (Colombo et al. 2015; Oldrati et al. 2016; Sandkühler and Bhattacharya 2008) by stressing the role played by the anterior cingulate cortex in establishing an emotional state favourable to this process (Subramaniam et al. 2008).

When focusing on the *connecting* operation, the correlation between creativity and intensity of activation of the brain network (Hines 1991; Hoppe and Kyle 1990) is supported by the observation that in split-brain patients creative activity is reduced

(Hoppe 1994). This link is also clarified by the results of experiments showing that the ability to find non-trivial associations requires the suppression of dominant associations, a process that is related to a specific neural activity with precise brain localizations (Kounios et al. 2006).

Finally, *reorganising* the mental field, like the operation required in certain insight problems, is related to the activation of the right anterior temporal gyrus (Jung-Beeman et al. 2004; Kounios and Beeman 2009) and to a specific modulation of the psychophysiological arousal (Antonietti et al. 2010).

4.3.2 The Creative Operations in Practice: From Testing to Training

The WCR model of creativity, which ties creativity to the three mental operations mentioned before, is validated not only on a conceptual level, but it is also validated by empirical data, showing that the abilities to perform the three operations are distinct, while all three correlating with general creativity. For instance, each mental operation follows a developmental trend which is different from the other ones (Andolfi et al. 2016) and pathologies, such as learning disorders (Cancer et al. 2016) or brain injuries (Colautti et al. 2018), affect such operations in a selective way, by enhancing the ability to perform one of them and by decreasing the capacity to apply the other ones.

4.3.2.1 The WCR Test

The WCR model has been taken as a basis also to devise a test to evaluate the creative ability (Pizzingrilli et al. 2015a). The test is available in six versions corresponding to different age levels.

In the first sub-test (*Widening*) the respondents are asked to choose, according to their preference, an answer among possible alternatives, which gradually vary from the obvious meaning to an unexpected one that implies a high level of mental transformation of the stimulus. For example: "A desk can be used for different goals other than writing. Choose one response among the following: to write; to grab an object on high shelf; as a bookshelf; as a shelter, in the event of an earthquake, if you crouch under it".

In the second sub-test (*Connecting*) the respondents are asked to choose, from a given list of words or pictures, the elements that they would associate with the given situation and to justify their choice. Options have been arranged according to a different degree of conceptual closeness with the stimulus, ranging from obvious associations to remote ones. For instance: "What does a backpack remind you of?

Choose one response among the following: school; books; pocket; colors; homework; walking; bus".

In the third sub-test (*Reorganising*) the respondents, faced with a hypothetical situation, are asked to select an answer from alternatives that vary in originality. For instance: "What would happen if we could only see in black-and-white? Choose one response among the following: We could not perceive colors; We could not appreciate the colors of the Harlequin costume; All would be more sad; Matching colors for our daily outfits would be not a problem; Painters would have only two colors on their palette; It would be as living in an old movie".

The scoring system of the WCR test is based on the assumption that the choice of responses endorsed by a small percentage of subjects within the normative sample reveals that the respondent processed the situation described in the item in a highly original way. Hence, it receives a high creativity score. On the contrary, the selection of an option that was frequently chosen in the normative sample is representative of the tendency to rely on common ways of thinking: For this reason, a low creativity score is attributed.

The application of the WCR test to different samples allowed to verify that it does discriminate individuals according to their creative potential, without any gender influence. It was also found that each of the three sub-tests contributes to the total score of creativity that can be obtained from the test. However, each one measures an aspect of creativity that is positively correlated to those measured by the other sub-tests, but does not overlap.

4.3.2.2 Training Programmes Inspired by the WCR Model

The model has been further validated by the application of two training programmes based on the WCR model of creative thinking (Antonietti et al. 2020b). The first training (Antonietti et al. 2011) targets primary school students and it is divided into three sections, each promoting one of the three operations (widening, connecting, reorganising). Since the application of a single creative operation seldom occurs in practice, while it is more likely that different operations actually coexist, the training programme also includes a fourth section, entitled multi-process, where the activities require the simultaneous application of two or more operations. The training is structured in the form of a series of activity cards. Each card reports an activity that can be carried out on the card itself.

The second training program (Pizzingrilli et al. 2015b) targets students from kindergarten (junior version) to high school (senior version). Trainees are presented with some situations related to either scholastic or personal life where some characters act displaying use of resources and also their limits. The focus is on positive and negative aspects that every person/situation has, by suggesting that the student has to know both to be ready to act adequately under different kinds of circumstances. Each activity included in the training program refers to some scholastic-related contents (mathematics, science, history, music, visual arts, and so on) that can be addressed by the teacher during class time. For instance, in one of the activities students are asked to think about why a peeled orange sinks, while it floats when it has the skin on. This leads to understand that the peel is waterproof and prevents water from entering the fruit and sinking it. For another activity, students have to debate to understand why Paul Cezanne painted five different versions of the same painting, *The Card Players*. The practical activities embedded in the episodes of the story are aimed at leading the students to apply widening, connecting, and reorganising operations in one of three possible settings. In the *modelling* setting, a prototypical, paradigmatic way of reasoning is presented so to motivate the students to imitate it by inviting them to assimilate it and to transform it, if the situation needs that. In the *research* setting, a problem-solving request is proposed, which stimulates individuals to find unconventional answers. Finally, in the *interrogation* setting, students are asked to discover possible questions implicated in a given situation (problem finding).

Both training programs were indirectly inspired by a previous educational tool devised to promote creativity in kindergarten and primary school children, which has been validated in a series of intervention studies involving several hundred students (Antonietti 1997). This training consists of a story where two kids have to discover the secret of an extinct volcano. In their journey within the volcano they are tutored by three pets who impersonate, respectively, the free production of abundant ideas (widening), the ability to find analogies and similarities (connecting), and the predisposition to consider situations from an opposite point of view (reorganising).

4.4 Creativity and Metacognition

In order to enhance the creativity level of individuals, we could trigger the activation of the three processes mentioned before by inviting trainees to apply them to a variety of situations, in different disciplinary areas. However, when we want to enhance a certain skill in people, it is not enough to make them do a series of exercises, as usually occurs in the traditional training programs. It is also recommended that the individuals reflect on the mental processes that they activate in order to carry out those exercises so to learn to control those processes autonomously. For example, they could identify the appropriate strategies for the task, evaluate how they can put them into practice, predict the effort that will be required, and consider how motivated and happy they are while carrying out that task (Antonietti et al. 2000).

Bransford et al. (1987) have pointed out that the most frequent difficulty when facing a problem is not the lacking of the cognitive tools to solve it, but not knowing where to look for them. Therefore, to develop creativity, it could be useful to adopt a metacognitive approach, which would help to manage the relevant cognitive strategies. After all, many great artists have stated that they produced better creations when they were engaged in metacognitive processes that required special attention to the strategies for performing the task concerning self-instruction, self-monitoring, and self-assessment (Kozbelt 2011). The claim that a metacognitive approach can foster creativity is however a conjecture that is waiting to be supported adequately (Armbruster 1989; Feldhusen 1995; Jaušovec 1994).

4.4.1 Metacognitive Knowledge

The first aspect of metacognition which is worth taking into account here concerns the beliefs that people have regarding the creative process. Some studies led to cast doubts about the adequacy of laypersons' opinions about the creative process by showing that naïve "theories" of creativity are wrong, if compared to what experts currently maintain. For instance, people continue to brainstorm in groups in work settings, since they believe that working together will spark their creativity, even though research demonstrated that it is an ineffective method to enhance creativity (Nijstad 2009). In the same vein stereotypes according to which creativity can be developed in specific educational areas—playful and artistic—but not in others (such as the scientific ones) that involve more structured thinking skills are still widespread.

It could be expected that some categories of professionals should share beliefs which are more consistent with what researchers found. For instance, teachers should be more sensitive to the psychological aspects of creativity because they sometimes engage students in creative activities. However, even teachers' naïve conceptions fail to match claims which are consistent with scientific theories and empirical studies. For instance, teachers share the belief that creativity is innate or that letting children free from constraints in school settings promotes creativity (Chan and Chan 1999; Dawson et al. 1999; Diakidoy and Kanari 1999; Fleith De Souza 2000; Fryer and Collings 1991; Odena and Welch 2007; Runco et al. 1993). Laypeople's conceptions of creativity change according to the cultural context (Lim and Plucker 2001; Runco and Johnson 2002), but if persons are asked to express their understanding of the cognitive functioning with respect to specific situations and strategies (Antonietti et al. 2020a; Colombo and Antonietti 2017; Pizzingrilli and Antonietti 2010), their beliefs about the creative process are not so far from the scientific understanding.

Studies on the metacognitive knowledge of creative thinking highlighted two interrelated aspects. First, knowing the implicit theories allows researchers to better understand the nature of a complex construct as creativity is. Secondly, educational issues related to teaching creativity in schools highlight the need to provide specific training to work on the mental mechanisms involved in the creative process and also on the implicit theories in order to promote the use of divergent thinking and eradicate trainers' and trainees' misconceptions (Howard-Jones et al. 2008).

4.4.2 *Metacognitive Awareness*

The second aspect of metacognition to be addressed in relation to creativity is awareness, which, according to Efklides (2009), is linked to metacognitive experience, namely, the set of feelings and judgments related to the features of the task, the underlying mental processes, and their outcome. Are people conscious of what is occurring in their own mind when they are engaged in a creative process?

Reconstructions of what happen to artists seem to support the notion that they are aware of a variety of facets of the creative process. For example, Kozbelt's (2007) analysis of Beethoven's assessments of his own work indicated a high level of self-awareness. In fact, his own evaluations of his compositions agreed with those of posterity. In addition, the accuracy of his self-criticisms improved over the course of his career, suggesting that accurate self-appraisal can be enhanced through experience. Self-monitoring led to improvements in the calibration process, namely, in the degree of fit between the subjective judgment of performance and the actual performance (Bol and Hacker 2012; Hacker et al. 2008). Moreover, the analysis of archives of larger samples of composers (Kozbelt 2008) suggested that the longitudinal improvement in creativity is rather pervasive, since it occurred to many composers.

Fayena-Tawil et al. (2011) studied the creative process in artists and non-artists and found that artists engaged in more metacognitive activities than non-artists did. Even though both artists and non-artists self-evaluated their work throughout, artists were more likely to monitor their progress. Moreover, artists often engaged in overt metacognition and evaluation while working and they did so at a reliably greater extent than non-artists did. More precisely, artists appeared to know when they have to stop working since the highest possible level of quality has been achieved (Kozbelt and Serafin 2009).

4.4.3 *Metacognitive Control*

As metacognitive control is concerned, Kozbelt (2011) found that artists whose artefacts were rated as more creative were more likely to revise and refine their drawings—demonstrating to exert control on their creative process—than those whose work was rated as less creative. Studies on advanced engineering and technology students showed that metacognitive processing (such as taking multiple perspectives or testing conceptual combinations) led to the creation of novel products (Zeng et al. 2011).

The relevance of metacognitive control is also stressed by acknowledging the fact that people should realise that the situation they face needs to be approached through creative processes or operations. For example, in a study where undergraduates were asked to visualise in their mind three geometrical shapes randomly chosen and try to combine them mentally to invent a new object, it was found that suggesting

Table 4.1 Distribution of children by grade and gender

Gender	Grade 3	Grade 4	Grade 5	Total
Males	28	31	17	76
Females	28	28	28	84
Total	56	59	45	160

Note: In some analyses missing data reduced the sample size

strategies to control the manipulation of the mental images led students to generate more creative outcomes (Antonietti and Martini 2000).

4.5 An Intervention Study to Assess the Impact of a Metacognitive Approach in Creativity Training

At this point, we could wonder about the degree of metacognitive awareness that naïve people possess when they are engaged in generating something which is new and meaningful. Is this awareness beneficial or not to increase the level of creativity of the processes themselves?

In order to try to answer these questions a study[1] has been designed, aimed at investigating the influence of metacognitive awareness on the development of creative skills. More precisely, the research questions were (i) whether a training focused on the three creative mental operations described above can increase children's creative skills and (ii) whether metacognitive prompts affect the effects of the training.

4.5.1 Participants

The study involved 160 children attending the third, fourth, and fifth grade in three primary schools in Milan (Italy) suburbs. The sample is described in Table 4.1.

4.5.2 Procedure

The study had three phases.

First Phase Students were administered the WCR test described in Sect. 4.3.2.1, aimed at evaluating children's creative skills on the basis of their propensity to

[1]The contribution of Claudia Scarantino is gratefully acknowledged. She implemented the training in the classes, collected and scored data.

Table 4.2 Overview of the activities constituting the training programme

Operation	First activity	Second activity
Widening	Children had to create four images using leaves of various shapes and sizes.	Children were asked to write and draw ideas and jokes which can make a character of a story laugh; children, after being rewarded with strawberries, should transform each strawberry into a wish.
Connecting	Children had to connect seven bubbles, some of which were empty, whereas others had labels on them; bubbles had to be filled and connected in order to create a story.	Children had to make associations starting from a given element (e.g., a ball, a rectangle, etc.), considering the connection between two associated elements through a feature they have in common.
Reorganising	Children had to define further configurations and/or uses of three given elements (a sheet, a glass, a folder).	Children were told a short story about the disappearance of pets; children had to generate ideas to solve the mystery.
Multi-process	Children had to define the effect that some magic potions can cause.	Children had to describe the appearance, personality, and work done by characters with particular names and then draw them.

perform three basic mental creative operations (widening, connecting, and reorganising).

The test consists of three sub-tests each investigating one of the three cognitive processes outlined in Sect. 4.3. Each sub-test consists of three items. The stimuli proposed in the items are both visual stimuli (pictures) and verbal stimuli (words and narratives).

Second Phase Students were engaged in a training program consisting of eight activities, which aimed at increasing the same creative skills investigated in the test. The eight activities were extracted from the toolkit described in Sect. 4.3.2.2 (Antonietti et al. 2011). The activities required the children to activate the three skills considered to be the basis of creativity, through manual activities like creating images with paper, free and structured drawing activities, and story writing. The activities were carried out in the classroom by providing the relevant card to each child, who worked individually. Activities were performed during the regular school hours with a bi-weekly work unit lasting each approximately 1 h. The eight proposed activities are described in Table 4.2.

Third Phase The WCR test was administered again in order to assess the influence of the training on creative skills.

Experimental Conditions During the training program half of the students (metacognitive group), randomly identified, were asked to fill in a questionnaire before each activity and immediately after finishing it. The questions were: (a) "How good do you think you are (before the activity)/were you (after the activity) at this task?" (*ability*); (b) "How much effort do you think this task will require (before the activity)/required (after the activity) you?" (*effort*); (c) How much do you think you will like (before the activity)/enjoyed (after the activity) carrying out this task?" (*liking*). The answers were given on a 10-points Likert scale.

The aim of the questions was to prompt children to reflect on the activity they were about to carry out, encouraging them to improve their ability to anticipate what would occur in their mind in relation to the three aspects under investigation (*prediction*), and to reconstruct, after the activity, what occurred in their mind when engaged in the task in order to stimulate the ability to recognise the previous mental states (*retrospection*). These questions can also be used as measures of calibration, that is, the matching of subjective judgments about one's performance and the real level of quality of the performance. The other half of the students (control group) were not administered the metacognitive questionnaire during the activities.

4.5.3 Results

4.5.3.1 Effects of the Training Programme

The mean scores obtained in the three sub-tests of the WCR test (Widening, Combining, Reorganising) in the pre-and post-training phases were calculated distinguishing among the three school grades (Table 4.3). Overall, the youngest children showed a higher ability to widen their mental field as compared to the other ones (Scheffé test: $p < .05$). An increase in the three creative dimensions assessed by the WCR test was found throughout the sample and at each school level. The ability to widen the mental field and to make connections between disparate elements increased significantly in the third and fourth grade. The ability to reorganise the mental field has instead developed more, thanks to the training, in the fifth grade.

As Table 4.4 shows, being assigned to the metacognitive or non-metacognitive group failed *per se* to affect performance in the WCR test. However, significant interaction effects, as assessed through ANOVAs, occurred in the Widening and Connecting sub-tests. The students assigned to the metacognitive group showed a greater increase in widening the mental field and a smaller increase in the reorganisation capacity than the controls did. The ability to make connections between disparate elements was enhanced similarly in the two sub-samples.

4.5.3.2 Calibration Across the Training Programme

Under-Confidence and Over-Confidence

By analysing the answers given to the questions concerning prediction and retrospection, a progressive increase of accuracy emerged. The improvement from the first to the eighth work session was noticed in the recognition of the ability and the

Table 4.3 Mean scores (SD in parentheses) in the WCR test in the pre- and post-training phases according to the grade

WCR sub-test	Grade	Phase		Effects		
		Pre	Post	Phase (pre vs post)	Grade (3 vs 4 vs 5)	Phase × grade
Widening	3	4.00 (1.68)	4.85 (2.01)	$F_{1,132} = 8.23$ $p < .005$	$F_{2,132} = 3.56$ $p < .05$	$F_{1,132} = 0.78$ n.s.
	4	3.63 (1.38)	4.02 (1.61)			
	5	3.76 (1.23)	4.11 (1.63)			
Connecting	3	18.57 (2.07)	20.26 (4.25)	$F_{1,132} = 14.15$ $p < .001$	$F_{2,132} = 0.26$ n.s.	$F_{1,132} = 0.27$ n.s.
	4	18.72 (2.58)	19.82 (3.56)			
	5	18.36 (2.51)	19.64 (4.14)			
Reorganising	3	8.36 (1.09)	9.70 (2.10)	$F_{1,140} = 58.63$ $p < .001$	$F_{2,140} = 2.04$ n.s.	$F_{1,140} = 0.21$ n.s.
	4	8.60 (2.10)	10.11 (2.03)			
	5	7.84 (1.83)	9.51 (2.21)			

effort required to carry out the training activities (prediction), which tended to match the reconstruction of what occurred in the mind during the activities previously carried out (retrospection). The improvement was measured by calculating the difference, within each activity, between the scores given before the activity (prediction) and those attributed afterwards (retrospection). On the basis of this difference, children can be categorised as *over-confident* if prediction over-scored retrospection, as *adequate estimators* if prediction matched retrospection, and as *under-confident* if retrospection over-scored prediction.

At the beginning of the training (first activity) prediction scores differed from the retrospective ones (in most cases revealing that children tended to overestimate their ability and pleasure, while they underestimated the effort). With the exception of the liking score, at the end of the training (eighth activity) the rates referred before the activity coincided with those after the activity at a larger extend, indicating an increase in the ability to anticipate the mental processes that would be activated (Table 4.5).

Correlations Between Prediction and Retrospection Ratings

More detailed analyses of the relationships between prediction and retrospection were provided by computing Pearson's r coefficients. As far as the metacognitive ratings in the *first activity* of the training program are concerned, ability scores

Table 4.4 Mean scores (SD in parentheses) in the WCR test in the pre- and post-training phases according to the sub-sample

Phase	Sub-test					
	Widening		Connecting		Reorganising	
	Without metacognitive reflections	With metacognitive reflections	Without metacognitive reflections	With metacognitive reflections	Without metacognitive reflections	With metacognitive reflections
Pre	3.87 (1.48)	3.62 (1.11)	18.27 (2.08)	19.12 (2.75)	8.16 (1.90)	8.64 (1.90)
Post	4.19 (1.67)	4.65 (2.02)	19.78 (3.80)	20.23 (4.15)	9.91 (2.04)	9.60 (2.20)
Effects						
Phase (pre vs post)	$F_{1,132} = 11.67, p < .001$		$F_{1,132} = 12.57, p < .001$		$F_{1,141} = 40.37, p < .001$	
Group (metacognitive vs non-metacognitive)	$F_{1,132} = 0.21$, n.s.		$F_{1,132} = 2.01$, n.s.		$F_{1,141} = 0.09$, n.s.	
Phase × group	$F_{1,132} = 3.22, p < .05$		$F_{1,132} = 0.29$, n.s.		$F_{1,141} = 3.46, p < .05$	

Table 4.5 Numbers (percentages in parentheses) of students in the whole metacognitive group who underestimated, estimated correctly, and overestimated ability, effort, and liking by moving from the first to the eighth activity

Metacognitive judgment	Comparison between prediction and retrospection	First activity	Last activity
Ability	Under-confidence	23 (29)	38 (48)
	Coincidence	30 (37)	37 (46)
	Over-confidence	27 (34)	5 (6)
Effort	Under-confidence	37 (46)	30 (37)
	Coincidence	18 (23)	30 (37)
	Over-confidence	25 (31)	21 (26)
Liking	Under-confidence	5 (6)	31 (39)
	Coincidence	59 (74)	39 (49)
	Over-confidence	16 (20)	14 (17)

correlated positively with liking scores ($r = .40$, $p < .001$) and negatively, although non significantly, with effort scores ($r = -.11$, n.s.), whereas no relation between effort and liking emerged ($r = .05$, n.s.). This means that if persons assess themselves as skilled in performing the task to be carried out, they anticipate that they will like the task and it will need less effort; the opposite occurs if they perceive themselves as lacking of the skills required by the task. Ratings concerning ability, effort, and liking provided before the task were correlated with the corresponding rates provided after the task (ability: $r = .34$, $p < .05$; effort: $r = .38$, $p < .01$; liking: $r = .46$, $p < .001$), suggesting that rates tend to be rather stable across the activity. However, correlations were higher in the retrospection phase (ability-effort: $r = -.38$, $p < .01$, ability-liking: $r = .54$, $p < .001$; effort-liking: $r = -.33$, $p < .04$). Hence, it appears that children's ratings were more coherent in retrospection than in prediction.

If we focus on the data at the end of the training (namely, in the *eighth activity*), we notice that the negative association between ability and effort increased from prediction to retrospection (respectively, $r = -.01$, n.s.; $r = -.30$, $p < .05$) as at the beginning of the training, but the connection between ability and liking in the prediction phase ($r = .59$, $p < .001$) was stronger at the end of the training than at the beginning (and remained quite constant in the retrospection phase: $r = .58$, $p < .001$). The same was true of the correlations between effort and liking in the prediction ($r = -.34$, $p < .05$) and retrospection ($r = -.21$, n.s.) phases. Also rating concerning ability, effort, and liking provided before the task correlated with the corresponding rates provided after the task (ability: $r = .44$, $p < .01$; effort: $r = .42$, $p < .01$; liking: $r = .59$, $p < .001$) in the last activity of the training programme at a larger extent than in the first activity. Overall, an improvement of the predictive skills across the training programme emerged.

4.5.3.3 Correlations Between Prediction and Retrospective Ratings and Actual Performance

Following the procedure usually adopted in creativity tests, responses given by the students in the first and eighth activity were scored according to criteria usually employed to evaluate originality (namely, in terms of rarity of the response within the reference sample) in order to attribute an overall creativity score to the performance. Spearman's rho coefficients between prediction and retrospection and actual performance were computed.

The capacity to *predict* the level of ability requested by the subsequent task improved from the beginning ($r = -.02$, n.s.) to the end ($r = .19$, n.s.) of the training even though correlation coefficients were not statistically significant: The higher was the performance, the higher should be the ability requested to succeed in the task and this tended to appear in the last activity of the training programme. The same was true of the prediction of the degree of liking perceived during the task, which increased from the first ($r = .29$, $p < .05$) to the eighth activity ($r = .88$, $p < .001$). If we assume that the higher was the performance, the higher should be the enjoyment experienced in succeeding in the task, we realise that such relation became stronger across the training. No evident change occurred in the relationships between prediction of effort by moving from the first ($r = -.12$, n.s.) to the eighth ($r = -.09$, n.s.) activity.

The correspondences between the *retrospective* judgements and the actual performance increased across the training as well. The correlation between ability rates and actual performance was higher in the eighth activity ($r = .33$, $p < .05$) than in the first activity ($r = -.02$, n.s.). The same was true of effort (first activity: $r = -.27$, $p < .05$; eighth activity: $r = -.25$, $p < .05$) and liking (first activity: $r = .23$, n.s.; eighth activity: $r = .19$, n.s.), even though in the last case coefficients were not statistically significant.

To summarise, it was found that metacognitive awareness is internally consistent. Metacognitive ratings were correlated in the expected directions: a positive relation between ability and liking and a negative relation between ability and effort and between liking and effort. Metacognitive ratings were correlated with actual performance in different directions: Ability showed positive relations and effort negative relations. Prediction was generally correlated with retrospection and children's ratings were more coherent in retrospective than predictive evaluations. At the beginning of the training metacognitive judgments were poorly associated to the actual performance but this picture improved at the end of the training. In fact, higher correlations (in five out of six measures) between prediction/retrospection and performance emerged after the training. Also, the relations between effort and liking changed after the training: Predictions showed higher negative correlations and retrospections lower negative correlations.

4.6 Conclusions

In a creative task, if people can apply more than one mental operation, they have to decide which operation is better depending on the situation. In addition, they should realise whether they are applying the chosen operation in the right way in order to achieve the goal. Hence, metacognitive control is required to plan the application of strategies aimed at supporting the generation of novel and original ideas. Planning is associated to calibration, since individuals should anticipate how good they will be in implementing the chosen strategy and how they will feel when doing so in order to predict the expected outcome. They also have to be introspective in order to be able to reflect on the process that occurred in their mind. This is necessary to assess retrospectively the quality of the process itself and to prepare themselves to face a similar task in the future and perform better.

The results of the intervention study reported in Sect. 4.5 showed first of all that the training enabled children to increase their creative skills. Secondly, it showed that metacognitive abilities, if stimulated, can be progressively refined when creative activities are involved. Finally, it appeared that the metacognitive approach favours only one aspect of creativity, i.e., the widening of the mental field, whereas it is counterproductive for reorganisation. This is consistent with the literature on the solution of insight problems (Wilson and Schooler 1991), which are similar to situations requiring the restructuring of the cognitive field, where reflection results to be detrimental.

It is important to stimulate children to reflect about the mental processes involved in the activity they are about to perform or have just finished performing as this can be useful to increase attention to the task and improve performance (Fasko 2001). However, metacognition can be useful to enhance only some of the skills required to perform a creative task. So, it is up to the teacher to diversify the methodology of work (metacognitive or non-metacognitive) according to the tasks and objectives to be reached.

Because the topic of the relationship between metacognition and creativity has been poorly investigated, further research is needed in order to get a clear picture of when and how metacognition can be beneficial to support the generation of novel and meaningful ideas. It may be that also in this domain, as in the other ones where the metacognitive approach has a long-lasting tradition, new approaches—as Anastasia Efklides showed in her forward-looking research—might allow researchers to acquire a more precise understanding. For instance, the possibility of different levels of metacognition, as Efklides (2008) suggested, has to be taken into account also in the field of creativity. Implicit measures of metacognition can be useful given the fact that creative process cannot be fully introspected and verbalised. Moreover, the affective aspects of metacognition might be considered. Finally, different aspects of metacognition—metacognitive knowledge, metacognitive awareness, and metacognitive control—should be distinguished when applied to creativity.

Perhaps a metacognitive approach is not, *per se*, neither beneficial nor detrimental to the creative process. Enhancing the sensibility about what occurs in the mind while engaged in a task requiring originality can improve the quality of some processes involved in creativity but might inhibit other processes. Therefore, it would be relevant to explore and understand the specific circumstances under which reflecting about how creative ideas develop can be an added value and a goal for education (Efklides 2009).

References

Andolfi, V. R., Valenti, C., Cesa-Bianchi, M., & Cristini, C. (2016). Creatività e tempo libero in età senile: un'indagine delle relazioni tra propensione al pensiero divergente e passatempi praticati [Creativity and leisure time in the elderly: A study of the relations between divergent thinking propensity and practised hobbies]. *Ricerche di Psicologia, 39*, 498–513.

Antonietti, A. (1997). Unlocking creativity. *Educational Leadership, 54*, 73–75.

Antonietti, A., & Colombo, B. (2013). Three creative operations. In A.-G. Tan (Ed.), *Creativity, talent development, and excellence* (pp. 13–26). New York: Springer.

Antonietti, A., & Colombo, B. (2016). Creative cognition: How culture matters. In V. Glaveanu (Ed.), *Handbook of creativity and culture* (pp. 101–124). Basingstoke: Palgrave Macmillan.

Antonietti, A., & Martini, E. (2000). Suggesting strategies improves the creative visual synthesis. *Perceptual and Motor Skills, 90*, 364–366.

Antonietti, A., Ignazi, S., & Perego, P. (2000). Metacognitive knowledge about problem-solving methods. *British Journal of Educational Psychology, 70*, 1–16.

Antonietti, A., Colombo, B., De Santis, S., & Fabio, R. A. (2010). Psychophysiological correlates of different kinds of insight problems. *Frontiers in Neuroscience*. https://doi.org/10.3389/conf.fnins.2010.11.00022.

Antonietti, A., Giorgetti, M., & Pizzingrilli, P. (2011). *Io penso creativo). Valutare e potenziare gli aspetti creativi del pensiero [I think creatively. Assessment and enhancement of creative thinking]*. Florence: Giunti.

Antonietti, A., Bonacina, S., Colombo, B., & Iannello, P. (2020a). Identifying the creative act in advertising. A study on naïve people's awareness of restructuring. *Journal of Creative Behavior*. https://doi.org/10.1002/jocb.389.

Antonietti, A., Pizzingrilli, P., & Valenti, C. (2020b). *Enhancing creativity through story-telling. Innovative training programmes for school settings*. Palgrave Macmillan: Cham.

Armbruster, B. B. (1989). Metacognition in creativity. In J. A. Glover, R. R. Ronning, & C. R. Reynolds (Eds.), *Handbook of creativity* (pp. 177–182). New York: Plenum Press.

Batey, M. (2012). The measurement of creativity: From definitional consensus to the introduction of a new heuristic framework. *Creativity Research Journal, 24*, 55–65.

Bol, L., & Hacker, D. J. (2012). Calibration research: Where do we go from here? *Frontiers in Psychology, 3*, 1–6. https://doi.org/10.3389/fpsyg.2012.00229.

Bransford, J. D., Sherwood, R. D., & Sturdevant, T. (1987). Teaching thinking and problem solving. In J. B. Baron & R. J. Sternberg (Eds.), *Teaching skills: Theory and practice* (pp. 161–182). New York: Freeman.

Cancer, A., Manzoli, S., & Antonietti, A. (2016). The alleged link between creativity and dyslexia: Identifying the specific process in which dyslexic students excel. *Cogent Psychology, 3*, 1–13. https://doi.org/10.1080/23311908.2016.1190309.

Chan, D. W., & Chan, L. K. (1999). Implicit theories of creativity: Teachers' perception of student characteristics in Hong Kong. *Creativity Research Journal, 12*, 185–195.

Colautti, L., Baldissini, D., Colombo, V., Mottura, S., Sacco, M., Sozzi, M., Corbo, M., Rusconi, M. L., & Antonietti, A. (2018). CREC: The role of serious games in improving flexibility in thinking in neuropsychological rehabilitation. *British Journal of Educational Technology, 49*, 717–727.

Colombo, B., & Antonietti, A. (2017). The role of metacognitive strategies in learning music: A multiple case study. *British Journal of Music Education, 34*, 95–112.

Colombo, B., Bartesaghi, N., Simonelli, L., & Antonietti, A. (2015). The combined effects of neurostimulation and priming on creative thinking: A preliminary tDCS study on dorsolateral prefrontal cortex. *Frontiers in Human Neuroscience, 9*, 1–12. https://doi.org/10.3389/fnhum.2015.00403.

Dacey, J. S., & Lennon, K. H. (1998). *Understanding creativity. The interplay of biological, psychological, and social factors*. San Francisco: Jossey-Bass.

Dawson, V. L., D'Andrea, T., Affinito, R., & Westby, E. L. (1999). Predicting creative behavior: A reexamination of the divergence between traditional and teacher-defined concepts of creativity. *Creativity Journal Research, 12*, 57–66.

De Stobbeleir, K. E. M., Ashford, S. J., & Buyens, D. (2011). Self-regulation of creativity at work: The role of feedback-seeking behavior in creative performance. *Academy of Management Journal, 54*, 811–831.

Diakidoy, I. A., & Kanari, E. (1999). Student teachers' beliefs about creativity. *British Educational Research Journal, 25*, 225–243.

Efklides, A. (2008). Metacognition: Defining its facets and levels of functioning in relation to self-regulation and co-regulation. *European Psychologist, 13*, 277–287.

Efklides, A. (2009). The role of metacognitive experiences in the learning process. *Psicothema, 21*, 76–82.

Efklides, A. (2011). Interactions of metacognition with motivation and affect in self-regulated learning: The MASRL model. *Educational Psychology, 46*, 6–25.

Efklides, A., & Misailidi, P. (Eds.). (2010). *Trends and prospects in metacognition research*. New York: Springer.

Efklides, A., Kuhl, J., & Sorrentino, R. M. (Eds.). (2001). *Trends and prospects in motivation research*. Dordrecht: Kluwer.

Erbas, A. K., & Bas, S. (2015). The contribution of personality traits, motivation, academic risk-taking and metacognition to the creative ability in mathematics. *Creativity Research Journal, 27*, 299–307.

Fasko, D. (2001). Education and creativity. *Creativity Research Journal, 13*, 317–327.

Fayena-Tawil, F., Kozbelt, A., & Sitaras, L. (2011). Think global, act local: A protocol analysis comparison of artists' and nonartists' cognitions, metacognitions, and evaluations while drawing. *Psychology of Aesthetics, Creativity, and the Arts, 5*, 135–145.

Feldhusen, J. F. (1995). Creativity: A knowledge base, metacognitive skills, and personality factors. *Journal of Creative Behavior, 29*, 255–268.

Fleith De Souza, D. (2000). Teacher and student's perceptions of creativity in the classroom environment. *Roeper Review, 22*, 148–158.

Fryer, M., & Collings, J. A. (1991). Teachers' view about creativity. *British Journal of Educational Psychology, 61*, 207–219.

Hacker, D. J., Bol, L., & Keener, M. C. (2008). Metacognition in education: A focus on calibration. In J. Dunlosky & R. Bjork (Eds.), *Handbook of memory and metacognition* (pp. 429–455). New York: Psychology Press.

Hargrove, R. A. (2013). Assessing the long-term impact of a metacognitive approach to creative skill development. *International Journal of Technology and Design Education, 23*, 489–517.

Hargrove, R. A., & Nietfeld, J. L. (2015). The impact of metacognitive instruction on creative problem solving. *Journal of Experimental Education, 83*, 291–318.

Hines, T. (1991). The myth of right hemisphere creativity. *Journal of Creative Behavior, 25*, 223–227.

Hong, E., Peng, Y., & Wu, J. (2010, August). *Effects of explicit instruction, metacognition, and motivation on creative performance*. San Diego, CA: American Psychological Association.

Hong, E., Neil, H. F. O., & Peng, Y. (2016). Effects of explicit instructions, metacognition, and motivation on creative performance. *Creativity Research Journal, 28*, 33–45.
Hoppe, K. D. (1994). Affect, hemispheric specialization, and creativity. In M. P. Shaw et al. (Eds.), *Creativity and affect* (pp. 185–212). Westport: Praeger.
Hoppe, K. D., & Kyle, N. L. (1990). Dual brain, creativity, and health. *Creativity Research Journal, 3*, 150–157.
Howard-Jones, P. A., Winfield, M., & Crimmins, G. (2008). Co-constructing an understanding of creativity in drama education that draws on neuropsychological concepts. *Educational Research, 50*, 187–201.
Jaušovec, N. (1994). Metacognition in creative problem solving. In M. A. Runco (Ed.), *Problem finding, problem solving, and creativity* (pp. 77–95). Westport: Ablex Publishing.
Jia, X., Li, W., & Cao, L. (2019). The role of metacognitive components in creative thinking. *Frontiers in Psychology, 10*, 1–11. https://doi.org/10.3389/fpsyg.2019.02404.
Johnson-Laird, P. N. (1988). *The computer and the mind*. London: Collins.
Jung-Beeman, M., Bowden, E. M., Haberman, J., Frymiare, J. L., Arambel-Liu, S., Greenblatt, R., et al. (2004). Neural activity when people solve verbal problems with insight. *PLoS Biology, 2*, 500–510.
Kounios, J., & Beeman, M. (2009). The Aha! Moment. The cognitive neuroscience of insight. *Current Directions in Psychological Science, 18*, 210–216.
Kounios, J., Frymiare, J. L., Bowden, E. M., Fleck, J. I., Subramaniam, K., Parrish, T. B., & Jung-Beeman, M. (2006). The prepared mind: Neural activity prior to problem presentation predicts subsequent solution by sudden insight. *Psychological Science, 17*, 882–890.
Kozbelt, A. (2007). A quantitative analysis of Beethoven as self-critic: Implications for psychological theories of musical creativity. *Psychology of Music, 35*, 144–168.
Kozbelt, A. (2008). Longitudinal hit ratios of classical composers: Reconciling "Darwinian" and expertise acquisition perspectives on lifespan creativity. *Psychology of Aesthetics, Creativity and the Arts, 2*, 221–235.
Kozbelt, A. (2011). Dynamic evaluation of high- and low-creativity drawings by artist and nonartist raters: Replication and methodological extension. *Psychology of Aesthetics, Creativity and the Arts, 5*, 350–359.
Kozbelt, A., & Serafin, A. (2009). Dynamic evaluation of high- and low-creativity drawings by artist and nonartist raters. *Creativity Research Journal, 21*, 349–360.
Lim, W., & Plucker, J. A. (2001). Creativity through a lens of social responsibility: Implicit theory of creativity with Korean samples. *Journal of Creative Behavior, 35*, 115–130.
Lizarraga, M. L. S. D. A., & Baquedano, M. T. S. D. A. (2013). How creative potential is related to metacognition. *European Journal of Educational Psychology, 6*, 69–81.
Martindale, C. (1999). Biological bases of creativity. In R. J. Sternberg (Ed.), *Handbook of creativity* (pp. 137–152). Cambridge: Cambridge University Press.
Nijstad, B. A. (2009). *Group performance*. New York: Psychology Press.
Odena, O., & Welch, G. F. (2007). The influence of teachers' backgrounds on their perceptions of musical creativity: A qualitative study with secondary school music teachers. *Research Study in Music Education, 28*, 71–81.
Oldrati, V., Patricelli, J., Colombo, B., & Antonietti, A. (2016). The role of dorsolateral prefrontal cortex in inhibition mechanism: A study on cognitive reflection test and similar tasks through neuromodulation. *Neuropsychologia, 91*, 499–508.
Perkins, D. N. (1988). The possibility of invention. In R. J. Sternberg (Ed.), *The nature of creativity* (pp. 362–385). Cambridge: Cambridge University Press.
Pizzingrilli, P., & Antonietti, A. (2010). Implicit theories of creativity in school children. An exploratory study. *Procedia - Social and Behavioral Sciences, 2*, 4732–4736.
Pizzingrilli, P., Valenti, C., Cerioli, L., & Antonietti, A. (2015a). Creative thinking skills from 6 to 17 years as assessed through the WCR test. *Procedia - Social and Behavioral Sciences, 191*, 584–590.

Pizzingrilli, P., Valenti, C., Cerioli, L., & Antonietti, A. (2015b). *Sviluppare il pensiero flessibile. Percorsi interdisciplinari nella scuola primaria [Developing creative thinking. Interdisciplinary activities for primary school]*. Trento: Edizioni Erickson.
Preiss, D. D., Cosmelli, D., Grau, V., & Ortiz, D. (2016). Examining the influence of mind wandering and metacognition on creativity in university and vocational students. *Learning and Individual Differences, 51*, 417–426.
Rothenberg, A. (1979). *The emerging goddess: The creative process in art, science, and other fields*. Chicago: University of Chicago Press.
Runco, M. A., & Johnson, D. J. (2002). Parents' and teachers' implicit theories of children's creativity: A cross-cultural perspective. *Creativity Journal Research, 14*, 427–438.
Runco, M. A., Johnson, D. J., & Bear, P. K. (1993). Parents' and teachers' implicit theories on children's creativity. *Child Study Journal, 23*, 91–113.
Sandkühler, S., & Bhattacharya, J. (2008). Deconstructing insight: EEG correlates of insightful problem solving. *PLoS One, 3*, e1459. https://doi.org/10.1371/journal.pone.0001459.
Schank, R. C. (1988). *The creative attitude: Learning to ask and answer the right questions*. New York: Macmillan.
Simonton, D. K. (1999). *Origins of genius: Darwinian perspectives on creativity*. New York: Oxford University Press.
Subramaniam, K., Kounios, J., Parrish, T. B., & Jung-Beeman, M. (2008). A brain mechanism for facilitation of insight by positive affect. *Journal of Cognitive Neuroscience, 21*, 415–432.
Weisberg, R. W. (1993). *Creativity. Beyond the myth of genius*. New York: Freeman.
Wilson, T. D., & Schooler, J. W. (1991). Thinking too much: Introspection can reduce the quality of preferences and decisions. *Journal of Personality and Social Psychology, 60*, 181–192.
Zeng, L., Proctor, R. W., & Salvendy, G. (2011). Fostering creativity in product and service development: Validation in the domain of information technology. *Human Factors, 53*, 245–270.

Part II
Metacognition and Affect in Self- and Co-regulation

Chapter 5
Socially-Shared Metacognitive Regulation in Collaborative Science Learning

Marja Vauras, Simone Volet, and Tuike Iiskala

Abstract Socially shared metacognitive regulation (SSMR) has substantially expanded our understanding of metacognitive regulation in collaborative learning environments, as documented in intensifying research over the past 15 years. Designing new, innovative collaborative learning environments in science fields is thriving, but more empirically grounded evidence is needed to fully understand the demands for regulation of the joint effort of all the participants to reach the intended goals in science learning. As a highly challenging disciplinary area, science offers an intriguing window to unveil metacognitive processes emerging in social contexts. This chapter discusses some conceptualization issues of social regulation of cognition found in the literature, particularly those in need of deeper understanding through empirical scrutiny. Further, through illustrations from studies—empirical evidence of social forms of metacognitive regulation in collaborative science learning, the role played by SSMR in different collaborative science learning environments is discussed. Discussed gaps in current empirical evidence offer grounds to future directions in SSMR research.

Keywords Socially-shared metacognitive regulation · Collaborative learning · Science learning

5.1 Introduction

> Metacognition is seen as a sine-qua-non constituent of social interaction and of co-regulation and other-regulation of behavior—(Efklides 2008, p. 277)

M. Vauras (✉) · T. Iiskala
Department of Teacher Education and Center for Research in Learning and Instruction, University of Turku, Turku, Finland
e-mail: marja.vauras@utu.fi

S. Volet
School of Education, Murdoch University, Murdoch, WA, Australia

D. Moraitou, P. Metallidou (eds.), *Trends and Prospects in Metacognition Research across the Life Span*, https://doi.org/10.1007/978-3-030-51673-4_5

Anastasia Efklides made this strong statement on the necessity of metacognition in social interaction in one of the first conceptual articles, entitled, *Metacognition: Defining its facets and levels of functioning in relation to self-regulation and co-regulation,* that addressed the social level of metacognition beyond other-regulation. She presented, from a psychological perspective, a multifaceted and multilevel model of metacognition, which offered the first theoretically coherent framework that integrated individual and social levels of metacognition. She wrote (p. 283):

> This level [social level] comprises only metacognitive judgments about one's own and others' ME, MK, and MS; it is informed by information received from the ongoing interaction with others. Monitoring at this level is explicit and can take the form of reflection. It leads to a socially-shared and negotiated representation of the person-in-context. Control at this level is exercised in a conscious analytic mode and its access to one's own and cognition and affect at the object level is through the personal-awareness level of the interacting persons.

At the time her insightful conceptual article was published, the notion of socially-shared metacognition with supporting empirical evidence had only been introduced in the scientific literature (Iiskala et al. 2004; Vauras et al. 2003), and it was conceptually analyzed for the first time from an educational viewpoint a year after (Volet et al. 2009b). However, at this stage, sustained empirical evidence was still waiting to be collected. Looking back, after more than 15 years of active research on the social nature of metacognition and metacognitive regulation, Efklides' insights are now easy to see and appreciate.

In our chapter, after a brief look back, we discuss some conceptualization issues of social regulation of cognition found in the literature, particularly those in need of deeper understanding through empirical scrutiny. In light of the growing body of empirical studies conducted in the context of collaborative science learning environments, we focus our discussion on the research in that applied context. The choice of collaborative science learning as research site for the study of socially shared metacognitive regulation is not surprising. As a highly challenging disciplinary area, science offers an intriguing window to unveil metacognitive processes in social contexts. Processes such as question posing, hypothesis generation and design, collection and synthesis of data, and the development and testing of models (Duschl and Hamilton 2011) characterize learning in science, and all these processes represent cognitively demanding complex reasoning and meaning making. Although not yet typical of all school science curricula, more and more contemporary science learning is taking place at the frontiers of and across disciplines. This creates new challenges for integrating meaningfully core, domain-specific knowledge from different disciplines.

Further, in the context of higher education, there is a heightened need for actively promoting the integration of complex core scientific knowledge with professional practice during the university study. This is particularly important in applied science disciplines, such as medicine or engineering (e.g., medicine and veterinary sciences programs are now inducing the development of clinical reasoning and problem-solving skills that explicitly build upon scientific knowledge) (see Duschl and

Hamilton 2011; see also, Lajoie and Lu 2012; Vauras et al. 2019). From a situated-cognitive point of view (see e.g., Hmelo-Silver et al. 2007), three core aspects concerning the nature and contexts of science learning include issues of authenticity, collaboration and inquiry (see e.g., Duschl and Hamilton 2011; de Jong 2019; Vauras et al. 2019). *Authenticity* focuses on embedding the learning within the learners' everyday world and the practice of the discipline. C*ollaboration* encourages the sharing and contrasting of ideas with other individuals sharing similar aims. *Inquiry* -playing a fundamental role within science, invites students to engage in problem-solving activities that require planning, synthesis and evaluation skills as well as relevant domain-specific content knowledge. Overall, it is reasonable to argue that the nature and contexts of science learning are challenging, and therefore demand regulation of behavior, whether at individual or social level.

5.1.1 From Individual to Social Regulation in Collaborative Learning

The significance of individual regulation of thinking and reasoning for effective cognitive performance is well established in the seminal literature on metacognition and self-regulation (Brown 1987; Flavell 1979; Winne and Perry 2000) and self-regulated learning (Boekaerts et al. 2000; Schunk and Zimmerman 1997). In the context of contemporary educational environments, characterized by a growing emphasis on the value of collaborative, cooperative and small group learning activities, regulatory constructs have been extended to include shared processes of regulation of cognition. Different theoretical groundings are noticeable in this research, including:

- *Metacognition theory* (e.g., Vauras et al.'s 2003; Iiskala et al. 2004, 2011 notion of shared metacognition and regulation); this grounding captures the overlap of metacognition and self-regulation (e.g., Dinsmore et al. 2008), and extends it to socially shared metacognition and socially shared regulation;
- *Situative perspective* inspired by Greeno's (2006) case for emphasizing the system in which activities take place and therefore studying learning in activity (e.g., Volet et al. 2009a proposed continuum from individual, solo regulation to co-regulation to capture the social nature of joint regulation in collaborative learning contexts);
- *Socio-cognitive perspective* (e.g., Hadwin et al. 2011; Rogat and Linnenbrink-Garcia 2011 on co-regulated and socially shared regulation, as well as Volet et al. 2013; Iiskala et al. 2015, on socially shared metacognitive regulation).

Schoor et al.'s (2015) article provide a comprehensive, critical review of the range of terms and concepts that have been generated in research on regulation in cooperative and collaborative learning. The authors note that although there are variations in subcategories of regulation, there is general agreement that social regulation can be accepted as "*an umbrella term for modes of regulation during cooperative and collaborative learning*" (p. 111). However, the term socially shared regulation can embrace more than regulation of cognition and also, include other objects of regulation during collaborative learning, such as regulation of motivation and emotions.

In this chapter, we concentrate on the concept of socially shared metacognitive regulation (SSMR), which focuses exclusively on social regulation of cognition.

5.2 Conceptualizations of Social Regulation of Cognition in Collaborative Learning Environments

The literature on social regulation of cognition features two distinct situations, in terms of the relational characteristics among participants involved in social forms of learning, therefore social regulation processes, namely situations where participants are in asymmetrical or symmetrical relations.

Social regulation featuring participants in *asymmetrical relations* typically takes place in developmental or instructional situations where the intended purpose of social regulation is for more able individuals (e.g., parents, teachers or more able peers) to guide the development of self-regulation of cognition in others. Schoor et al. (2015) suggested using the term co-regulation as an umbrella term for all situations of unequal relationships, where the purpose of social regulation is to scaffold an individual's appropriation of self-regulation. This proposal is consistent with Järvelä and Hadwin's (2013) use of the term co-regulation to represent the entire process by which a more able individual initially regulates the cognition of a less able other (other-regulation at that starting point). While regulating the cognition of the less able other, the more able individual proactively creates a transition process where the less able person is induced through modelling and scaffolding to gradually take part in the regulation process (thus co-regulation), until that person is able to self-regulate their cognition autonomously.

In contrast, social regulation among participants in *symmetrical relations* is found in collaborative learning environments, where peers (of equal status since all are learners) engage together in a joint activity aimed at achieving the same group goals or producing a collective outcome. The identification and naming of the process by which group members genuinely share the regulation of their joint, goal-directed cognitive activity was initially grounded in research on metacognition and thus called socially shared metacognition (Iiskala et al. 2004; Vauras et al. 2003). It was subsequently renamed socially shared metacognitive regulation (SSMR; Volet et al. 2013; and used e.g. by Iiskala et al. 2015; de Bakker et al. 2015) in order to make it explicit that the focus is on the regulatory component of metacognition (Brown 1987; Flavell 1979). To be more specific, SSMR represents socially shared regulation of cognition that takes place interactively and dynamically during collaborative learning. Since in real-life situations groups consist of individuals with diverse background characteristics, learning histories, personal goals, expectations, motivation, and level of commitment, asymmetrical relations among peers are created during collaborative learning activities, even among peers of equal status. Therefore, the social regulation of cognition is not always genuinely shared. Episodes of other-regulation of cognition can emerge, for example, when one individual takes over temporarily the metacognitive regulation process of one peer. Another example is when one individual regulates on behalf of the group, ideally in a facilitative mode that enables task progress and the group enhanced conceptual understanding, thus leading to peers' confidence to further contribute to SSMR. Volet et al. (2009a) found evidence of the importance of social regulation processes that invite further contribution of peers, for example, through asking questions that seek explanations of content knowledge and displaying tentativeness of explanations. Dysfunctional processes of other regulation of cognition among peers in symmetrical relations are sometimes observed when one member adopts a directive, controlling mode of other regulation, which prevents peers to participate in SSMR because it involves other-regulation toward own goal and not toward the group goal (e.g., Rogat and Adams-Wiggins 2014; Rogat and Linnenbrink-Garcia 2011).

In the next section, we scrutinize the empirical evidence of SSMR in collaborative learning with illustrations, by discussing in turn the focus of SSMR, the functions of SSMR, the triggering factors leading to SSMR, the interplay and shifts between SSMR and other forms of metacognitive regulation in collaborative learning, and the relationship of SSMR to learning outcomes.

5.3 Empirical Evidence of Social Forms of Metacognitive Regulation in Collaborative Learning and Illustrations from Studies

5.3.1 Focus of SSMR

Research on SSMR has evolved from identifying episodes of SSMR to research where the role of SSMR, such as its focus and function, in collaborative learning is scrutinized in more detail. To determine the *focus* of SSMR is important since research on SSMR (e.g., Khosa and Volet 2014; Iiskala et al. under revision) has shown that the manifestation of SSMR itself is not crucial in successful science learning as such, the essential issue being what SSMR focuses on. In addition, to support the claim that SSMR is critical when it focuses on understanding conceptual aspects and not when applied to less important issues, the learning task should not be too easy to solve (e.g., Iiskala et al. 2011).

As empirical evidence of the relationship between the focus of SSMR and the task difficulty, Iiskala et al. (2011) studied the focus of SSMR in mathematical word problem-solving by considering different categories: the situation model (i.e., understanding); the operations (i.e., strategies); and incidental matters (i.e., irrelevances)

Table 5.1 Summary of the focus of task-related SSMR according to different studies

Focus of SSMR study	Conceptual understanding	Activity orienting	Inessential items
Iiskala et al. (2011)	Situation model	Operation	Incidental matter
Grau and Whitebread (2012)	Fundamental aspects	Organization	Surface level
Khosa and Volet (2014) and Volet et al. (2009a)	Knowledge co-construction	Task co-production	–

(see Table 5.1). In that study, although fourth grade high-achieving dyads' SSMR had all these different foci, they regulated incidental matters more often when the problems were easy and, by contrast, situation models more often when the problems were difficult. These findings suggested that collaborative tasks should be difficult enough to get students to focus their SSMR on understanding. The same categories were applied to small group's Computer-Supported Collaborative inquiry Learning (CSCL) in a science learning context, as illustrated in the following example (published by Iiskala et al. 2015, pp. 91–92, but here re-analyzed from the viewpoint of focus). In this example, a small group comprising four 12-year-old girls was working in asynchronous[1] computer-supported collaborative inquiry learning in science. The group had already set up their research question "*How can it be concluded that an asteroid will hit the earth, and what will then happen to the earth?*", and were now constructing a hypothesis to address that question (more details are provided in Iiskala et al. 2015). As the excerpt reveals, the focus of SSMR is on understanding. Specifically, the girls were jointly regulating their understanding of how it can be known that a crash will happen. In their written notes, the girls often demonstrated evidence of regulating their own and each other's cognitive processes, such as knowing and remembering as well giving reasons for their thinking (*"I think so because..."*, *"I think that it is possible to know because..."*). Some examples revealed that the girls had become aware of their lack of knowledge (*"I don't know much about this topic"*, *"I don't know if it..."*, *"I don't know anything of it, it was just an assumption"*, *"if it is wrong? Let's check this"*, *"Let's think other possibilities"*). These students' social regulation was based on reciprocity and the flow of regulation, where students reacted to each other's regulative acts by constructing SSMR together, as evidenced in their notes (the underlined text specifically highlighting metacognition):

Iina: *I think... It has been calculated that... they [asteroids] would crash in the year... <u>I think so because</u>... <u>how can it be concluded that</u>...?*
Piia: *... <u>I think that it is possible to know that because if</u>...*
Julia: *<u>how can it</u> last so long a time? ...years?*
Sonja: *It has probably... estimated... <u>I don't know much about this topic</u>...*
Piia: *<u>but how has it been found out</u>* that how...?

[1]In asynchronous learning, the unit of analysis is a thread, not a continuous episode. This is discussed in detail by Iiskala et al. (2015).

Julia: *maybe Iina is right that... if I remember right... then it was...*
Julia: *no... it can't be so!? or can it?*
Iina: *Because... But I don't know if it is*
Julia: *I don't know anything of it, it was just an assumption...*
Julia: *If they* [scientists] *have made a mistake in these interpretations*??
Iina: *So what is the end result?*
Julia: *if it is wrong? Let's check this...*
Sonja: *It's not necessary to find the end result right now. We still have time... Let's think other possibilities...*

In the same vein, Grau and Whitebread (2012) have distinguished between different foci of SSMR in face-to-face science learning context. One could be the fundamental aspects of the task (such as knowledge and understanding), and others the organizational aspects of the group work, or surface inessential-level features. A focus of SSMR on fundamental aspects refers to regulation that directs discussion and problem-solving to relevant processes and knowledge in view of task and learning goals. In contrast, a focus of SSMR at the surface level is directed towards the more contingent aspects of the task. Their empirical study showed that 8–9 years old children were already able to jointly regulate different aspects of their collaborative cognitive activity but their regulation generally focused on the surface level aspects. That study further revealed that these students' SSMR processes focused more on fundamental aspects of regulation than their other forms of regulation (i.e., self- and co-regulation).

The focus of SSMR has also been investigated with university learners, for example, small groups of veterinary medicine students' in face-to-face collaborative learning (Khosa and Volet 2014; Volet et al. 2009a, 2013). In that environment, it was found that SSMR focused on high- or low-level task co-production or on high- or low-level knowledge co-construction. Task co-production involved joint cognitive activity directed at the completion of the expected tangible task outcome, while knowledge co-construction featured joint cognitive activity focusing on content information related to the clinical case. Furthermore, and regardless of whether students were focusing on the completion of the task or on content knowledge related to the clinical case, high-level cognitive activity always included explicit conceptual justifications and attempts at meaning making, whereas low-level activity mainly dealt with gathering and sharing information relevant to the case. Consistent with other studies (Iiskala et al. 2011; Grau and Whitebread 2012), Khosa and Volet's (2014) study also highlighted the important role of the focus of SSMR, since the episodes of SSMR of the veterinary student groups with high learning outcomes were more often focused on high-level knowledge co-construction and task completion than low-level knowledge co-construction and task co-production. Overall, although conceptualizations of the focus of SSMR differ among studies (Grau and Whitebread 2012; Iiskala et al. 2011; Khosa and Volet 2014; Volet et al. 2009a), they share some important commonalities (see Table 5.1). In all these studies, conceptual understanding features as one of the foci of SSMR and in each study its importance is highlighted for quality learning outcomes. Furthermore, all these studies made an explicit distinction between "doing the task", such as activity orienting or task production, and higher level foci, such as meaning making and conceptual understanding. Iiskala et al. (2011) and Grau and Whitebread (2012) also analyzed instances where task-related SSMR focused on inessential aspects of the task that were not crucial to regulate for a collaborative group striving towards a learning goal (e.g., in Iiskala et al. study, when the dyad discussed whether it should write 90 cm or 90.0 cm even though it is not relevant in that case). These researchers concluded that when SSMR focuses on inessential items, it takes students' mind off the SSMR focusing on conceptual understanding.

5.3.2 *Functions of SSMR*

Besides the focus, the functions of SSMR have been established as important in the monitoring and controlling of cognition. Unlike in the case of individual regulation, though, the functions of SSMR in collaborative learning are assumed to affect the shared problem space and the shared cognitive processes applied to the task at hand. Thus, the functions of SSMR can be conceived as facilitating the building of shared conceptual understanding by confirming what has been consensually reached, or alternatively by activating processes that can lead to understanding (i.e., facilitation function of SSMR: confirm and activate) (Iiskala et al. 2011). According to Iiskala et al. (2011), another function of SSMR is to represent the execution of control processes, in which case SSMR would be used appropriately to inhibit inappropriate conceptualization and understanding (i.e., inhibition function of SSMR: slow down, change, and stop).

The facilitate and inhibit functions of SSMR have been found in different science learning contexts (e.g., Iiskala et al. 2015; Lajoie et al. 2015; Lee et al. 2017). For example (originally published by Iiskala et al. 2015, but rephrased here), in the case study of 12-year-old girls' asynchronous computer supported collaborative inquiry learning, SSMR threads were found to play both facilitative and inhibitive functions. Importantly, though, the main function was to inhibit the perceived inappropriate direction of the ongoing cognitive process (Iiskala et al. 2015, p. 96). The following example (originally discussed in Iiskala et al. (2015), and included shortened here) describes the inhibitive, especially changing, function of SSMR: One small group were summarizing their findings and drawing conclusions to their question of "*how it can be concluded that an asteroid will hit the earth, and what will then happen to the earth*". The SSMR thread indicated that the girls had become aware of the mismatch between their question and their findings, and consequently, inhibited the continuation of this mismatch, changed the direction of the process, and finally, changed their question (see below).

Sonja: *We have a rather extensive problem because there are so many sub-problems. We have more answers to sub-problems than to the main problem.*

Julia: *So could we take one sub-problem and substitute it for a main problem? So, such* [a sub-problem] *of which much knowledge is known*

Sonja: *Our problem could be change a bit...*

Julia: *so we change the* [main] *problem into a sub-problem?? Any suggestions for the sub-problem?*

Sonja: *We could combine sub-problems so that they form a main problem?*

Iina: *Yes! A really good thing! To this we have answers already! Yet, the hypothesis should be changed.*

Julia: *Maybe it's not use changing it because then the hypothesis must be changed as well, perhaps some changes could be made to it as well??*

Iina: *I think that the problem needs to change because it's much better in that new form. Changing the hypothesis may not be so difficult here in the networking...*

The functions of SSMR have also been identified in medical students' interaction in an online synchronous problem-based learning (see Lajoie et al. 2015[2]; Lee et al. 2017). Their results revealed that the medical students were able to generate deep understanding through regulating the process together since the most frequently occurring functions were activation and confirming the process. In addition, when needed, these medical students were also able to change the direction of their thinking process through SSMR (see Lajoie et al. 2015; Lee et al. 2017).

In sum, the functions of SSMR are important in collaborative learning because SSMR can affect to the direction of the cognitive learning process. Thus, a small group can construct a deep understanding so that this activation process is regulated together by the members of the group. Also, the small group can confirm by SSMR that the chosen direction of the process towards the learning goal is on the rails. In contrast to the facilitation functions of SSMR, it is also important to inhibit inappropriate direction of the process. The slowing down function of SSMR makes it visible that the small group regulates the process and is aware of the possible cognitive dissatisfaction. Further, by SSMR the inappropriate direction can be changed or stopped.

5.3.3 Triggering Factors Leading to SSMR

Previous research on SSMR has dominantly concentrated on scrutinizing SSMR *during* the collaborative learning process. As a consequence, one largely unexplored area refers to the kinds of factors that may trigger SSMR in a collaborative learning.

[2]Note that Lajoie et al. used the term 'co-regulation', but in light of their descriptions, it can be interpreted as representing SSMR.

To date, we have only scarce empirical evidence of the kinds of activities that precede SSMR. The shortage of research on the triggers of SSMR has practical consequences as it makes it difficult to give support to activities which could promote high-level SSMR in a collaborative learning process. Based on some prior research, metacognitive experiences (ME), (socio)cognitive conflict, and effort feedback have been identified as possible triggers of SSMR.

Metacognitive Experiences ME (Flavell 1979) are seen as the product of online monitoring of cognitive processing (Efklides 2001, 2009), that is, what the person experiences during the cognitive processing of the task at hand (Efklides 2001). Thus, they can be seen as a person's subjective cognitive or affective experiences (Efklides 2001), some kind of self-reactions in the cognitive domain (Efklides and Tsiora 2002). ME monitor the interaction between the person and the task (Efklides 2001). Their role can be seen as two-fold: On the one hand, ME make the person aware of disruptions of processing and/or, on the other hand, they make the person aware of the deviation from the standard (e.g., learning goal) in which case control processes take over to restore the processing (Efklides and Dina 2004).

ME have mostly been investigated in an individual's learning context using self-reports (e.g., Efklides 2014; Salonen et al. 2005). However, as Efklides (2006, 2008) points out, research on the dynamic nature of ME during the learning process is needed because ME are essential for individuals to regulate their own learning and the collaborative learning process. For example, if an individual lacks ME in a collaborative learning process, it can have a negative affect or generate conflict (Salonen et al. 2005). Importantly, ME have also been identified as triggers to SSMR in high-achieving dyads' mathematical word problem solving process (Iiskala et al. 2011). In that study, there was evidence of ME at the beginning of the SSMR episodes in over the half of the cases. Thus, turns such as *"We have had a rather similar problem earlier"*, *"I'm confused."* or *"I'm not sure if this is correct."* were important triggers for SSMR. Further, when there were observable ME at the beginning of the SSMR episode, the episode focused more often on situation models.

Similar evidence of ME as triggers of an SSMR episode aimed at conceptual understanding were found in Khosa and Volet's (2014) study of veterinary students building a concept map of a clinical case, for example, "*Yep, but I'm not sure about Polydipsia*", "*A double arrow you reckon? Weight loss wouldn't cause azotemia*" or "*Are you happy with the hypertension story? Like, yeah, you know how it like feeds in first of all you get the um, not causing each other they actually make it into renal failure and… Do you think it's kind of demonstrated there?*" These findings suggest that observable ME are crucial triggers especially when the focus of SSMR is to build a situation model (Iiskala et al. 2011) or develop conceptual understanding (Khosa and Volet 2014). Khosa and Volet also found evidence, in the conversation of a high performing group that the start of one of their episode of SSMR aimed at conceptual understanding, had been triggered by one group member's realization that there were different conceptualizations of the notion of "anorexia" within the group, and that her peers had misconceptions. This suggests that in collaborative learning, metacognitive experiences can extend to observed and inferred experiences of others. To date, research on ME in relation with other aspects of metacognition such as SSMR is still limited and, consistent with Efklides' earlier call (2014), we propose to strengthen that line of study in the future.

(Socio)cognitive Conflict Based on Piagetian conceptualization of (dis)equilibrium, cognitive conflict refers to discrepancy between a person's own view of the world and new information that conflicts with the person's existing view. Cognitive conflict can also arise from social interaction while jointly pondering new information, and then the concept of socio-cognitive conflict is used (see Tudge and Rogoff 1999). In the process of (socio)cognitive conflict, metacognition can be seen as an important factor because it covers a persons' awareness of their own and scientific conceptions. Thus, metacognition is assumed to help a person recognize that there is a gap between his/her existing concept and the new scientific concept and, in this way, it supports a person's conceptual understanding (Mason et al. 2017; Mikkilä-Erdmann and Iiskala 2020).

Cognitive conflict can be triggered, for example, when a teacher presents information that contradicts students' ideas, beliefs or theories (Limón 2001). In a collaborative learning context, students can produce (socio)cognitive conflicts within the group by presenting conflicting ideas (Tudge and Rogoff 1999). As an example of this, Ucan and Webb (2015) reported that experienced conflicting viewpoints initiated SSMR processes among seventh grade students (aged 12) engaged in small group's collaborative science inquiry. For example, after experiencing cognitively conflicting ideas, students started to co-construct new knowledge by means of SSMR. Thus, their conflicting ideas were facilitated by SSMR. In other cases, though, conflicting ideas had an inhibitive function in the following SSMR processes. For example, conflicting viewpoints triggered SSMR, which slowed down the continuation of the (inappropriate) cognitive process. However, it is important to note, as Limón (2001) reminded us, that conflicting ideas do not necessarily automatically enhance a person's cognitive conflict. Related to this point, Iiskala (2015) also expressed concern that, in collaborative learning, students can also co-construct misconceptions. In spite of some evidence of a connection between metacognition, such as SSMR, and (socio)cognitive conflict and conceptual change, there is still limited empirical research on this relationship (Mikkilä-Erdmann and Iiskala 2020). To increase our understanding of the role of (socio)cognitive conflict in SSMR as well the role of SSMR in conceptual change, more empirical evidence is needed. One interesting question for future research is whether the conceptual change process could also be shared in collaborative learning (so-called socially-shared conceptual change) and what is the role of SSMR in that process (see Mikkilä-Erdmann and Iiskala 2020).

Error Feedback As shown in previous research (e.g., Iiskala et al. 2004; Vauras et al. 2003), students receive feedback from each other during the collaborative learning process. For example, in Iiskala et al. (2004) study of a high-achieving dyad's (fourth graders) collaborative mathematical word problem solving, it was found that the collaborating students had become aware of their reciprocal influence in the joint effort. This was made evident in the subsequent stimulated recall interview (p. 165), when the researcher asked the two boys Jaakko and Kalle to describe their collaboration. The two boys displayed an awareness of the role SSMR had played in their common solution by declaring that the problem solution would have been incorrect if they had worked alone.

Jaakko: *... in the beginning Kalle realized that... and after that I realized that we should have counted...*

Jaakko (a bit later): *If we had each worked alone, the solution would have been incorrect...,*

Kalle: *...I would have counted that.... I wouldn't have discovered those ... so it would have been wrong...*

The same degree of awareness was evident in Vauras et al.'s (2003, p. 29) study, where high-achieving girls described their collaboration.

Titta: *We were thinking together, and then when we both agreed, we didn't have disagreements...*

Jonna: *...you could always do better and better, you came along with each other, that if we always work here together...*

And later, when the teacher asked "*How did you recognize that your collaboration went well?*", Titta replied: *Because, when one notices something, the other began to think ... we told the other ... told aloud ... and she noticed the other one is of a different opinion, then we pondered is it quite like this or that ... and then we figured it out ...*

Error feedback may also affect students' metacognitive behavior, that is, it has been assumed that students may act differently depending on knowing whether their solution to some, for example, mathematical problem is correct or incorrect (Iiskala et al. 2004). Thus, it would be important to scrutinize the role of error feedback provided by other group members, a teacher or some other source (e.g., computer program) in collaborative learning context. For example, different kinds of feedback and their role as a trigger factor for more accurate monitoring and control decisions in SSMR should be studied. To date, this kind of research in SSMR is still lacking.

5.3.4 Relationship of SSMR to Learning Outcomes

The evolving SSMR processes in collaborative inquiry among students, and the effects of these processes on the cultivation of content understanding and on desired learning outcomes are not yet well established in the empirical research. Theoretical assumptions, though, signpost the positive relation between SSMR, deep understanding and high-level outcomes (see e.g., Iiskala et al. 2011, 2015; Schoor et al. 2015). This assumption stems logically from the evidence of monitoring and controlling of cognitive activity to achieve desired learning goals in individual learning situations (e.g., Kinnunen and Vauras 2010). However, existing empirical findings in social learning contexts are somewhat contradictory, with some studies reporting partly positive (e.g., Järvelä et al. 2016; Volet et al. 2013) and others non-existent (e.g., Schoor and Bannert 2012) associations. After new, although yet scarce, empirical evidence, the relations between SSMR and desired learning outcomes seem more intricate in collaborative learning contexts, though.

Therefore, it is plausible to assume that several mediating factors appear to contribute to the actual causal effect of SSMR to learning outcome, but due to the lack of research explicitly focusing on these factors, only tentative relations can be discussed presently. As discussed earlier, the frequency, focus and functions of SSMR can vary considerably, depending, for example, on task demands and characteristics, mutual understanding and agreement of learning goals, interest and engagement in the task. The frequency of SSMR itself does not seem to explain the level of learning outcomes well (e.g., Volet et al. 2013; see also, Khosa and Volet 2014). For example, the study by Khosa and Volet (2014, see also Volet et al. 2013) showed no significant difference in the relative time spent on SSMR processes between the high- and low-outcome groups. These empirical outcomes indicate that the relation between SSMR processes and learning outcome is mediated by other factors. Some of these factors illustrated by empirical observations are briefly discussed below.

First, *the type of task*, e.g., in terms of novelty or complexity, expected answers or solutions, seem to determine if and when SSMR is present and needed for adequate or high-level outcome (Iiskala et al. under revision). For example, Badia and Becerril (2015) reported differences in the impact of shared regulation across task types, such as listing information, interpreting information, and performing conceptual tasks. Their findings indicated that in a more complex task (i.e., interpreting information) shared task regulation was significantly related to learning outcomes but not in the other two tasks. Molenaar et al. (2014) and Lajoie and Lu (2012) showed that different collaborative learning tasks and contexts may demand or afford different degrees (i.e., amount, quality) of metacognitive regulation.

For example, the study of Iiskala et al. (2004) showed that there is no need for SSMR if the task is very easy because these can be solved as a matter of routine without any difficulties. Thus, the type of the task plays a role in triggering SSMR. The following example of two high-achieving fourth-grade girls solving a novel-type, moderately difficult, mathematical word-solving problem, indicates how the difficulty of the task forced the girls to monitor and regulate their problem solving (see Iiskala et al. 2011, p. 386). This problem demanded counting how many different routes a boatman can choose to transport students from the Ferry Bank to the school (a map and task specifying six routes from the Ferry Bank to Middle Island, from there two routes to Beaver Fall, and from there four routes to the Beaver Lake school). First, the girls did not understand how to solve this problem but as they clearly shared a common goal, their reasoning evidenced reciprocity of regulation, leading finally to correct solution.

Sofia: *How is it even possible to count…but?*
Paula: *Hmm*

Sofia: *There are 6 (with emphasis) routes…*
Paula: *I draw here, 2, 3, …6…*(begins to draw)
Sofia: *How many routes, what, there's a terrible number to count, so 6, how can one go different routes, oh dear* (begins to draw)
Paula: *Here is Lake Beaver, the Beaver Fall* (Sofia looks at the notebook) …
Sofia: *No, no, the Ferry Bank…* (looks at the notebook)
Paula: *Oh, aah*
Sofia: *1, 2, …6*
Paula: *This is the Middle Island* (draws)
Sofia: *What on earth are you doing, the Middle Island?* (looks at the notebook)
Paula: *Look now, 6 safe routes…* (points with her finger at the computer screen, both draw)
Sofia: *Okay, the Middle* (both draw)
Paula: *4, 5…12* (count from her own notebook)
Sofia: *It can't be so* (looks at Paula)
Paula: *Oh boy…*
Sofia: *But let's look …* (looks at Sofia)
Paula: *Then it goes here, then from here…*

Second, the *focus* of SSMR plays an important role in determining which aspects of learning (such as creating understanding, performing operations, producing outcomes) the joint regulation is targeted. It is important to note that during a typical group learning process, all these phases need to be addressed, and therefore, the level of cognitive effort and level (low or superficial vs. high or deep) on which the group works and discusses during these phases may determine the magnitude of the effect of SSMR. As evidenced in the recent research, SSMR may take place at different levels of cognitive activity (e.g., low or high), and resulting in very different learning outcomes as a consequence (Volet et al. 2013, 2017). This means that SSMR is critical when groups engage in high-level cognitive activity in order for it to support their achievement of high-level cognitive outcome, and it can be claimed to be particularly applicable when the tasks are cognitively demanding, but yet within the scope of students' competence. Support for the importance of regulating high-level cognitive activity was also found at the individual level. In the research with university students in veterinary medicine (Volet et al. 2017) there were significant differences between higher and lower performing groups. This was found both in the overall distribution of their group members' contributions to SSMR, and in the range of individual contributions to SSMR aimed at conceptual understanding between the two higher performing groups (2 to 19 and 4 to 24 contributions) in comparison to the lower performing groups (1 to 7 and 0 to 10 contributions).

Third, if the *functions* of SSMR are ill-timed ill-placed or inadequate in a particular situation, they, in turn, may essentially influence the effect of SSMR despite the frequency of regulatory processes. An example of two high-school students working on a challenging science task illustrates an ill-timed regulation, since at the stage where the students should already write a presentation of their study, they start regulating their thinking. This should have taken place much earlier, at the stage they were actually planning their study and formulating their hypotheses.

Anna: *First there is like planning…*
Emma: *planning of the study*
Anna: *I don't even know, what this is about…*
Emma: *Messy*
Anna: *There are so many things…*

These problems seemed to stem from the girls' earlier, rather superficial and interrupted, attempts to regulate their joint reasoning, exemplified here with a short episode while formulating hypotheses.

Emma: *… something like…the lower the pH, the lower the temperature, but we do not kind of know how… how to happens… we do not know, sort of that needs…*
Anna: *… a little more material and deeper knowledge, but if something should be… on the basis of that so… perhaps from temperature.*

Although the students seemed to be totally lost in the task and had to even spend some time consulting the literature, they soon, without sorting out their understanding, rushed forward to formulate the hypothesis as Anna commanded: "*We need to go ahead*".

Fourth, and closely related to the previously mentioned factors, *interruptions* or *abrupt shifts* of the SSMR processes (e.g., shifting focus from high to low level activity or from facilitating to inhibiting regulation, or other type of regulatory processes are triggered) may hamper the collective discussions. For example, enough time is not devoted to solve the problem at hand or reach common conceptual understanding. This was already seen in the previous example already exemplified this, and the study of SSMR in veterinary students' joint construction of a concept map of a clinical case illustrates it further (Khosa and Volet 2014). Khosa and Volet found frequent evidence of shifts in SSMR processes between regulating the group understanding of the case clinical condition and regulating the completion of the set task, namely the concept map itself. In the excerpt below, four students (Blanca, Winnie, Thea and Mark), were trying to understand how Amoldipine medication relates to retinal detachment and hypertension in a cat in order to decide how to place their concept cards and draw arrows between them on their developing map. In contrast, one other student (Renee) showed evidence of almost exclusive focus on the production of the map, through initially seeking necessary information from her peers and then interrupting their emerging, tentative high-level conceptual talk, in order to move on with drawing links between concept cards on the map. She clearly ignored her peers' apparent motivation to engage in SSMR of their conceptual understanding of the cat's condition and management.

Renee: *And then Retinal detachment we're also going with* (indicates a possible arrow from Retinal detachment to Amoldipine) *Amoldipine as well as arrows, both ways?* (Turns to look at Thea)
Blanca: *The Amoldipine wouldn't fix the Retinal detachment*
Winnie: (shakes head to indicate no)
Thea: *No to fix the Hypertension which is why xxx* (inaudible)
Winnie: *It can also prevent Retinal detachment* (at the same time as Renee is drawing a line from Retinal detachment to Hypertension)
Blanca: *Yeah*
Thea: *Yeah*
Mark: *It prevents further* ... (unable to continue as Blanca steps in)
Blanca: *Cos if the hypertension* ... (interrupted by Renee)
Renee: *So, I'm going like this?* (indicating a line from Amoldipine to Retinal detachment)

(Note: The terms 'Retinal detachment, Hypertension, Amoldipine, Blood pressure measurement' are capitalized as they refer to the cards that students could select to build their concept map.)

In the same study, however, there were also occasions, where the group was actively engaged in SSMR of the completion of their conceptual map, when one student suddenly interrupted the flow of task co-production by asking a fundamental conceptual question: "*but what is Azotaemia*?" This triggered the start of an SSMR episode focusing on knowledge co-construction, which was itself interrupted too early by another student who brought back the focus on the implications of that unfinished conceptual talk for the pursuit of their map.

5.4 Concluding Remarks

More than 15 years of active research of SSMR has established it as an important and integral component of productive engagement in learning. However, as Volet et al. (2009a) argued, in real time collaborative learning, individuals and social entities should be conceptualized as self-regulating and co-regulated systems at the same time. Already early observations of young high-achieving student dyads (Iiskala et al. 2004; Vauras et al. 2003) indicated that although high awareness and regulation of one's own thinking, self-regulation, seemed to be the bottom line in dyads' collaboration, the social level regulation often took place in students' communication. This could be seen in the form of other-regulation, e.g., via peer tutoring or asymmetric development of ideas and understanding. At times, symmetric, equal contributions to the group discourse aimed at understanding or solving the task were also observed. These contributions were in the form of socially shared regulation directed at the group collective activity (see also, Grau and Whitebread 2012; Whitebread et al. 2009).

Yet today, in spite of different levels and forms having been emphasized in models on regulation in collaborative learning contexts (e.g., Efklides 2008; Volet et al. 2009a) as well as included in coding systems and observed in empirical studies (e.g., Iiskala et al. 2004; Grau and Whitebread 2012; Iiskala et al. under revision), their concurrent interplay is yet to be established. Further, as transactional cognitive partnerships always require sophisticated social and communication skills, such as listen actively, understand the partner's point of view, and communicate one's own views unambiguously (see Ding and Flynn 2000; Vauras et al. 2003), developmental studies aimed at unveiling the complex and subtle interplay among these regulation processes are further necessary.

In addition, in line with the claims of Efklides (2011), another intriguing line of potential research is to extend the metacognitive analyses to include affective reactions as part of the SSMR process. For example, external feedback could trigger epistemic emotions to one or more of the collaborating students, and through affect, shape the process of SSMR (see Touroutoglou and Efklides 2010). Considering that the impact of affective reactions in the context of SSMR appears important on the ground that such impact depends on the complex interplay among emotions, task demands and individual conditions (Pekrun 2018). For such interplay to be productive requires effective monitoring processes and control decisions to be informed by the outcome of monitoring processes. When considering the impact of affect on the process of SSMR different types of negative and even positive affect would need to be distinguished, given evidence that experiences of positive achievement emotions (such as joy) do not have the same function on subsequent engagement in learning as positive epistemic emotions (such as interest) (Volet et al. 2019). The philosophical question as to whether epistemic emotions are metacognitive in nature may not need to be addressed (Carruthers 2017), if the main issue at stake is to establish their function in the process of SSMR.

While acknowledging the big steps already made in understanding regulation processes in collaborative learning, this chapter has identified several important gaps in research of socially shared metacognitive regulation. As the corpus of extant research has focused on the manifestations of SSMR during collaborative learning, knowing what actually triggers SSMR remains relatively unknown, although some potential candidates, such as metacognitive experiences, error feedback and cognitive conflict, have been discussed in the context of self-regulation and also identified in the case of SSMR. Other gaps raised here, e.g., in terms of foci, function, interruptions and shifts, concern the relation and meaning of SSMR for learning outcomes. Moreover, scientific problems are complex and often need collaborative effort. SSMR may play an important role in collaborative problem solving in science and in science learning context, but more research is needed to understand its role.

Future research related to SSMR in collaborative science learning (and beyond), would no doubt benefit from a solid grounding in Efklides (2008) multifaceted and multilevel model of metacognition. As stated by Efklides (2009, p.14), the potential of the model "*lies in the unifying framework it provides and the predictions it allows regarding the components of each level and the interactions with those of the other levels*". Regardless of whether the applied focus is on the interactions of participants in symmetrical or asymmetrical relations, both individual and social regulation processes play a part and need to be acknowledged, since by today evidence undeniably confirms the nature of metacognition as *"a sine-qua-non constituent"* (Efklides 2008, p. 277) of social interaction and regulation in collaborative learning.

References

Badia, A., & Becerril, L. (2015). Collaborative solving of information problems and group learning outcomes in secondary education. *Journal for the Study of Education and Development, 38*, 67–101.

Boekaerts, M., Pintrich, P. R., & Zeidner, M. (Eds.). (2000). *Handbook of self-regulation*. San Diego: Academic Press.

Brown, A. (1987). Metacognition, executive control, self-regulation and other more mysterious mechanisms. In F. E. Weinert & R. H. Kluwe (Eds.), *Metacognition, motivation and understanding* (pp. 65–116). Hillsdale: Lawrence Erlbaum.

Carruthers, P. (2017). Are epistemic emotions metacognitive? *Philosophical Psychology, 30*, 58–78.

de Bakker, L., van Keer, H., & Valcke, M. (2015). Exploring evolutions in reciprocal peer tutoring groups' socially shared metacognitive regulation and identitying its metacognitive correlates. *Learning and Instruction, 38*, 63–78.

de Jong, T. (2019). Moving towards engaged learning in STEM domains; there is no simple answer, but clearly a road ahead. *Journal of Computer Assisted Learning, 35*, 153–316.

Ding, S., & Flynn, E. (2000). Collaborative learning: An underlying skills approach. In R. Joiner, K. Littleton, D. Faulkner, & D. Miell (Eds.), *Rethinking collaborative learning* (pp. 3–18). London: Free Association Books.

Dinsmore, D. L., Alexander, P. A., & Loughlin, S. M. (2008). Focusing the conceptual lens on metacognition, self-regulation, and self-regulated learning. *Educational Psychology Review, 20*, 391–409.

Duschl, R., & Hamilton, R. (2011). Learning science. In R. Mayer & P. Alexander (Eds.), *Handbook of research on learning and instruction* (pp. 78–107). New York: Routledge.

Efklides, A. (2001). Metacognitive experiences in problem solving; cognition, affect, and self-regulation. In A. Efklides, J. Kuhl, & R. Sorrentino (Eds.), *Trends and prospects in motivation research* (pp. 297–323). Dordrecht, The Netherlands: Kluwer.

Efklides, A. (2006). Metacognition and affect: What can metacognitive experiences tell us about the learning process? *Educational Research Review, 1*, 3–14.

Efklides, A. (2008). Metacognition: Defining its facets and levels of functioning in relation to self-regulation and co-regulation. *Educational Psychologist, 13*, 277–287.

Efklides, A. (2009). The new look in metacognition: From individual to social, from cognitive to affective. In B. C. Larson (Ed.), *Metacognition: New research developments* (pp. 137–151). New York: Nova Science.

Efklides, A. (2011). Interactions of metacognition with motivation and affect in self-regulated learning: The MASRL model. *Educational Psychologist, 46*, 6–25.

Efklides, A. (2014). How does metacognition contribute to the regulation of learning: An integrative approach. *Psychological Topics, 23*, 1–30.

Efklides, A., & Dina, F. (2004). Feedback from one's self and from the others: Their effect on affect. *Hellenic Journal of Psychology, 1*, 179–202.

Efklides, A., & Tsiora, A. (2002). Metacognitive experiences, self-concept, and self-regulation. *Psychologia: An International Journal of Psychology in the Orient, 45*, 222–236.

Flavell, J. H. (1979). Metacognition and cognitive monitoring: A new area of cognitive-developmental inquiry. *American Psychologist, 34*, 906–911.

Grau, V., & Whitebread, D. (2012). Self and social regulation of learning during collaborative activities in the classroom: The interplay of individual and group cognition. *Learning and Instruction, 22*, 401–412.
Greeno, J. G. (2006). Learning in activity. In R. K. Sawyer (Ed.), *The Cambridge handbook of the learning sciences* (pp. 79–96). New York: Cambridge University Press.
Hadwin, A. F., Järvelä, S., & Miller, M. (2011). Self-regulated, co-regulated, and socially shared regulation of learning. In B. J. Zimmerman & D. H. Schunk (Eds.), *Handbook of self-regulation of learning and performance* (pp. 65–84). New York: Taylor & Francis.
Hmelo-Silver, C., Duncan, R., & Chinn, C. (2007). Scaffolding and achievement in problem-based and inquiry learning: A response to Kirschner, Sweller, and Clark (2006). *Educational Psychologist, 42*, 99–107.
Iiskala, T. (2015). *Socially shared metacognitive regulation during collaborative learning processes in student dyads and small groups*. Doctoral dissertation. Turku: University of Turku.
Iiskala, T., Vauras, M., & Lehtinen, E. (2004). Socially-shared metacognition in peer learning. *Hellenic Journal of Psychology, 1*, 147–178.
Iiskala, T., Vauras, M., Lehtinen, E., & Salonen, P. (2011). Socially shared metacognition of dyads of pupils in collaborative mathematical problem-solving processes. *Learning and Instruction, 21*, 379–393.
Iiskala, T., Volet, S. E., Lehtinen, E., & Vauras, M. (2015). The emergence of socially shared metacognitive regulation and students' participation in asynchronous computer supported collaborative learning. *Frontline Learning Research, 3*, 77–111.
Iiskala, T., Volet, S., Jones, C., Koretsky, M., & Vauras, M. (under revision). Significance of forms and focus of metacognitive regulation in collaborative science learning across contexts: Comparison of low- and high-outcome groups.
Järvelä, S., & Hadwin, A. (2013). New frontiers: Regulating learning in CSCL. *Educational Psychologist, 48*, 25–39.
Järvelä, S., Malmberg, J., & Koivuniemi, M. (2016). Recognizing socially shared regulation by using the temporal sequences of online chat and logs in CSCL. *Learning and Instruction, 42*, 1–11.
Khosa, D., & Volet, S. E. (2014). Cognitive activity and metacognitive regulation during collaborative learning: Can it explain differences in conceptual understanding? *Metacognition and Learning, 9*, 287–307.
Kinnunen, R., & Vauras, M. (2010). Tracking on-line metacognition: Monitoring and regulating comprehension in reading. In A. Efklides & P. Misailidi (Eds.), *Trends and prospects in metacognition research* (pp. 209–229). New York: Springer.
Lajoie, S. P., & Lu, J. (2012). Supporting collaboration with technology: Does shared cognition lead to co-regulation in medicine? *Metacognition and Learning, 7*, 45–62.
Lajoie, S. P., Lee, L., Poitras, E., Bassiri, M., Kazemitabar, M., Cruz-Panesso, I., & Lu, J. (2015). The role of regulation in medical student learning in small groups: Regulating oneself and others' learning and emotions. *Computers in Human Behavior, 52*, 601–616.
Lee, L., Lajoie, S. P., Poitras, E. G., Nkangu, M., & Doleck, T. (2017). Co-regulation and knowledge construction in an online synchronous problem-based setting. *Education and Information Technologies, 22*, 1623–1650.
Limón, M. (2001). On the cognitive conflict as an instructional strategy for conceptual change: A critical appraisal. *Learning and Instruction, 11*, 357–380.
Mason, L., Baldi, R., Di Rondo, S., Scrimin, S., Danielson, R. W., & Sinatra, G. M. (2017). Textual and graphical refutations: Effects on conceptual change learning. *Contemporary Educational Psychology, 49*, 275–288.
Mikkilä-Erdmann, M., & Iiskala, T. (2020). Developing learning and teaching practices for adults – Perspectives from conceptual change and metacognition research. In E. Kallio (Ed.), *Development of adult thinking: Interdisciplinary perspectives on cognitive development and adult learning*. New York: Routledge.
Molenaar, I., Sleegers, P. J. C., & van Boxtel, C. A. M. (2014). Metacognitive scaffolding during collaborative learning: A promising combination. *Metacognition and Learning, 9*, 309–332.

Pekrun, R. (2018). Control-value theory: A social-cognitive approach to achievement emotions. In G. A. D. Liem & D. M. McInerney (Eds.), *Big theories revisited 2: A volume of research on sociocultural influences on motivation and learning* (pp. 162–190). Charlotte: Information Age Publishing.

Rogat, T. K., & Adams-Wiggins, K. R. (2014). Other-regulation in collaborative groups: Implications for regulation quality. *Instructional Science, 42*, 879–904.

Rogat, T. K., & Linnenbrink-Garcia, L. (2011). Socially shared regulation in collaborative groups: An analysis of the interplay between quality and social regulation and group processes. *Cognition and Instruction, 29*, 375–415.

Salonen, P., Vauras, M., & Efklides, A. (2005). Social interaction-what can it tell us about metacognition and coregulation in learning? *European Psychologist, 10*, 199–208.

Schoor, C., & Bannert, M. (2012). Exploring regulatory processes during a computer-supported collaborative learning task using process mining. *Computers in Human Behavior, 28*, 1321–1331.

Schoor, C., Narciss, S., & Körndle, H. (2015). Regulation during cooperative and collaborative learning: A theory-based review of terms and concepts. *Educational Psychologist, 50*, 97–119.

Schunk, D., & Zimmerman, B. J. (1997). Social origin of self-regulatory competence. *Educational Psychologist, 32*, 195–208.

Touroutoglou, A., & Efklides, A. (2010). Cognitive interruption as an object of metacognitive monitoring: Feeling of difficulty and surprise. In A. Efklides & P. Misailidi (Eds.), *Trends and prospects in metacognition research* (pp. 171–208). Boston: Springer.

Tudge, J., & Rogoff, B. (1999). Peer influences on cognitive development: Piagetian and Vygotskian perspectives. In P. Lloyd & C. Fernyhough (Eds.), *L. Vygotsky: Critical assessments: The zone of proximal development* (pp. 32–56). New York: Routledge.

Ucan, S., & Webb, M. E. (2015). Social regulation of learning during collaborative inquiry learning in science: How does it emerge and what are its functions? *International Journal of Science Education, 37*, 2503–2532.

Vauras, M., Iiskala, T., Kajamies, A., Kinnunen, R., & Lehtinen, E. (2003). Shared-regulation and motivation of collaborating peers: A case analysis. *Psychologia, 46*, 19–37.

Vauras, M., Volet, S., & Nolen, S. (2019). Supporting motivation in collaborative learning: Challenges in the face of an uncertain future. In E. Gonida & M. Lemos (Eds.), *Motivation in education at a time of global change: Theory, research, and implications for practice. Advances in motivation and achievement* (pp. 187–203). New York: Emerald.

Volet, S. E., Summers, M., & Thurman, J. (2009a). High-level co-regulation in collaborative learning: How does it emerge and how is it sustained? *Learning and Instruction, 19*, 128–143.

Volet, S. E., Vauras, M., & Salonen, P. (2009b). Self- and social regulation in learning contexts: An integrative perspective. *Educational Psychologist, 44*, 215–226.

Volet, S. E., Vauras, M., Khosa, D., & Iiskala, T. (2013). Metacognitive regulation in collaborative learning: Theoretical advances and methodological contextualizations. In S. Volet & M. Vauras (Eds.), *Interpersonal regulation of learning and motivation: Methodological advances* (pp. 67–101). London: Routledge.

Volet, S., Vauras, M., Salo, A.-E., & Khosa, D. (2017). Individual contributions in student-led collaborative learning: Insights from two analytical approaches to explain the quality of group outcome. *Learning and Individual Differences, 53*, 79–92.

Volet, S., Seghezzi, C., & Ritchie, S. (2019). Positive emotions in student-led collaborative science activities: Relating types and sources of emotions to engagement in learning. *Studies in Higher Education, 44*, 1734–1746.

Whitebread, D., Coltman, P., Pino Pasternak, D., Sangster, C., Grau, V., Bingham, S., Almeqdad, Q., & Demetriou, D. (2009). The development of two observational tools for assessing metacognition and self-regulated learning in young children. *Metacognition and Learning, 4*, 63–85.

Winne, P. H., & Perry, N. E. (2000). Measuring self-regulated learning. In M. Boekaerts, P. R. Pintrich, & M. Zeidner (Eds.), *Handbook of self-regulation* (pp. 531–566). San Diego: Academic Press.

Chapter 6
The Role of Social Emotions and Co-regulation of Learning During Complex Math Problem Solving

Cara A. Singh and Krista R. Muis

Abstract We investigated the antecedents and consequences of social emotions in the context of mathematics problem solving within a cooperative learning situation with elementary students. Twenty-nine fifth grade students were asked to solve a complex mathematics problem in groups. Measures of task value, perceived control, and basic needs satisfaction were collected. After problem solving, interviews were conducted to obtain a richer picture of students' experiences. A think aloud protocol was used to capture co-regulatory processes. Results revealed that task value, control and basic needs were antecedents to the social emotions that students experienced. Social emotions subsequently mediated feelings of relatedness and functional co-regulatory strategies.

Keywords Co-regulation of learning · Metacognition · Social emotions · Collaboration

6.1 Introduction

Collaborative learning is a promoted staple of the classroom-learning environment and requires special consideration of the way it is implemented by educators and received by students (Slavin 2015). Jones and Isroff (2005) noted that collaboration and conversation have the potential to generate positive emotions and foster motivation, which in turn supports beneficial communication and collaboration, and reinforces commitment to the co-construction of understanding (Jones and Isroff 2005). Moreover, the satisfaction of an individual's basic needs of autonomy, relatedness, and competence via positive social relationships has been shown to lead to an increase in self-determined motivation for learning. This results in increased academic enjoyment, interest, and effort (Ryan and Connell 1989).

C. A. Singh · K. R. Muis (✉)
Department of Educational and Counselling Psychology, McGill University, Montreal, QC, Canada
e-mail: krista.muis@mcgill.ca

D. Moraitou, P. Metallidou (eds.), *Trends and Prospects in Metacognition Research across the Life Span*, https://doi.org/10.1007/978-3-030-51673-4_6

However, it is also important to note that these same circumstances may bring about negative emotions and produce unique motivational barriers for students when their personalities, objectives, ability levels, or ideas clash (Järvelä et al. 2000; Kreijns et al. 2003).

Importantly, as Pekrun and colleagues (Pekrun 2006; Pekrun et al. 2002) suggested, emotions may facilitate or constrain self-regulated learning (SRL). Similarly, in her Metacognitive and Affective Model of SRL (MASRL), Efklides (2011) proposed that motivation, perceptions of control over a learning task, and value for learning in relation to the task predict an individual's metacognitive knowledge and their use of metacognitive skills. Despite a rich literature on the role of emotions in educational contexts (Pekrun and Linnenbrink-Garcia 2014), social emotions, which arise in the context of social situations, have been largely overlooked (Pekrun and Stephens 2012). As such, the aims of this study are to explore the antecedents and consequences of social emotions, and to assess whether these emotions predict co-regulation strategies and learning outcomes in the context of solving complex mathematics problems in a collaborative learning environment with elementary school students. Prior to delineating our specific research questions and hypotheses, we elaborate relevant theoretical and empirical work.

6.1.1 Social Achievement Emotions

Emotions are defined as, "...sets of coordinated psychological processes including affective, cognitive, physiological, motivational and expressive components" (Pekrun and Stephens 2012, p. 4). In the context of learning, emotions affect a student's attentional resources, motivation to learn, the quality and effectiveness of learning strategies, and the regulation of learning (Pekrun and Stephens 2012). For example, when students experience negative emotions such as anger, frustration, or anxiety in relation to a learning experience, they may begin to engage in off-task thinking where they worry about their ability to successfully complete an exam. These feelings of nervousness can reduce the dedication of attentional resources for the task, and ultimately undermine intrinsic motivation for learning (Pekrun and Stephens 2012).

Indeed, given the negative effects that anxiety can have on learning processes and learning outcomes, a rich literature on test anxiety has dominated research on emotions in education over the past 50 years (see Zeidner 1998). However, recent research suggests that a variety of emotions play an important role in learning. To take into consideration how other emotions might relate to learning in achievement situations, Pekrun (2006; Pekrun and Perry 2014) proposed the control-value theory of achievement emotions. Achievement emotions are emotions that are tied to any achievement activity or achievement outcome (e.g., the emotions one anticipates based on future and/or reflective emotions related to an achievement task) and may occur in academic situations, but may also occur in other achievement settings, like sports- or work-related achievement outcomes.

According to Pekrun (2006), emotions may be categorized by their valence (positive, negative), activation (activating, deactivating), and object focus (e.g., topic emotions, epistemic emotions, social emotions). For example, positive activating emotions (e.g., enjoyment, pride, hope) are predicted to increase learner readiness to perform an academic activity, strengthen perseverance, increase the use of creative and flexible learning strategies, and help focus attention (Pekrun and Stephens 2012). In contrast, negative activating emotions (e.g., anger, frustration) are thought to consume cognitive resources, result in task-irrelevant thinking, and limit intrinsic motivation. Conversely, these same emotions may boost extrinsic motivation to avoid failure (Pekrun and Stephens 2012).

With regard to object focus, of particular relevance to our study are social emotions. Social emotions are emotions directed at or experienced in relation to interactions with teachers and peers, as well as emotions that are the result of socially constructed guidelines of the environment, curriculum, and/or learning task (i.e., content and/or goals of the curriculum/learning task). Social emotions may include envy, contempt, schadenfreude, gratitude, empathy, shame, pride, jealousy, embarrassment, and guilt (Immordino-Yang et al. 2009; Pekrun and Stephens 2012).

6.1.2 Antecedents and Consequences of Emotions

Pekrun (2006) posited that the experience of achievement emotions is related to the perceived appraisals of control and value in relation to the learning task and other personal and environmental factors (i.e., beliefs, goals, cognition, motivation, and the cultural and social environment). Thus, control and value serve as antecedents to the achievement emotions experienced in relation to a learning task. Control refers to the amount of controllability one perceives in relation to the achievement task, whereas value refers to the amount of perceived importance and utility of the achievement activity itself along with the outcome of the activity. Both control and value are said to interact to predict the kinds of emotions individuals experience during learning. For example, high perceptions of control and high perceptions of value for a task interact to predict higher levels of enjoyment during task engagement. Conversely, perceptions of low control and low value may bring about frustration and anger. Anxiety may result from high perceived value but low control over the learning task. Lastly, boredom may result from overly challenging learning situations where control and value are perceived as being low.

Theoretically, Pekrun (2006) proposed that emotions, driven by appraisals of control and value, predict the cognitive and metacognitive processes students employ in a learning context. Although perceived control and value are likely key antecedents to social emotions, the social environment, such as the amount of autonomy support, goal structures and expectations, and feedback in terms of competence, may play a role in predicting the social emotions students experience during learning (Frenzel and Stephens 2013). For instance, Ahmed et al. (2010) found that competence, as experienced within a supportive peer environment, had a significant mediating effect on mathematics achievement. Efklides et al. (2018) discussed how a sense of competence not only informs one's self-efficacy, but one's entire self-concept (which includes self-perceptions, self-efficacy and self-esteem). Collaboration on a task may bring about emotions that are a consequence of personal and/or social relations experienced in the group. These emotions may have the capacity to affect mood-states, which in turn could impact the effectiveness of co-regulation of learning (Efklides 2011). Therefore, the motivational effects of a supportive peer group may be an additional antecedent to the social emotions students experience within a collaborative context.

Given the link to autonomy, support and competence, Ryan and Deci's (2000) self-determination theory (SDT) may provide some insight into the antecedents and consequences of social emotions. Specifically, SDT posits that human motivation is based on the fulfillment of three basic innate psychological needs (BPN), a sense of competency, autonomy and relatedness, to function at and grow towards a psychologically optimal level, as well as experience social and personal well-being. That is, within a social context, the degree to which individuals feel that they are in charge of their own behavior (i.e., autonomy), are efficacious within their environment (i.e., competence), and are connected to others and being cared for (i.e., relatedness), determines the level of quality of an individual's motivation. The quality of motivation, in turn, directly impacts goals and outcomes and the regulatory processes involved in pursuing goals and outcomes. This, in turn, predicts how the individual performs within a given task (Deci and Ryan 2010). For instance, within a collaborative context, if students feel that their behavior is constrained, feel ineffective and/or disconnected from their peers, they may experience frustration or anger towards their group, which may negatively impact the quality of co-regulatory processes and ultimately impact task achievement. Conversely, students who feel valued, effective, and connected to their group may experience enjoyment and pride during the collaborative task, thus facilitating beneficial co-regulatory processes and ultimately result in higher achievement on the task.

Research in the area of SDT and BPN has demonstrated that self-determined motivation is related to task-related enjoyment and better performance (Miserandino 1996). In contrast, less self-determined motivation has been linked to higher instances of negative activating emotions such as anxiety (Ryan and Connell 1989). Hareli and Parkinson (2008) have also claimed that social emotions are connected with specific social behaviors. They argued that social behaviors are those in which an 'other' is the focus of behavior (i.e., experiencing anger or happiness in relation to another) and/or influences the nature of the interaction with the 'other' (i.e., inhibiting or extending help). For example, anger appears to be associated with the withdrawal or abstinence of helping behavior (Weiner 1985), whereas happiness appears to facilitate helping behavior (Isen 1987). As well, Ryan and Deci (2000) contended that social contexts, and the extent to which these contexts support members' psychological needs, provide an influential milieu through which an individual's commitment to a task, performance, and effort may be encouraged or constrained.

De Dreu and Weingart (2003) conducted a meta-analysis of research on the connections between team relationships and satisfaction and relationships and task conflict, and found that in a social learning context, interpersonal conflict experienced within a group was more detrimental to team member satisfaction than conflict associated with the task. The researchers posited that because interpersonal disagreements are more emotional in nature (as compared to emotions related to a learning task), they tend to produce more intense instances of negative affect (De Dreu and Weingart 2003). Within the aforementioned dynamic, it is important to note that emotion has the potential to encourage and provoke both learning *and* social behavior (Pekrun 2006). As well, it appears that the social affect experienced between group members has a larger impact on the individual group member than do feelings associated with the actual learning task (De Dreu and Weingart 2003). However, the details of this relationship as it relates to co-regulated learning have not been explored. Therefore, an individual's experienced affect and subsequent behavior within a collaborative learning context not only has the ability to constrain or potentially bring about co-regulatory processes but may also influence performance and achievement.

Given that positive social relations between collaborative group members have the potential to influence members' motivation and impact emotions related to the learning task, it is important to consider the role of satisfaction of basic psychological needs in the context of social and collaborative learning. In the same way that consequences of emotions serve to predict the regulation of learning at the individual level (Pekrun 2006), it is important to consider the way in which social emotions may facilitate or constrain the co-regulation of learning at the cooperative level.

6.1.3 Regulation of Learning in Collaboration

From a socio-cognitive perspective, SRL is defined as the "... strategic and metacognitive behavior, motivation, and cognition aimed toward a goal" (Hadwin and Oshige 2011, p. 243). That is, individuals are active in their own learning processes in that they engage in the recursive processes of planning, goal setting, performing and evaluating in relation to their learning task (Muis 2007; Winne 2018). However, SRL is also socially influenced in that the strategies individuals employ, along with their thoughts and behaviors, are acquired via social influence, modelling, and feedback (Hadwin and Oshige 2011; Schunk 1998). Hadwin et al. (2011, 2018) have proposed three primary modes of learning regulation that occur in collaborative learning contexts: self-regulated learning (SRL), [socially] shared regulation of learning (SSRL), and co-regulated learning (CoRL). Given the focus of co-regulated learning for this study, we briefly define the first two types of regulation and then fully elaborate our primary focus: co-regulated learning.

6.1.3.1 Self-Regulated Learning

SRL refers to an individual's ability to independently engage in regulating behavior, motivation, emotion and cognition during completion of an academic task (Hadwin et al. 2018). Most SRL theorists propose four phases of learning regulation that are recursive and weakly sequenced (Puustinen and Pulkkinen 2001) and five areas for regulation. The four phases include: (a) task definition; (b) planning and goal setting; (c) enactment; and, (d) evaluation. The five areas for regulation include: (a) cognition, (b) motivation, (c) affect, (d) behavior (e.g., effort expenditure, help seeking); and, (e) context (e.g., resources, instructional cues, social context) (Muis 2007; Muis et al. 2018). Additionally, some theories situate the social context as being at the center of SRL (Corno and Mandinach 2004; Winne 1989, 1997; Zimmerman 1989). Although SRL is an individual process, it is socially influenced in that a learner's self-regulation may be influenced as a consequence of working within a social context (Hadwin et al. 2011).

6.1.3.2 Shared Regulation of Learning

Socially shared regulation of learning (SSRL) is, "...a group's deliberate, strategic, and transactive planning, task enactment, reflection, and adaptation" (Hadwin et al. 2018, p. 86). During SSRL, groups must collectively engage in metacognitive control of a learning task by negotiating cognitive, motivational, behavioral and emotional situations when required. Iiskala et al. (2011) argued that socially shared metacognition is best assessed during episodes of collaborative work that is particularly challenging, like during complex mathematics problem solving, and can be reliably identified by observers via discourse analysis. For example, in their own research, they found that mathematics problem difficulty increased episodes—in instances and duration—of socially shared metacognition. That is, the more difficult the problem, the more socially shared metacognition occurred. Episodes were identified by increases in instances of function (e.g., facilitation or inhibition) and focus (e.g., situational model, operation, or incidental matter). Socially shared metacognition also contributed to increased instances of metacognition and to the facilitation of problem solving.

6.1.3.3 Co-regulated Learning

Co-regulation of learning (CoRL) in a collaborative context is defined by Hadwin et al. (2018) as the liaison between self-regulation and the shared regulation of cognition, behavior, emotion and motivation. CoRL includes self-motivated metacognitive processes with means aimed at bringing about or constraining the oscillation of regulatory ownership (i.e., between self-regulation and social regulation). Co-regulation involves the temporary and transitional support amongst group members where goals, beliefs, and progress about a given learning task are shared, and where the monitoring and regulation of cognition, behavior, emotion and/or motivation are provisionally offloaded to another group member. In this way, CoRL encourages the use of SRL and SSRL (Hadwin et al. 2018).

Factors involved in successful instances of CoRL in collaborative learning are beginning to emerge. To assess whether CoRL predicts individuals' ability to self-regulate their learning, Hadwin et al. (2005) investigated how scaffolding unfolds naturally between teachers and graduate students during instances of dialogue over students' research portfolios. Qualitative discourse analysis revealed that there were observable changes in responsibility and ownership over learning from teacher to student over the course of a year. They interpreted that teachers directly regulated student learning through instances of explicit teacher-led regulation (i.e., telling students what to do next), and indirectly regulated student learning more subtly (i.e., through prompts and questioning). Students gradually took increased ownership over their regulation over time and this increase was mediated by indirect teacher and student regulation.

In another study, Lee et al. (2016) investigated the way in which CoRL supports the collaborative construction of knowledge in the context of an on-line problem-based learning activity with four medical students. Using Iiskala et al.'s (2011) amalgamated conceptualization of the function (Iiskala et al. 2011) and focus (Cummins et al. 1988) of CoRL, the researchers coded discourse for the function of co-regulatory processes that facilitates or inhibits the collaborative process, along with the corresponding focus of the function (i.e., whether the situation model, the operation, or an incidental matter was the focus of the CoRL function). They found a strong relationship between instances of CoRL and metacognitive statements and episodes of overt inquiry or questioning. This research suggests that co-regulatory episodes foster individual metacognitive processes, aid group members, and facilitate monitoring of progression of the cooperative learning process. Taken together, research has shown important links between emotions and learning processes but has not simultaneously taken into consideration antecedents and consequences of social emotions during collaborative learning.

In sum, research on the antecedents and consequences of achievement emotions has provided support for Pekrun's (2006) control-value theory of achievement emotions and their role in self-regulated learning (Muis et al. 2015b). However, what is not clear is what the antecedents are for social emotions during collaborative work, and how these emotions facilitate or constrain CoRL. As such, the purpose of this study was to explore the antecedents and consequences of social emotions during complex mathematics problem solving during collaborative group work. Complex problem solving has the capacity to stimulate and evoke emotion. The ill-structured nature of complex problems set the stage for a myriad of emotions to take place during learning (i.e., confusion, frustration, joy, boredom, anxiety) (Muis et al. 2015b). Additionally, difficult problems produce more instances of CoRL (Iiskala et al. 2011). Complex problem solving within a collaborative setting also affords additional challenges in that the affective dynamics between group members can serve to bring about or inhibit motivation for learning (Järvelä et al. 2000; Jones and Isroff 2005; Kreijns et al. 2003). Using a triangulated, mixed-methods approach of self-reports, discourse analysis, and individual interviews, we explored the following research questions: (a) Do students' perceptions of control, value and basic needs predict the social emotions they experience within the collaborative context? (b) What are the relations between social emotions and learning processes across the two functions and four phases of regulation of learning during complex mathematics problem solving in a collaborative context? (c) Do learning processes experienced within the collaborative setting predict achievement in mathematics problem solving? (d) Do emotions mediate the relationship between perceptions of control, value and basic psychological needs, and CoRL processes and achievement?

6.2 Methodology

6.2.1 Participants

Thirty-one fifth grade students from an elementary school in the Montreal area ($n = 17$ girls) in a single classroom were invited to participate. One of the students was on an individualized education program and followed a separate math program and was not able to participate in the study. A second student was absent on the day of the data collection. Consequently, twenty-nine fifth grade students ($n = 17$ girls) participated. The mean age of the sample was 11.38 years ($SD = .45$). Parental consent and student assent were attained prior to the study.

6.2.2 Materials

6.2.2.1 Prior Knowledge

Students' mathematics grade on their most recent report card served as a measure of students' prior knowledge. Grades were based on complex situational problems, formal exams, teacher observation, project-based activities, mathematics homework, in-class worksheets, and mathematics warm-up activities. Considering the breadth and variety of assessments used to calculate students' math grades, reported mathematics grades served as a reliable estimate of prior mathematics knowledge.

6.2.2.2 Academic Control

Students' perceived control for learning mathematics content and engaging in the problem-solving activity was measured using Perry et al.'s (2001) Academic Control Scale, modified for elementary school students by Muis et al. (2015b). The Academic Control Scale is an eight-item questionnaire that measures two dimensions of control (i.e., action and outcome) on a five-point Likert scale ranging from "completely disagree" (rating of one) to "completely agree" (rating of five). Question examples include, "*There is little I can do about my math grade*" and "*When I do poorly in math, it's usually because I haven't given it my best effort*". In line with previous research (see Muis et al. 2015a, b) all items were summed and averaged to obtain an overall control score. The greater the score, the greater the amount of perceived control for learning mathematics content. Cronbach's alpha reliability estimate was.66.

6.2.2.3 Task Value

Students' task value for learning and problem solving in mathematics was measured using Pekrun and Meier's (2011) Task Value Measure, which was adapted from a similar measure created by Eccles et al. (1993). The task value measure is a seven-item questionnaire that measures three dimensions of perceptions regarding mathematics learning (i.e., interest, utility, and importance) along a five-point Likert scale ranging from "not at all true of me" (rating of one) to "very true of me" (rating of five). Question examples include, "*In general, learning about math is useful*" (utility), "*In general, I find learning about math very interesting*" (interest), and "*I feel that, to me, learning more about math is very important*" (importance). All seven questionnaire items were summed and averaged to obtain a global value score for each student, with higher scores representing greater perceived task value. Cronbach's alpha reliability estimate was .87.

6.2.2.4 Activity Emotions

The Epistemically-Related Emotions Scales (EES) (Pekrun et al. 2016), modified for elementary students (see Muis et al. 2015b) was used to measure the emotions students experienced during the problem-solving session (i.e., surprise, curiosity, joy, confusion, anxiety, frustration, boredom). The EES is a single-item adjective questionnaire (e.g., "curious") that includes a five-point Likert scale wherein participants are instructed to indicate the extent to which they experienced each of the emotions. Response options ranged from "Not at all" (a rating of one) to "Very strong" (a rating of five). Social emotions were also added to the EES (i.e., embarrassment, guilt, shame, envy, jealousy, empathy and pride). Because both activity emotions and more traditional social emotions could be experienced during problem solving, students were also asked to indicate the object focus of the emotion (i.e., whether the emotion was directed at themselves, members of their group, or both).

6.2.2.5 Basic Needs Satisfaction

To assess the degree to which participants' needs were met in the group context, an adaptation of La Guardia et al. (2000) Basic Psychological Needs Scale–Relationship Domain (BPNS-R) was administered subsequent to the problem-solving activity. The BPNS-R assesses an individual's needs related to the group experience along three dimensions: the degree to which an individual felt a sense of belonging, relatedness, and perceived competency within the group. This particular questionnaire was adapted to reflect language and vocabulary appropriateness given the age of the participants, and to make it specific to the learning task. The BPNS-R is measured along a seven-point Likert scale ranging from "not at all true" (rating of one) to "very true" (rating of seven). Examples include, "*When I was solving the math problems with my group, I felt like I could be myself*" (autonomy), "*When I was solving the math problems with my group, I often felt like I didn't know how to do the work or can't do the work*" (competence), and "*When I was solving the math problems with my group, I felt a lot of closeness and kindness*" (relatedness). Previous research has established the validity and reliability of the BPNS (Vlachopoulos and Michailidou 2006). Cronbach's alpha reliability estimate was .62 for autonomy, .58 for competence and .72 for relatedness, with an overall scale reliability of .79.

6.2.2.6 Complex Problem

The complex problem, *The Dragon's Desserts,* required students to collaboratively calculate the bill totals of four families' orders at an ice cream store. Each family member's order was described and, using a price list, students were required to tally each individual's order, and subsequently each family's total bill. A 15% tax rate was also calculated where students were required to convert percentages to decimals and calculate the tax rate accordingly for each bill total. Lastly, an end of the day cash-out was required so as to provide the total sales for the day, before and after taxes.

The complexity of the problem stems from the fact that there was no clear pathway to a solution. Students had to rely on previously learned concepts and apply various strategies to solve the problem. Complex mathematics problem solving was a staple of the current classroom curriculum, therefore, the students in this study had previous experience working through similar problems to the one presented for the purposes of this study. The classroom teacher and primary investigator worked collaboratively to develop the complex problem to ensure that the mathematical concepts needed to solve the problem had been previously reviewed in class. Additionally, the complex problem was reviewed for level of difficulty to ensure that the problem would be challenging, but achievable. A rubric was developed to assess the achievement score on the task.

6.2.3 Procedure

Prior to the study, parental consent and participant assent were collected, along with basic student demographic information (i.e., age, gender, first language spoken). The study was conducted over a period of two sessions. In the first session, students responded to questionnaires used to measure academic control for learning mathematics (*Academic Control Scale*), and their task value for mathematics (*Task Value Measure*). Students also received think-aloud training where the primary investigator modelled examples of how to think out loud. Students were asked to verbalize everything that they would normally say to group members while solving the problem, just like they would normally solve a problem as a group. To ensure that students were continuously thinking aloud, the primary investigator along with one research assistant and the classroom teacher verbally prompted groups to continue talking aloud if they were silent for more than 10 s. Subsequently, in groups of three, students were asked to solve a simple mathematics problem (i.e., *Kim can walk 3 km in 1 h, how many kilometers can Kim walk in 2.5 h?*) while being audio recorded. The first session lasted approximately 40 min.

In the second session, which occurred on a separate day from session one, the class was divided up into groups of two, three or four students. Groups were comprised of students of the same gender for control purposes, but of mixed ability. Student ability was determined by the classroom teacher (based on students' achievement to date) and, as such, the classroom teacher was also responsible for devising the groups so that ability was varied. Groups were then given one iPad per group (for audio-recording purposes) as well as the complex mathematics problem, *The Dragon's Desserts*, to solve collaboratively. Students were told that the activity was comparable to, and should be considered with the same importance as, any other mathematics activity that they do during their mathematics class. Students were instructed to place their group's iPad face-up in the middle of their table and press the "record" button once they were ready to begin. During this time, CoRL was measured during task engagement via audio-recording.

Students worked on the problem for their 75-min mathematics class, and all groups completed the problem within that time frame. Once students completed the problem, they were asked to individually complete the EES, and the Basic Psychological Needs Satisfaction in Relationships Scale (BPNS–R). Subsequent to the completion of the complex problem, the primary researcher applied a prior-to-feedback, open-ended, semi-structured interview with six students selected by the classroom teacher. The interviews were conducted individually, audio-recorded, and transcribed verbatim. Interview questions focused on the emotions that students experienced during the collaborative problem session and the circumstances surrounding the experience of discrete emotions (i.e., happy, curious, bored, proud, confused). The interviewer prompted students for further elaboration/clarification responses when their answers were short or lacking detail.

6.2.4 *Coding and Scoring*

6.2.4.1 Co-regulatory Processes

A Type 1, concurrent, think aloud protocol was used (see Ericsson and Simon 1998; Kuusela and Pallab 2000) to capture students' co-regulatory processes as they collaboratively solved the complex mathematics problem. A concurrent protocol, as opposed to a retrospective (or Type 2) protocol, was used as it allows for fluidity of thoughts or achievement without constrain or interruption, and offers an accurate evaluation of students' co-regulatory processes as they occur during problem solving when compared to self-report questionnaires that are retrospective in nature (see Winne et al. 2002). Think-alouds were then transcribed verbatim by two research assistants and the primary investigator. The transcribed think-alouds ranged in time from 25 min and 2 s to 55 min and 47 s and generated 316 double-spaced pages of transcriptions (38,885 words).

Discourse analysis focused on identifying the function and phase of co-regulatory processes. The function coding scheme was borrowed from a study conducted by Iiskala et al. (2011) as they coded for the facilitative or inhibitory episodes of socially shared metacognition. The coding scheme was reconceptualized for co-regulatory processes in accordance with Hadwin et al.'s (2011) characterization as facilitating group member learning (see Lee et al. 2016). Four categories of co-regulatory functioning were used in our coding scheme (i.e., activate, confirm, slow, and change). Functions of CoRL fulfill one of two roles; that is, they facilitate CoRL processes or inhibit CoRL processes. Facilitative CoRL functions can be delineated by whether they are activating (i.e., the activation of a new construct that is in line with the previous direction of understanding) or confirming (i.e., confirming whether the previous line of understanding is correct). Inhibitory CoRL functions can be delineated by whether they are slowing (i.e., attempts to slow down the processes of the previous direction) or changing (i.e., changing the direction of the previous activity) (Iiskala et al. 2011).

Muis et al.'s (2015b) and Muis (2007) coding scheme was employed for identifying the phase during which the functional CoRL episodes took place: task definition (e.g., *recognizing critical information*), planning and goal setting (e.g., *making a plan*), enactment (e.g., *summarizing or rereading*), and monitoring/evaluation (e.g., *questioning oneself*). Instances of co-regulated learning were organized within the same dimensions as outlined above. An initiation of a co-regulation was marked by a group member verbally directing group attention relating to the problem in the quest for a solution, and were maintained through cooperative instances that represent evolving interactions between group members, the adjustment of support for peers for self-regulatory purposes, mediation techniques that guide or support self-regulation or the group process, and encouraging and prompting group members to self-regulate their learning (Hadwin et al. 2011). The primary investigator spent 8 weeks examining the transcripts to identify instances of CoRL episodes, which were then categorized into 16 function-phase processes across the four phases of

SRL: facilitation-activate, facilitation-confirm, inhibit-slow, and inhibit-change. A research assistant independently coded 10% of the transcripts. Agreement was 96%, with discrepancies resolved through discussion. Details of the coding scheme can be found in Table 6.1.

6.2.4.2 Achievement Scoring

To determine each group's achievement score on the mathematics problem, a rubric was developed by the primary investigator. Five criteria were assessed (i.e., evidence of mathematical concept use, evidence of mathematical reasoning, strategy use, percentage of mathematical errors, problem completion) on a four-point scale that ranged from one (low demonstration) to four (full demonstration). The total number of points possible was 20, with zero points given for no evidence of the criteria, to partial points awarded for some evidence of the criteria, to full points awarded for complete demonstration of the criteria. The primary investigator and a research assistant scored one group's solution together. Agreement was 100%. The primary investigator then scored the remaining solutions. The research assistant blindly re-scored two solutions to establish inter-rater agreement. Agreement was 93%, with discrepancies resolved through discussion.

6.3 Results

6.3.1 Preliminary Analyses

Values of skewness and kurtosis were examined for normality prior to carrying out analyses. Skewness results showed that achievement on the complex problem was within range (−.64). All antecedents were also within the normal range: control (−.56), value (−.85), along with the three dimensions of BPN, competence (−.60), autonomy (−.57), and relatedness (−.07). For the episodes of CoRL, all were within the normal range for skewness (i.e., highest absolute value was for inhibition-change during the enactment phase of learning at 2.62).

6.3.2 Path Analyses

To model the antecedents and consequences of emotions during complex mathematics problem solving, Hayes and Preacher (2013) PROCESS SPSS macro (v. 2.16) was used to test the mediation model presented in Fig. 6.1. The PROCESS macro is recommended as it allows for more complex path modelling appropriate for smaller sample sizes using a single command feature (Hayes and Preacher 2013). A bootstrapping technique was used given the small sample size ($n = 29$) and

Table 6.1 Function and phases of CoRL: definitions, codes and examples

Function (*phase*)	Definition	Code	Example
Facilitate: Activate	The direction of the activity continues in the same way as previous and strengthens during the episode by activating a new construct in-line with the previous direction.	F-AC	
Task definition	Perception of a task, context, and the group is generated.	F-AC-TD	S1: "So first we have to figure out what 15% is." S2: "15% for taxes is, like, every dollar you have..." S1: "You add fifteen cents." S3: "You add 15 cents."
Planning and goal setting	Creation of a plan to solve the problem. Creation of goals related to the problem.	F-AC-PG	S1: "So how about we add, what was the answer for that..." S2: "That if we add them all up it's $11.90." S1: "Then we have to get the percentage for that." S2: "For that whichhhhh..." S1: "'Cause then we have to add 15% of $11.90." S2: "So what we do is 11 point 90 divided by 15."
Monitoring and evaluation	Evaluate the success or failures of each phase or products.	F-AC-ME	S1: "Okay, so now we do..." S2: "Do we continue? I don't think we have to continue." S1: "So we just have to add on $0.65..." S3: "Ya." S1 (writing): "...So $9.80 plus $0.65... $10.45."
Facilitate: Confirm	The direction of the activity continues in the same way as previous and strengthens during the episode by confirming that the previous direction is correct.	F-CO	
Task definition	Perception of a task, context, and the group is confirmed.	F-CO-TD	S1: "What's 15% off?" S2: "15% off?" S1: "15% off of $11.90." S2: "15% off... 15 cents off?" S1: "No, 15%." S2: "Oh, 15%!"
Planning and goal setting	Confirmation of a plan to solve the problem. Confirmation of goals related to the problem.	F-CO-PG	S1: "I got one regular scoop in waffle... in a waffle cone." S2: "Ya, you do one regular scoop in a waffle cone. $3.00, you do one kiddie scoop in a regular cone. Okay? Kiddie scoop, regular cone, okay, you got it? S3, do one kiddie scoop in a regular cone."

(continued)

Table 6.1 (continued)

Function (*phase*)	Definition	Code	Example
			S1: "One regular scoop in a waffle cone is what I've got, okay?" S2: "One regular scoop in a waffle cone is what you have, good! I have two regular scoops in a cup with sprinkles."
Enactment	Work on the task by confirming strategies or tactics.	F-CO-E	S1: "So in the cup..." S1 & S2: "...with sprinkles, in the cup." S3: "So that's a cup times two." S1: "Yes." S3: "Or one cup. So that's zero... one point thirty...in a cup..." S2: "0.35." S3: "0.35 for the sprinkles." S2: "Ya! For the sprinkles."
Monitoring and evaluation	Confirm the success or failures of each phase or products.	F-CO-ME	S1: "How is it 145?" S2: "It's 15." S3: "It's 15 times 9..." S2: "So 120..." S3: "5 times 9 is 45, 9 times 1 is 9, times 4 is..." S1: "Wouldn't it be... ummmm... 135? 'Cause..." S3: "We'll use that, yes, sorry." S2: "So 9, then 135." S1: "Yes."
Inhibit: Slow	The direction of the previous activity is interrupted during the episode by slowing down a continuation of the previous direction.	I-SL	
Task definition	Perception of a task, context, and the group is slowed by the group.	I-SL-TD	S1: "Wait, what do they mean, 'costs'? What's the 'subtotal'?" S2: "'Subtotal' is the total before the task." S1: "Okay so then what's 'costs'?!" S2: "It's costs."
Planning and goal setting	The slowing of devising a plan to solve the problem or establishing goals in-line with the problem.	I-SL-PG	S1: "Wait. Wait, wait, wait... we should write the goal." S2: "You guys, guys... write the goal at the bottom." S3: "Goal is to..." S1: "Find out how much money we've earned at the end of the day."

(continued)

Table 6.1 (continued)

Function (*phase*)	Definition	Code	Example
Enactment	Slowing the progression of performing strategies or tactics.	I-SL-E	S1: "Wait, so let's do..." S2: "...wait, wait, wait, wait! 15..." S1: "...let's do 30% then." S2: "15..." S3: "S1, let's do...1-...S1, come on, you're rushing ahead of the group! S1, we're a group here, you're not by yourself. S1, you're not by yourself!" S2: "No, you're not by yourself!" S1: "So 15 times 11.90."
Monitoring and evaluation	Evaluation of the success or failures of each phase or products is slowed by the group.	I-SL-ME	S1: "Okay, hold on, I didn't write this, like, properly." S2: "Okay sure." S3: "Are you done?" S1: "Okay... sorry." S3: "No, it's okay, it's fine."
Inhibit: Change	The direction of the previous activity is interrupted during the episode by changing the direction of a previous activity.	I-CH	
Task definition	Perception of a task, context, and the group is changed by the group.	I-CH-TD	S1: "So now we have to add the 15..." S2: "percent." S3: "So we do a 'divided by' (inaudible)." S1: "Divide by what though? (laughing)." S3: "Divided by 15! Divided 11.90 by 15." S2: "No. No, not (inaudible)." S1: "Wait, to do percent we need a fraction..."
Planning and goal setting	The changing of a plan to solve the problem or establishing goals in-line with the problem.	I-CH-PG	S1: "What did I miss? I say we all do it just to make sure." S2: "... 1.20... no, let's not all do it then otherwise it's a waste of time." S3: "Sprinkles, uh, okay." S1: "Wait, so..." S2: "Brownstone family..." S1: "You know you don't have to do that." S2: "I know, but we might as well all do it in case we take them..." S1 (interrupts): "Ya, but then we're wasting time 'cause we

(continued)

Table 6.1 (continued)

Function (*phase*)	Definition	Code	Example
			could do another part of it." S2: "Okay, true."
Enactment	Changing the progression of performing strategies or tactics.	I-CH-E	S1: "So, 15 goes into a 140... so let's do it... 15 times 6... (writing)." S2: "Stop, we know that it's probably 9." S3: "Times 9, it's times 9, ya, we said 9." S2: "Because we know..." S1: "You do 9, I'll do 10."
Monitoring and evaluation	Evaluation of the success or failures of each phase or products is changed by the group.	I-CH-ME	S1: "Wait, S2, can you double check this fast?" S2: "wait, so that's... $11.90 plus $9.80." S1: "No, it's (inaudible). Eleven dollars... wait, what are you doing?" S2: "No, I'm going down... I'm going... look. We're adding up totals..." S1: "No, add $11.90 plus $9.80 plus $7.00 and..." S2: "No, you have to add the total amounts." S1: "Ya, we do that next."

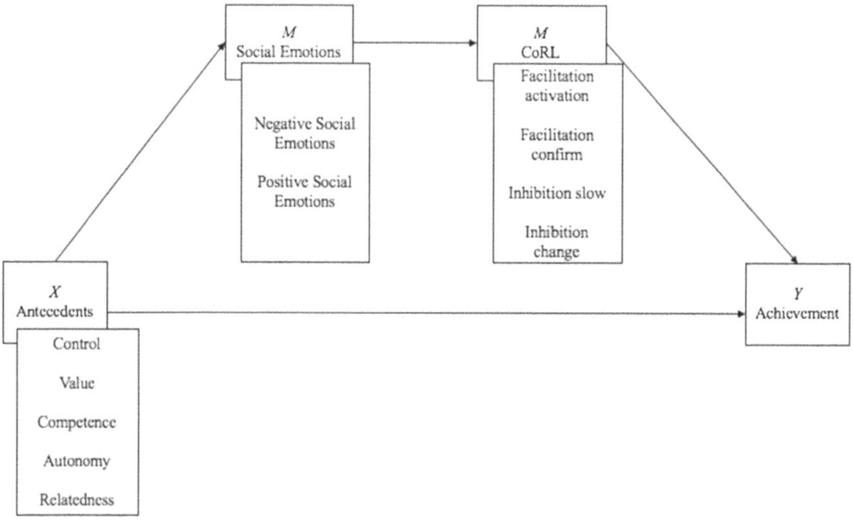

Fig. 6.1 Hypothesized mediation model of antecedents and consequences of social emotions

associated low power to detect statistically significant paths in the model (Hayes and Preacher 2013). The random resampling of the bootstrapping technique (i.e., 10,000 times) allows for an increase in the amount of power and enables for more precision in translating the estimates of the effects. However, due to low power, results must be interpreted with caution.

6.3.3 Interview Data

Interviews were qualitatively analyzed for themes relating to emotions experienced during the collaborative problem-solving session and the circumstances under which these emotions arose. Discrete emotions surfaced in relation to various facets of the learning task, or in response to collaborating with other members of the group, for all six of the students interviewed. Two overarching themes emerged in the interviews that provide support for the quantitative results of RQ1 and RQ2. Specific results of the interviews are discussed in conjunction with the quantitative results below.

RQ 1. Do students' perceptions of control, value and basic needs predict the social emotions they experience within the collaborative context?

Results revealed that perceptions of control positively predicted global positive social emotions ($\beta = .31, p = .09$). Control was also found to negatively predict feelings of jealousy ($\beta = -.46, p = .02$), and boredom ($\beta = -.32, p = .07$). Reports of competency in the group negatively predicted hopelessness ($\beta = -.35, p = .05$), as did competency and confusion ($\beta = -.50, p < .01$). Competency did not predict global positive or negative social emotions, but significantly predicted pride ($\beta = .38, p = .04$). Similarly, reports of autonomy negatively predicted hopelessness ($\beta = -.39, p = .03$), and confusion ($\beta = -.46, p = .01$). Autonomy did not predict negative social emotions, but significantly predicted positive social emotions ($\beta = .35, p = .07$), and specifically, feelings of pride ($\beta = .50, p = .01$). Lastly, perceptions of relatedness within the group positively predicted positive social emotions ($\beta = .40, p = .04$). Specifically, perceptions of relatedness positively predicted pride ($\beta = .47, p = .01$), and negatively predicted jealousy ($\beta = -.36, p = .07$) and boredom ($\beta = -.47, p = .01$).

Qualitative results revealed that pride was mentioned most in relation to group functioning. All six interviewees confirmed that they experienced feelings of pride during the problem-solving session, and that their feelings of pride were in relation to appraisals associated with compatible group functioning: "I was proud when, umm…, when, when, when we were…, when [we] finished it, I was proud that we were able to finish it, and that we were able to do the math together and not like argue like this and that and this and that." (*Interviewee 1*).

Additionally, students expressed instances of pride in reference to successful group accomplishments, and the collaborative completion of the problem: "Well, as I said, I felt proud when we finished the problem because it looked really hard and we actually managed to finish it. And we were the first ones to finish." (*Interviewee 2*). "...we started to get the same answers, and we were pride, we were proud of the answers.", "Well, [I] was proud of everybody..." (*Interviewee 3*). Two of the six students expressed positive emotions, namely enjoyment, in relation to their belief that their group was capable of solving the problem: "I knew we were going to solve it." (*Interviewee 1*). "I knew we could do it." (*Interviewee 2*).

Negative social emotions were cited as negatively impacting appraisals of relatedness and overall communication and in turn, CoRL processes. Four out of the six interviewees mentioned that experiences of frustration and anxiety occurred in relation to either perceptions of task difficulty, or when communications broke down amongst group members. When asked to provide an example of when interviewee 4 felt frustrated, the student responded:

> Uhh... probably when we were doing the task 'cause what we decided to do was we each take one item that the family bought, and we add that and add that together so sometimes we were a bit panicking because we didn't know what the total was for one ice cream so we could add it.

RQ 2. What are the relations between social emotions and learning processes across the two functions and four phases of regulation of learning during complex mathematics problem solving in a collaborative context?

Results revealed that overall global positive social emotions did not predict either of the CoRL functions across the four phases of learning regulation. However, empathy positively predicted the facilitative-confirmation function during the task definition ($\beta = .33$, $p = .09$), and monitoring and evaluation phases of learning ($\beta = .41$, $p = .03$). Global negative social emotions positively predicted the inhibition-change function of CoRL during the planning and goal setting phase of learning regulation ($\beta = .38$, $p = .05$). Specifically, reported feelings of guilt and jealousy positively predicted the inhibition-change function of CoRL during the planning and goal setting phase ($\beta = .49$, $p = .02$ and $\beta = .34$, $p = .07$, respectively). Moreover, frustration and anxiety negatively predicted the facilitation-activation function during the monitoring and evaluation phase ($\beta = -.41$, $p = .03$ and $\beta = -.48$, $p = .01$, respectively). Frustration and anxiety also negatively predicted the facilitation-confirmation function during the enactment phase ($\beta = -.42$, $p = .03$ and $\beta = -.37$, $p = .06$, respectively). Lastly, boredom negatively predicted the inhibition-change function during the monitoring and evaluation phase ($\beta = -.42$, $p = .05$).

Qualitative analysis revealed that interviewees expressed that emotions influenced group relations and subsequently group communication and collaboration:

> It was a little bit like stressful because, um, we didn't all understand and then we got into this like, feeling like, to not talk to each other and then we would just work like independently and because we had, weren't sure what to do and we were mad at each other…'cause well we were stressed out so we didn't really communicate as much as we did in the beginning so, yeah. (*Interviewee 6*).

RQ 3. Do learning processes experienced within the collaborative setting correlate to achievement in mathematics problem solving?

Results from path analysis revealed that the inhibition-slow function during the planning and goal setting phase positively predicted achievement ($\beta = .32, p = .03$). Additionally, facilitation-activation and inhibition-slow functions at the monitoring and evaluation phases positively predicted achievement on the complex problem ($\beta = .61, p < .01$ and $\beta = .38, p = .01$, respectively).

RQ 4. Do social emotions mediate the relationship between task value, control, and BPN, and the functions of CoRL and achievement?

A mediation analysis was conducted to investigate whether global social positive emotions (i.e., empathy and pride) and global social negative emotions (i.e., envy, jealousy, shame, embarrassment and guilt) mediated the relationship between control, value, basic psychological needs (i.e., competence, autonomy, and relatedness) and the two functions of CoRL at all four phases of learning regulation and achievement. Results indicated that social emotions did not mediate the relationship between antecedents and achievement. However, global positive social emotions ($B = 2.70$, 90% CI $= -.70$ to -8.43), and global negative social emotions ($B = 1.63$, 90% CI $= -2.87$ to -2.34) fully mediated the relationship between relatedness and CoRL. Specifically, relatedness was no longer a significant predictor of CoRL after controlling for the mediators of positive and negative social emotions, consistent with full mediation analysis.

6.4 Discussion

The aim of the study was to investigate the antecedents of social emotions (i.e., control, value, and the three dimensions of basic psychological needs), and whether social emotions predicted the functions of CoRL across the two functions and four phases of learning regulation. Consequently, we explored whether specific CoRL processes related to achievement on the complex problem. Lastly, we examined whether emotions mediated relations between the antecedents, and learning processes inherent in CoRL. We discuss these results as a function of each research question followed by theoretical and educational implications.

6.4.1 Control, Value and Basic Psychological Needs as Antecedents of Social Emotions

The first research question addressed whether higher perceptions of control, value, and the three dimensions of basic psychological needs (i.e., competence, autonomy, and relatedness) positively predicted students' positive social emotions, and negatively predicted negative social emotions. The findings presented help support Pekrun's (2006) control-value theory and extend the implications of perceptions of control beyond achievement emotions to social emotions. Pertaining to the study's focus on social emotions, the findings echo Muis et al. (2015b) results that perceptions of control and value serve as important antecedents to the kinds of epistemic and activity emotions students experienced during mathematics problem solving. Specifically, higher perceptions of control over the learning task, and value for what is being learned, related to lower reports of experienced boredom in relation to the group problem solving task. In this way, control and value served as important buffers against disengagement, or avoidance motivation (i.e., trying to flee a given situation) (Pekrun et al. 2014).

As well, students' reported feelings of control over learning, and the outcome of learning, were negatively associated with feelings of jealousy within the collaborative setting. Jealousy is an emotion thought to be experienced by an individual when they conclude a gap between a social comparison and their self-perception (Salovey and Rodin 1984). Social comparisons have been found to take place during instances of self-doubt, and with the hopes of reaffirming or boosting one's sense of competence. It follows then, that when individuals hold high self-perceptions of competence [a control-related appraisal (Frenzel et al. 2007)], there is little practice of social comparisons that could result in feelings of jealousy, thus corroborating the finding in this study.

Outcomes of this research also demonstrate that social emotions are preceded by specific social appraisals above and beyond control and task value. Consequently, these appraisals were shown to affect the kinds of regulatory processes that group members used while engaged in a collaborative learning situation. Pekrun (2006) explained that the influence of emotions associated with functioning within a social setting is mediated by control and value appraisals. However, as demonstrated by the findings of this study, the impact on affect as a result of the social environment is also related to social appraisals, such as the degree to which an individual feels competent, autonomous, and related to, within the social context. Findings from this study demonstrate that feelings of relatedness correlated with positive and negative global social emotions. This is in line with theoretical suppositions by Leary (2001), who explained that in a social context, positive social emotions arise when people experience feelings of being valued in relation to a social situation. Additionally, negative social emotions arise as a consequence of *relational devaluation*, or when an individual perceives that a social relationship with another is not important, of value, or close.

Consistent with research by Hareli and Weiner (2002), who found that hopelessness is the result of a learner's perception of low ability, our findings demonstrated that reports of competency and autonomy negatively related to feelings of hopelessness and confusion. That is, when the collaborative context contributed to an individual's perception of personal ability and increased feelings of self-governance in relation to the learning activity, the less the individual experienced hopelessness. The same relationship was also found between competency and autonomy in relation to confusion. Confusion, according to D'Mello and Graesser (2014), is the result of a learner's inability to resolve cognitive incongruity, with the resolution of confusion requiring strategic regulation on the part of the learner. As previously mentioned, satisfaction of the dimensions of BPN relates to the quality of motivation, and consequentially, motivation is found to directly impact the goals and outcomes, and the regulatory processes involved in pursuing those goals and outcomes. It may then be the case that the satisfaction of the two dimensions of BPN, as seen in this study, provides group members with the motivation, and in turn, the appropriate regulatory processes required to resolve the cognitive impasses, and refocus on the goal of the activity.

Interestingly, with regards to this study, all three dimensions of BPN were found to positively predict pride. Additionally, interview analysis corroborates these findings in that students' perceptions of competency, autonomy, and relatedness were reported to positively relate to feelings of pride during the problem-solving session. Fischer and Tangney (1995) describe pride as being an emotion that is experienced in relation to the evaluations made by others and/or social standards. Hareli and Weiner (2002) consider that peers express pride for others when an individual experiences success because of high ability and/or experiences success due to high effort. In addition, the experience of pride is an ego enhancement in that an individual seeks to maintain pride by either showcasing effort/ability and/or attempting to sustain feelings of worth (Ryan and Deci 2000). Although analysis of the object focus of the experience of pride (i.e., pride towards an individual, or pride towards oneself) was beyond the scope of this study, theoretically, experiencing pride in relation to feeling that the self or other group member are able, in charge, and valued within a group context is supported by the results of this study.

6.4.2 Relations Between Social Emotions and Learning Processes

The second research question addressed relations between social emotions and learning processes across the two functions and four phases of regulation of learning during complex mathematics problem solving in a collaborative context. In relation to CoRL, Furrer and Skinner (2003) found that students may experience enthusiasm when working with peers who they like, and who, in turn, express a like for them. This resulting positive affect may spur interest and motivation to learn and persevere but may also lead to lengthier episodes of high-level collaborative functioning (Volet et al. 2009). Additionally, feelings of relatedness within a social context are hypothesized to be a potential buffer for negative emotions (Furrer and Skinner 2003). Pekrun (2006) also explained that feedback from the social environment serves to provide the learner with information that in turn shapes their appraisals of control and task value, both of which influence emotions and in turn learning regulation and achievement.

In the present study, we found that empathy positively predicted the facilitative-confirmation function of CoRL at the monitoring and evaluation phase of learning regulation. Essentially, when one student understands another individual's feelings, the more likely students are to engage in more instances of confirming and reviewing the appropriateness of the goals, plans, and strategies that they collaboratively decided upon. A reason for this occurrence may be due to the desire of group members to alleviate the negative individual feelings (e.g., confusion) of a fellow group member by confirming that the plan or strategy employed to solve a section of the problem was indeed effective. Another reason for this occurrence may lie in the relationship between positive social emotions and instances of *high-level collaborative processes,* which are a kind of deep level processing in the collaborative context where group members share inferences, justifications, elaborations, thought-provoking inquiry, and point out relationships, which all serve to contribute to the co-construction of knowledge (Volet et al. 2009).

Conversely, *low-level collaborative processes* are shallower in nature and involve practices such as sharing information, reciting definitions, exchanges of ideas, and understanding without the occurrence of transformation of the information at hand (Volet et al. 2009). Volet et al. (2009) explained that the maintenance of high-level collaborative processes, which are processes akin to what group members experienced during the facilitative-confirmation function of CoRL during the monitoring and evaluation phase, may be in part sustained due to the experiencing of positive social emotions, like empathy.

Global negative social emotions positively correlated with inhibition-change functions of CoRL specifically during the planning and goal setting phase. Taken together, when feelings of shame, jealousy, embarrassment, guilt, and/or envy were experienced in the group context, the co-regulation that occurred was defined by greater instances of changing the goals of the problem and/or plan to solve the problem. Muis (2007) explains that phases can be reciprocal in nature and therefore, as it pertains specifically to the second and third phase of learning regulation, changes in enactment could call for changes in the kinds of goals or plans decided upon and vice versa.

Therefore, greater instances of negative social emotions experienced by group members are associated with an increase in changing the plans and goals while solving the mathematics problem.

In relation to discrete emotions, guilt and jealousy positively correlated with the inhibition-change function of CoRL during the planning and goal setting phase. Thus, it appears that reported experiences of guilt and jealousy are contributors of the negative social emotions that relate to higher instances of the inhibition-change function of CoRL during the second phase of learning regulation. Hareli and Weiner (2002) explain that guilt occurs when an individual recognizes that an *other* in the social group performs an admirable behavior that was not, but could have been performed by the individual themselves. As well, feelings of guilt stimulate behavior that serves to make up for the wrongdoing (see Weiner 1985). As previously mentioned, jealousy occurs when an individual determines a gap between a social comparison and their self-perception (Salovey and Rodin 1984). Social comparisons occur during moments of self-doubt with the intention of reaffirming one's sense of competence (Salovey and Rodin 1984). From these definitions, it can be concluded that both emotions are initiated by episodes of social comparison. Theoretically, it follows then, that the increased and overt changing of plans and strategies could in part be due to individuals noticing a gap between potential for their own demonstration of understanding, and/or needing to reaffirm a sense of competence by attempting to close the gap between self-doubt and the social comparison.

In the social context, reported feelings of frustration and anxiety were associated with lower instances of facilitating the activation of metacognitive monitoring and evaluation (i.e., the initiation of reflection or evaluation of the effectiveness of cognitive strategies). Additionally, frustration negatively correlated with the facilitation-confirmation function during the enactment phase, meaning that when group members experienced frustration, the less likely they were to confirm that the strategies they were using were appropriate. Interview analysis confirms this finding that frustration negatively related to effective group communication, specifically, the group's ability to facilitate the confirmation of strategy enactment and facilitate the activation of monitoring and evaluation (e.g., "...frustration and then I got tired, so I just left the answer as it was."—*Interviewee 5).*

According to Pekrun (2006) both frustration and anxiety result in the use of shallow cognitive strategies. Additionally, Pekrun and Perry (2014) explain that anxiety, in particular, carries the consequence of task-irrelevant thinking, which in turn, undermines cognitive resources required for the task at hand. It may be the case that these emotions experienced in a collaborative context serve to distract group members from the task and undermine intrinsic motivation to complete the task successfully, and instead boost extrinsic motivation to escape the learning situation (Pekrun et al. 2011).

Lastly, boredom negatively correlated with the inhibition-change function during the monitoring and evaluation phase. It appears that boredom experienced in the collaborative context decreases instances of metacognitive processes embedded in the fourth phase of learning regulation. Interestingly, this lack of metacognitive monitoring occurs specifically when in the inhibition-change function of CoRL. Inhibitory functions (i.e., slow and change) are mainly used by group members to control for inappropriate conceptualizations of the problem and offer possible alternatives to the problem representation. Therefore, boredom appears to be negatively associated with the metacognitive event of group members slowing or changing group function in order to rectify an individual's incorrect conceptualizations of the problem. A possible reason for this is that boredom is a negative deactivating emotion that negatively affects the learner(s) motivation to solve the problem and leads to the occurrence of shallow or superficial strategy use (Pekrun 2006), and may, in CoRL terms, lead to low-level collaborative processes.

6.4.3 Learning Processes and Achievement

The third research question addressed whether learning processes experienced within the collaborative setting predict achievement in mathematics problem solving. Muis et al. (2015b) found that both shallow and deep cognitive and metacognitive processes predicted achievement on a complex mathematics problem. Findings from this study demonstrated that the use of collaborative metacognitive processes involved in monitoring and evaluating cognitive strategies positively related to achievement outcomes on the complex problem. Therefore, results from this research study, at the CoRL level of learning regulation, corroborate findings by Muis et al. (2015b).

Specifically, we found a positive correlation between instances of inhibition-slow functions of CoRL during the planning and goal setting, and monitoring and evaluation phase of learning regulation, and achievement on the mathematics problem. Additionally, there was a positive correlation between instances of facilitative-activation functions of CoRL during the monitoring and evaluation phase of learning regulation and achievement outcomes on the complex problem. The function of the inhibition-slow CoRL process is to decelerate the continuance of the previous direction's thought or action, whereas the function of facilitative-activation is to initiate action in accordance with the previous direction. It is possible that this slowing down of collective thought or action, and the activation of the metacognitive practice of monitoring and evaluation could be considered a *high-level collaborative process* particularly if the reason for the deceleration or activation was due to questioning. The act of questioning is high-level in that it requires other members to display understanding rather than rehearse facts and information (Volet et al. 2009). Considering that high-level collaborative processes are analogous to metacognitive strategies in self-regulated learning, this is consistent with the typical finding that the more students engage in these processes, the higher their achievement (Volet et al. 2009). It is important to note that analyzing the CoRL functions for instances of questioning was beyond the scope of this study but would nonetheless be a fruitful line of inquiry.

6.4.4 Emotions as Mediators Between Control, Value and BPN, and Episodes of CoRL and Achievement

The final research question addressed whether social emotions mediate the relationship between task value, control, and BPN, and the functions of CoRL and achievement. Other studies have considered the role that social emotions may play in the regulation of learning (Muis et al. 2015b; Volet et al. 2009), but this study is the first of its kind to empirically test these suppositions. Results partially supported the hypothesis that emotions serve as a mediator between perceptions of control, task value, and BPN, and episodes of CoRL.

Internalization, or the "...process in which individuals attempt to transform socially sanctioned mores or requests into personally endorsed values and self-regulations" (Deci and Ryan 2000, pp. 235–236) is best facilitated through feelings of relatedness (Niemiec and Ryan 2009). Additionally, an individual is more likely to internalize the practices and values of those with whom they feel, or want to feel connected to, or within contexts where they experience a sense of belonging (Niemiec and Ryan 2009). Niemiec and Ryan (2009) further explain that the promotion of feelings of relatedness within the classroom environment aid specifically in the internalization of motivation to learn, regulation for the tasks required for learning to take place and increase self-governed behavior in relation to what they are learning. Results from this study revealed that positive and negative social emotions mediated the relationship between feelings of relatedness and total instances of CoRL across the two functions and all four phases of learning regulation. That is, relatedness, the degree to which one feels that they belong and are connected to others (Ryan and Deci 2000), above all other antecedents, predicted the use of facilitative and inhibitory co-regulatory processes across all four phases of learning regulation that the students engaged in as mediated by social emotions.

In our study, discrete emotions were the consequence of the appraisals relating to perceptions of competency, autonomy, and relatedness (in addition to appraisals of control and value). In turn, various emotions were correlated to specific CoRL functions and phases. Through mediation analysis, relatedness predicting CoRL processes is mediated, or explained by, the emotions experienced within the social context. Kreijns et al. (2003) who warns that the occurrence of social interaction should not be taken for granted, put forth that socially setting the stage is required for CoRL, but not enough to ensure that it happens. Findings from this study serve to partially support the aforementioned theorization, that is, relatedness on its own was not found to be a significant predictor of the use of CoRL processes. Therefore, feeling like a valued member within the group does not on its own predict the use of CoRL.

Lastly, perceptions of relatedness came up throughout the research study as being an influential consequence of, and having a rather influential effect on, the other variables analyzed. Contrary to theorizations made by Deci and Ryan (2000), who describe relatedness as being a more distal contributor to motivation as when compared to competency and autonomy, the findings presented in this study show that relatedness as an antecedent was found to share the most relationships with emotions, and was the only antecedent to have an effect in the mediation analysis. Therefore, although SDT theorizes that relatedness may be a background player in the maintenance of motivation, considering the findings presented, future studies that delve into collaborative learning and/or social emotions would be wise to consider the potential role played by feelings of relatedness.

6.4.5 Educational Implications

Findings from this study demonstrated that, in a collaborative learning context, educators need to be aware of two things when assigning an appropriately demanding task to a group. (a) Group member ability should be at the same level so that the task demands are appropriate for all members, *or* (b) should the group be of mixed ability, and task demands are appropriate for a high-to medium-ability learner with the intention that they will be able to successfully scaffold the lower-ability learner (s), and the lower-ability learner(s) will be active and receptive to the scaffolding/ assistance. Both contexts require that there has been enough performance information acquired to properly and appropriately formulate groups. That said, it is recommended that small group collaborative work should be low-stakes and short in duration for the first few weeks of school, until enough information about student ability and personality has been collected, so groups can be formulated with appropriate consideration. In both instances, but perhaps more imperative for the second context, explicit instruction of sufficient modelling and practice of scaffolding techniques by the students themselves should be conducted in a variety of collaborative learning contexts.

Considering the aforementioned, it is important that for students to appropriately engage in learning regulation, they need to know what SRL and CoRL look like behaviorally, and concretely. Järvelä and Hadwin (2013) explained that collaborative success based on collaborative experiences shape the kinds of regulation in which students engage. Zimmerman and Labuhn (2012) discuss that modeling learning regulation plays an important role in that it influences students' development of learning strategies. Additionally, strategies used to overcome instances of confusion have been shown that they can be successfully modeled and taught (MacArthur 2011). It is therefore suggested that teachers communicate to their students explicit SRL and CoRL protocols, and conduct SRL and CoRL protocol training. Clear training of this sort aimed at helping students remedy issues concerning obstructions, uncertainty, and conflict in learning would assist students in eventually being able to independently mediate collaborative roadblocks. Additionally, educators should not hesitate to be transparent and share with students the actual phases involved in learning regulation (i.e., task definition, planning and goal setting, enactment, and monitoring and evaluation) and explain how the model works.

6.5 Conclusion

In conclusion, our study offers an intriguing glimpse into relations that social emotions have with learning processes and achievement. The implications garnered from the results offer multiple suggestions for extending exploration in this field that have the possibility of leading to insightful future study. Kreijns et al. (2013) hazard against educators falling prey to the pedagogic falsehood, "*if you build it, they will come*", which implies that because an individual is simply involved in a collaborative task, they will socially interact, and CoRL will occur. It is our hope that the conclusions drawn from this research thwart the haphazard implementation of collaborative educational practices and, instead, inspire thoughtful pedagogical design that is affectively supportive, socially positive, and has the student's well-being residing at its heart.

Acknowledgments A portion of this chapter is from Cara A. Singh's MA thesis. Funding for this research was provided by a grant to Krista R. Muis from the Social Sciences and Humanities Research Council of Canada (grant # 435-2014-0155) and from the Canada Research Chairs program. We also wish to thank the administration, teachers and students for their participation in this research study.

References

Ahmed, W., Minnaert, A., van der Werf, G., & Kuyper, H. (2010). Perceived social support and early adolescents' achievement: The mediational roles of motivational beliefs and emotions. *Journal of Youth and Adolescence, 39*, 36–46.

Corno, L., & Mandinach, E. B. (2004). What we have learned about student engagement in the past twenty years. In D. Mclnerney& & S. Van Etten (Eds.), *Big theories revisited* (pp. 299–328). Greenwich: Information Publishing Age.

Cummins, D. D., Kintsch, W., Reusser, K., & Weimer, R. (1988). The role of understanding in solving word problems. *Cognitive Psychology, 20*, 405–438.

D'Mello, S. K., & Graesser, A. C. (2014). Confusion. In R. Pekrun & L. Linnenbrink-Garcia (Eds.), *International handbook of emotions in education* (pp. 289–310). New York: Routledge.

De Dreu, C. K., & Weingart, L. R. (2003). Task versus relationship conflict, team performance, and team member satisfaction: A meta-analysis. *The Journal of Applied Psychology, 88*, 741–749.

Deci, E. L., & Ryan, R. M. (2000). The "what" and "why" of goal pursuits: Human needs and the self-determination of behavior. *Psychological Inquiry, 11*, 227–268.

Deci, E. L., & Ryan, R. M. (2010). Self-determination. In I. B. Weiner & W. E. Craighead (Eds.), *The Corsini encyclopedia of psychology* (pp. 1–2). Hoboken, NJ: Wiley.

Eccles, J., Wigfield, A., Harold, R. D., & Blumenfeld, P. (1993). Age and gender differences in children's self-and task perceptions during elementary school. *Child Development, 64*, 830–847.

Efklides, A. (2011). Interactions of metacognition with motivation and affect in self-regulated learning: The MASRL model. *Educational Psychologist, 46*, 6–25.

Efklides, A., Schwartz, B. L., & Brown, V. (2018). Motivation and affect in self-regulated learning: Does metacognition play a role? In D. H. Schunk & J. A. Greene (Eds.), *Self-regulated learning and performance* (pp. 64–82). New York: Routledge.

Ericsson, K. A., & Simon, H. A. (1998). How to study thinking in everyday life: Contrasting think-aloud protocols with descriptions and explanations of thinking. *Mind, Culture, and Activity, 5*, 178–186.

Fischer, K. W., & Tangney, J. P. (1995). Self-conscious emotions and the affect revolution: Framework and overview. In J. P. Tangney & K. W. Fischer (Eds.), *Self-conscious emotions: The psychology of shame, guilt, embarrassment, and pride* (pp. 3–22). New York: Guilford.

Frenzel, A. C., & Stephens, E. J. (2013). Emotions. In N. C. Hall & T. Goetz (Eds.), *Emotion, motivation, and self-regulation: A handbook for teachers* (pp. 1–56). Bingley: Emerald.

Frenzel, A. C., Pekrun, R., & Goetz, T. (2007). Girls and mathematics—A "hopeless" issue? A control-value approach to gender differences in emotions towards mathematics. *European Journal of Psychology of Education, 22*, 497–514.
Furrer, C., & Skinner, E. (2003). Sense of relatedness as a factor in children's academic engagement and performance. *Journal of Educational Psychology, 95*, 148–162.
Hadwin, A., & Oshige, M. (2011). Self-regulation, co-regulation, and socially shared regulation: Exploring perspectives of social in self-regulated learning theory. *Teachers College Record, 113*, 240–264.
Hadwin, A. F., Wozney, L., & Pontin, O. (2005). Scaffolding the appropriation of self-regulatory activity: A socio-cultural analysis of changes in teacher–student discourse about a graduate research portfolio. *Instructional Science, 33*, 413–450.
Hadwin, A. F., Järvelä, S., & Miller, M. (2011). Self-regulated, co-regulated, and socially shared regulation of learning. In B. J. Zimmerman & D. H. Schunk (Eds.), *Handbook of self-regulation of learning and performance* (pp. 65–84). New York: Routledge.
Hadwin, A., Järvelä, S., & Miller, M. (2018). Self-regulation, co-regulation, and shared regulation in collaborative learning environments. In D. H. Schunk & J. A. Greene (Eds.), *Self-regulated learning and performance* (pp. 83–106). New York: Routledge.
Hareli, S., & Parkinson, B. (2008). What's social about social emotions? *Journal for the Theory of Social Behaviour, 38*, 131–156.
Hareli, S., & Weiner, B. (2002). Social emotions and personality inferences: A scaffold for a new direction in the study of achievement motivation. *Educational Psychologist, 37*, 183–193.
Hayes, A. F., & Preacher, K. J. (2013). Conditional process modeling: Using structural equation modeling to examine contingent causal processes. In G. R. Hancock & R. O. Mueller (Eds.), *Quantitative methods in education and the behavioral sciences: Issues, research, and teaching. Structural equation modeling: A second course* (pp. 219–266). Charlotte: IAP Information Age Publishing.
Iiskala, T., Vauras, M., Lehtinen, E., & Salonen, P. (2011). Socially shared metacognition of dyads of pupils in collaborative mathematical problem-solving processes. *Learning and Instruction, 21*, 379–393.
Immordino-Yang, M. H., McColl, A., Damasio, H., & Damasio, A. (2009). Neural correlates of admiration and compassion. *Proceedings of the National Academy of Sciences of the United States of America, 106*, 8021–8026.
Isen, A. M. (1987). Positive affect, cognitive processes, and social behavior. *Advances in Experimental Social Psychology, 20*, 203–253.
Järvelä, S., & Hadwin, A. F. (2013). New Frontiers: Regulating learning in CSCL. *Educational Psychologist, 48*, 25–39.
Järvelä, S., Lehtinen, E., & Salonen, P. (2000). Socio-emotional orientation as a mediating variable in the teaching–learning interaction: Implications for instructional design. *Scandinavian Journal of Educational Research, 44*, 293–306.
Jones, A., & Isroff, K. (2005). Learning technologies: Affective and social issues in computer-supported collaborative learning. *Computers and Education, 44*, 395–408.
Kreijns, K., Kirschner, P. A., & Jochems, W. (2003). Identifying the pitfalls for social interaction in computer-supported collaborative learning environments: A review of the research. *Computers in Human Behavior, 19*, 335–353.
Kreijns, K., Kirschner, P. A., & Veremeulen, M. (2013). Social aspects of CSCL environments: A research framework. *Educational Psychologist, 48*, 229–242.
Kuusela, H., & Pallab, P. (2000). A comparison of concurrent and retrospective verbal protocol analysis. *The American Journal of Psychology, 113*, 387–404.
La Guardia, J. G., Ryan, R. M., Couchman, C. E., & Deci, E. L. (2000). Within-person variation in security of attachment: A self-determination theory perspective on attachment, need fulfillment, and well-being. *Journal of Personality and Social Psychology, 79*, 367–384.

Leary, M. R. (2001). Affect, cognition, and the social emotions. In J. P. Forgas (Ed.), *Feeling and thinking: The role of affect in social cognition* (pp. 331–355). Cambridge: Cambridge University Press.

Lee, L., Lajoie, S. P., Poitras, E. G., Nkangu, M., & Doleck, T. (2016). Co-regulation and knowledge construction in an online synchronous problem based learning setting. *Education and Information Technologies, 1*, 1–28.

MacArthur, C. A. (2011). Strategies instruction. In K. R. Harris, S. Graham, & T. Urdan (Eds.), *Educational psychology handbook* (pp. 379–402). Washington: American Psychological Association.

Miserandino, M. (1996). Children who do well in school: Individual differences in perceived competence and autonomy in above-average children. *Journal of Educational Psychology, 88*, 203–214.

Muis, K. R. (2007). The role of epistemic beliefs in self-regulated learning. *Educational Psychologist, 42*, 173–190.

Muis, K. R., Pekrun, R., Sinatra, G. M., Azevedo, R., Trevors, G., Meier, E., & Heddy, B. C. (2015a). The curious case of climate change: Testing a theoretical model of epistemic beliefs, epistemic emotions, and complex learning. *Learning and Instruction, 39*, 168–183.

Muis, K. R., Psaradellis, C., Lajoie, S. P., Di Leo, I., & Chevrier, M. (2015b). The role of epistemic emotions in mathematics problem solving. *Contemporary Educational Psychology, 42*, 172–185.

Muis, K. R., Chevrier, M., & Singh, C. A. (2018). The role of epistemic emotions in personal epistemology and self-regulated learning. *Educational Psychologist, 53*, 165–184.

Niemiec, C. P., & Ryan, R. M. (2009). Autonomy, competence, and relatedness in the classroom: Applying self-determination theory to educational practice. *Theory and Research in Education, 7*, 133–144.

Pekrun, R. (2006). The control-value theory of achievement emotions: Assumptions, corollaries, and implications for educational research and practice. *Educational Psychology Review, 18*, 315–341.

Pekrun, R., & Linnenbrink-Garcia, L. (2014). Introduction to emotions in education. In R. Pekrun & L. Linnenbrink-Garcia (Eds.), *International handbook of emotions in education* (pp. 11–20). New York: Routledge.

Pekrun, R., & Meier, E. (2011). *Epistemic emotion scales (EES)*. Unpublished manuscript. Department of Psychology, University of Munich, Munich, Germany.

Pekrun, R., & Perry, R. P. (2014). Control-value theory of achievement emotions. In R. Pekrun & L. Linnenbrink-Garcia (Eds.), *International handbook of emotions in education* (pp. 120–141). New York: Routledge.

Pekrun, R., & Stephens, E. J. (2012). Academic emotions. In K. Harris, S. Graham, T. Urdan, S. Graham, J. Royer, & M. Zeidner (Eds.), *Individual differences and cultural and contextual factors. APA educational psychology handbook* (pp. 3–31). Washington: American Psychological Association.

Pekrun, R., Goetz, T., Titz, W., & Perry, R. P. (2002). Academic emotions in students' self-regulated learning and achievement: A program of qualitative and quantitative research. *Educational Psychologist, 37*, 91–105.

Pekrun, R., Goetz, T., Frenzel, A. C., Barchfeld, P., & Perry, R. P. (2011). Measuring emotions in students' learning and performance: The achievement emotions questionnaire (AEQ). *Contemporary Educational Psychology, 36*, 36–48.

Pekrun, R., Hall, N. C., Goetz, T., & Perry, R. P. (2014). Boredom and academic achievement: Testing a model of reciprocal causation. *Journal of Educational Psychology, 106*, 696–710.

Pekrun, R., Vogl, E., Muis, K. R., & Sinatra, G. M. (2016). Measuring emotions during epistemic activities: The epistemically-related emotion scales. *Cognition and Emotion, 31*, 1268–1276.

Perry, R. P., Hladkyj, S., Pekrun, R. H., & Pelletier, S. T. (2001). Academic control and action control in the achievement of college students: A longitudinal field study. *Journal of Educational Psychology, 93*, 776–789.

Puustinen, M., & Pulkkinen, L. (2001). Models of self-regulated learning: Review. *Scandinavian Journal of Educational Research, 45*, 269–286.

Ryan, R. M., & Connell, J. P. (1989). Perceived locus of causality and internalization: Examining reasons for acting in two domains. *Journal of Personality and Social Psychology, 57*, 749–761.

Ryan, R. M., & Deci, E. L. (2000). Self-determination theory and the facilitation of intrinsic motivation, social development, and well-being. *American Psychologist, 55*, 68–78.

Salovey, P., & Rodin, J. (1984). Some antecedents and consequences of social-comparison jealousy. *Journal of Personality and Social Psychology, 47*, 780–792.

Schunk, D. H. (1998). Teaching elementary students to self-regulate practice of mathematical skills with modeling. In D. H. Schunk & B. J. Zimmerman (Eds.), *Self-regulated learning: From teaching to self-reflective practice* (pp. 137–159). New York: Guilford Publications.

Slavin, R. E. (2015). Cooperative learning in elementary schools. *Education 3-13: International Journal of Primary, Elementary and Early Years Education, 43*, 5–14.

Vlachopoulos, S. P., & Michailidou, S. (2006). Development and initial validation of a measure of autonomy, competence, and relatedness in exercise: The basic psychological needs in exercise scale. *Measurement in Physical Education and Exercise Science, 10*, 179–201.

Volet, S., Summers, M., & Thurman, J. (2009). High-level co-regulation in collaborative learning: How does it emerge and how is it sustained? *Learning and Instruction, 19*, 128–143.

Weiner, B. (1985). An attributional theory of achievement motivation and emotion. *Psychological Review, 92*, 548–573.

Winne, P. H. (1989). Theories of instruction and of intelligence for designing artificially intelligent tutoring systems. *Educational Psychologist, 24*, 229–259.

Winne, P. H. (1997). Experimenting to bootstrap self-regulated learning. *Journal of Educational Psychology, 89*, 397–410.

Winne, P. H. (2018). Cognition and metacognition within self-regulated learning. In D. Schunk & J. A. Greene (Eds.), *Self-regulated learning and performance* (pp. 52–63). New York: Routledge.

Winne, P. H., Jamieson-Noel, D., & Muis, K. (2002). Methodological issues and advances in researching tactics, strategies, and self-regulated learning. *Advances in Motivation and Achievement: New Directions in Measures and Methods, 12*, 121–155.

Zeidner, M. (1998). *Test anxiety: The state of the art.* New York: Plenum Press.

Zimmerman, B. J. (1989). A social cognitive view of self-regulated academic learning. *Journal of Educational Psychology, 81*, 329–339.

Zimmerman, B. J., & Labuhn, A. S. (2012). Self-regulation of learning: Process approaches to personal development. In K. R. Harris, S. Graham, T. Urdan, C. B. McCormick, G. M. Sinatra, & J. Sweller (Eds.), *APA educational psychology handbook, Vol. 1. Theories, constructs, and critical issues* (pp. 399–425). Washington: American Psychological Association.

Chapter 7
Metacognition and Meta-emotion in Kindergarten: Is the Combination Necessary for Self-Regulation in Mathematical Problem Solving?

Bracha Kramarski, Meirav Tzohar-Rozen, and Zohar Gadasi

Abstract This study among kindergarten children ($n = 90$) investigated the necessity of combined self-regulated learning (SRL) programs relating to metacognition and meta-emotional support (MES) embedded in the "Interactive Storytelling" problem-solving environment, for enhancing SRL and mathematical problem solving at different levels of complexity. The MES program was compared to a single metacognitive support (MS) and a control group without SRL. Findings showed that the combined MES group approach induced the greatest change in the amount of metacognitive and emotional verbal regulation, while thinking aloud mathematical problems, as well as, success in routine and complex mathematical problems, both immediately and in lasting effect (2 months after). Whereas the control group didn't show any increased use of SRL and problem solving. Implications are discussed.

Keywords Metacognition and meta-emotion · Self-regulation · Math problem solving · Interactive storytelling · Kindergarten

7.1 Introduction

Mathematics is an inseparable part of daily life from childhood. Therefore, it is very important to develop mathematical knowledge and skills already at an early age (Organization for Economic Cooperation and Development [OECD] 2000). One of the most important challenges in the mathematics field is solving verbal problems

---

B. Kramarski (✉)
School of Education, Bar Ilan University, Ramat Gan, Israel
e-mail: Bracha.Kramarski@biu.ac.il

M. Tzohar-Rozen
Levinsky College of Education, Tel Aviv-Yafo, Israel

Z. Gadasi
Shanan College, Bar Ilan University, Ramat Gan, Israel

D. Moraitou, P. Metallidou (eds.), *Trends and Prospects in Metacognition Research across the Life Span*, https://doi.org/10.1007/978-3-030-51673-4_7

(National Council of Teachers of Mathematics [NCTM] 2000), which constitute a significant component of the mathematics curriculum both in kindergarten and primary school. Cultivating the ability to solve verbal mathematical problems is critical, since these problems focus on the link of mathematics to daily situations. However, research has shown that verbal mathematical problems are very demanding for children, because they require both cognitive knowledge (e.g., facts and processes) and metacognitive awareness about task requirements, strategy, adaptation, and performance evaluation. This complexity often leads to negative experiences and emotions (e.g., avoidance, fear) when solving such problems (NCTM 2000; Schoenfeld 1992).

One way to help children to cope with metacognitive and emotional experiences in solving verbal problems is to support self-regulated learning (SRL). SRL focuses on cognition, metacognition and affect referencing to motivation and emotional aspects of learning (Efklides 2011). SRL is defined as a process in which learners are responsible for their own learning, using their individual thoughts, feelings, and actions to achieve their personal goals (Zimmerman 2008). To date, most SRL intervention programs focused on school children and have mainly addressed the metacognitive component (Mevarech and Kramarski 2014; Pintrich 2000), whereas the affective emotional aspect remained neglected (Gidalevich and Kramarski 2017). Thus, we still do not know the added value of combined meta-level awareness support directed simultaneously to metacognition and meta-emotion, particularly for young kindergarten children. The current study aimed to fill this gap.

7.1.1 Self-regulated Learning-SRL

SRL is critical for productive engagement with real-life situations (OECD 2012; Zimmerman 2008). SRL involves cognition and its regulation, using metacognitive and affective aspects (motivation and emotions) of the learning context, so that it facilitates engagement with learning (Pintrich 2000). Cognition is the process involved in knowing, that includes strategies to encode or/and recall information and solution processing (Schraw et al. 2006). Metacognition is a second-order process, namely "thinking about thinking", that enables learners to understand and monitor their cognitive processes (Flavell 1976). Metacognition involves three aspects: knowledge of cognition, experiences as judgements and feelings about cognitive processing, and regulation of cognition (Pintrich 2000). Knowledge of cognition is comprised of declarative knowledge about strategy/task (what?), procedural knowledge used in various cognitive strategies (how?), and conditional knowledge (when? and why?) that is important for the flexible and adaptive use of various cognitive strategies (Schraw 1998). Compared to the static nature of the metacognitive knowledge aspect, metacognitive judgments are more process-related, reflecting metacognitive awareness/experiences and feelings in ongoing metacognitive activities that individuals may engage in as they monitor and control processes (Efklides 2008; Gidalevich and Kramarski 2017; Tzohar-Rozen and

Kramarski 2013, 2018). Metacognitive control refers to the selection and use of learning and thinking strategies to repair or correct a mistake (Nelson and Narens 1994).

Similar to metacognitive judgments, regulation of cognition skills refers to a *dynamic* strategic processing activity (Pintrich 2000) that helps control one's thinking or learning (Nelson and Narens 1994) through three phases. In the *planning* (forethought) phase, learners set goals and select a strategy for their own planning of specific activities, to complete a specific task. Next, in the *monitoring* (performance) phase, learners use their goals to monitor and control the process and move it along, using goals as progress checkpoints through tasks. Finally, in the *evaluation*) reflection) phase, learners use information gained from the completed task to improve performance on the next task: what worked, what did not work and why (Pintrich 2000; Zimmerman 2008).

Research shows that cultivation of metacognitive skills plays an important role in the development of mathematical thinking during early childhood (Ginsburg et al. 2008; Whitebread and Coltman 2010) and solving of verbal problems (Mevarech 1995). For example, Whitebread and Coltman (2010) found evidence for the presence of metacognitive skills in verbal and nonverbal behaviors of children aged 3–5 years, while being involved in mathematical activities designed for them. Among preschoolers aged 4–5 years, Mevarech (1995) found that metacognitive ability explained more variability in mathematical performance than children's general ability.

7.1.2 SRL and Emotions

SRL classical models focus mainly on metacognition and motivation (e.g., Pintrich 2000; Zimmerman 2008), whereas the role of non-cognitive processes, such as emotions, are less dominant. Although positive affective processes are essential for investigating resources for self-regulation and achievement performance (Boekaerts 2007; Pintrich 2000; Schunk and Zimmerman 2008), positive and negative emotions (e.g., happiness, sadness, anger, fear) have only recently been studied in relation to learning processes (Gidalevich and Kramarski 2017, 2018; Mega et al. 2014; Pekrun et al. 2018; Tzohar-Rozen and Kramarski 2013, 2018).

Findings indicate that emotions are significant predictors of students' SRL and achievement (e.g., Boekaerts 2007). It was found that children with high test anxiety had difficulty encoding information at the time of the test (Ahmed et al. 2013). On the other hand, positive emotional experiences promote cognitive processes such as organization and problem solving in situations that require flexibility, integration, and efficiency (Pekrun et al. 2018). Thus, it is important for learners to recognize negative emotions and know how to cope and regulate (Efklides 2011; Gross 2013; Kramarski et al. 2010; Pekrun et al. 2018; Tzohar-Rozen and Kramarski 2018).

Young children have difficulties in spontaneous emotional regulation. Efklides (2011) in her SRL model argued that metacognitive experiences are not only influenced by cognitive processing but they are also influenced by affect, so that the relations between metacognition and affect can be much deeper and can help in regulation of emotions (Efklides et al. 2017).

7.1.3 Metacognition and Emotional Regulation

Learning to regulate emotions has been identified as one of the most important tasks of early childhood (Cole et al. 2004; Eisenberg and Spinrad 2004). Emotional regulation has been broadly defined as the heterogeneous set of processes by which individuals influence the timing, experience, and expression of their emotions (e.g., Gross 2013).

The ability to promote thinking through the regulation of emotion can be conceived of as a metacognitive process (Pintrich 2000). Metacognitive emotional regulation strategies in learning contexts involve deliberately changing thoughts or goals to alleviate negative emotions and support learning. Adults commonly engage in this type of emotional regulation, but little is known about the developmental roots of this ability in kindergarten children (Davis et al. 2010; Duncan et al. 2018; Pekrun et al. 2002).

Findings are mixed with respect to the age at which children are aware of and able to generate metacognitive strategies to regulate emotions. For example, Flavell et al. (2001) and Pons et al. (2004) concluded that 5–6-year-olds are generally unaware that thoughts accompany feelings and can cause changes in feelings without any external input. In contrast, Davis et al. (2010) found in both of their studies that the majority of children can describe metacognitive emotional regulation strategies. Children were surprisingly sophisticated in their suggestions for how to cope with negative emotions, and tailored their regulatory responses to specific emotional situations. These descriptive SRL strategies described by young students raise the need for further investigating the effects of cultivating metacognitive and emotional abilities of kindergarten students (5–6 year-olds) in different conditions.

A review of the literature showed that the few programs that did include a metacognitive and emotional component in a combined manner, focused on children in primary school but not in kindergarten. For example, Tzohar-Rozen and Kramarski (2018) compared three different intervention programs with fifth grade students: *Metacognition, Motivational-Emotional, combined program* (*Metacognition and Motivational-Emotional*) for mathematical problem solving and SRL. The study showed that the group exposed to the combined program had higher gains than the other two with respect to mathematics problem-solving performance, metacognitive regulation and reduction of mathematics-related anxiety. Similar conclusions were reached by Hanin and Van Nieuwenhoven (2018) with sixth grade students. They found that among three intervention programs, namely, *Cognition* (heuristic strategies), *Emotion*, *Emotion and Cognition*, and *Control* group, only the combined group (*Emotion and Cognition* with heuristic strategies) succeeded in reducing negative emotions, stimulating positive emotions, and promoting the use of adaptive emotional regulation strategies.

To sum up, the above studies show that programs that include metacognitive and emotional awareness components have the potential to improve students' mathematics achievement at school by increasing metacognitive thinking and decreasing negative emotions. Moreover, these findings pose new challenges for SRL programs in the preschool years, since this is a critical time for children to lay the foundations for mathematics learning and its associated emotions.

7.1.4 Theoretical Foundations for Intervention Programs

Since there is a lack of mathematics-related metacognitive and emotional intervention programs for preschool children, in the present study two intervention programs were developed: the combined program that includes metacognitive and meta-emotional aspects, and the separate metacognition program. The theoretical framework underlying the intervention programs in a mathematical problem-solving context was based on Pintrich's (2000) theoretical framework to raise awareness about metacognition and meta-emotion across the SRL phases matched to solution processes (before, during, and after performance):

- Planning and activation-*Before* the solution the child is asked to understand the task and to select a strategy;
- Monitoring and Controlling-*During* the solution the child is asked to self-assess and re-select a strategy;
- Evaluation and reaction-*After* the solution the child is asked to evaluate his/her performance (see the Method section).

Two principles guided the design of the two SRL intervention programs: direct guidance for SRL and self-questioning prompts for supporting SRL embedded into an "Interactive Storytelling" activation in mathematics. *Direct guidance for SRL.* SRL is not an innate or naturally acquired skill (Zimmerman 2008). For this reason, educators should cultivate and teach SRL through explicit instruction (Dignath and Büttner 2008). Explicit teaching means that the preschool teacher purposely presents and models SRL-appropriate learning strategies for the children, emphasizing the significance and importance of each strategy. *Self-questioning prompts for supporting SRL.* Prompts are external stimuli, questions, or statements that indicate to learners *when* and *how* to engage in productive learning processes (Gidalevich and Kramarski 2018; Kramarski et al. 2010; Shilo and Kramarski 2019). Studies have shown that metacognitive self-questioning prompts lead to significant improvement in mathematics achievement and SRL among school children (Mevarech and Kramarski 1997, 2014). The self-questioning strategy has already been extended to the meta-emotional component of SRL in a study of fifth-graders (Tzohar-Rozen and Kramarski 2013, 2018). The present study aimed to further investigate the effects of self-questions among pre-primary children, for enhancing metacognitive and meta-emotion in the context of mathematical problem solving, using "Interactive Story telling".

Storytelling is a popular instrument used in kindergarten classrooms to enrich the learning experience (Casey et al. 2008). It is an authentic way of activating children and can serve as an effective means for learning mathematics in a meaningful context that enables children to better understand abstract mathematics contents at an earlier age. The story is constructed from a narrative text in a mathematical context that contains relations between quantities.

The story helps children connect with the world of numbers in which they live, and leads to an accurate internal representation of the meanings of mathematical processes such as subtraction, addition, multiplication and division. To avoid children listening passively to the story, it is suggested to activate children's learning by having teachers ask math questions and stimulate students to ask their own questions. See examples in Appendix A (Tale of Five Balloons). This approach is in line with the principles of meaningful learning, which emphasize the involvement of the child in constructing knowledge (OECD 2012).

It has been found (Casey et al. 2008) that an arithmetic story guided by mathematical questioning was a more effective pedagogical method for promoting problem solving in kindergarten children when compared to a control group. However, effects of metacognitive and meta-emotional questioning support embedded in the storytelling have not yet been investigated, particularly among kindergarten children.

7.1.5 Design of the Study and Main Objectives

A pre-/post with follow up and a control group intervention study was designed. We developed two SRL intervention programs for kindergarten children: (a) Combined metacognitive and meta emotional support (MES) and (b) Only metacognitive support (MS) that were compared to (c) the control group (CG) that received no SRL support.

The participants were pre-primary school children. The interventions were applied in the context of mathematical verbal problem solving using "Interactive Storytelling". Assessment of the two SRL and control groups took place *before* the intervention (T1), *immediately* after it (T2), and 2 months later (T3, follow up). The aim was to investigate the potential added value of the combined MES group compared to the other two groups on the tested variables: metacognitive and meta-emotional SRL skills (planning, monitoring, controlling and evaluation statements) and performance on mathematical problem solving: routine verbal tasks (similar to trained tasks) and complex verbal tasks (non-trained tasks). We formulated two hypotheses:

Hypothesis 1 (H1) The combined meta-emotional support group (MES) will develop higher SRL skills (metacognitive and meta-emotional statements across the three phases) than the metacognitive support (MS) group. The lowest skills will be found in the control group (CG), as compared to the other two groups;

Hypothesis2 (H2) The MES group will show higher performance, compared to the MS and CG, in mathematical verbal problem solving, particularly in complex untrained problems demanding sense making relating to "understanding of a situation, context, or concept by connecting it with existing knowledge or previous experience" (NCTM 2000, p. 4).

7.2 Method

7.2.1 Participants

The sample comprised 90 children (51.1% boys; 48.9% girls), from three kindergartens in Northern Israel. Their ages ranged from 5 to 6 years. The kindergartens were from the same area and at similar SES level (according to Ministry of Education criteria). Each of the kindergartens was randomly assigned to one of the three study groups: the MES group ($n = 30$), the MS group ($n = 30$), and the CG group ($n = 30$). The groups were similar on gender distribution ($x^2(2) = 1.16$, $p = 0.561$) and official background measures of students' mathematical and general language ability [$F(2,87) = 0.35, p = 0.704$. $\eta_p{}^2 = 0.01$ $F(2,87) = 1.30, p = 0.278$. $\eta_p{}^2 = 0.03$, respectively, see elaboration in the measures section]. Three female teachers participated in the study. They were similar on their educational degrees and years of teaching experience.

7.2.2 Measures

7.2.2.1 General Mathematical Knowledge Test

The General Mathematical Knowledge Test is based on the contents of the mathematics curriculum—preschool (Ministry of Education 2010), and consists of 15 items that included: 6 assignments relating to the *sequence of numbers*; 3 tasks relating to *basic concepts*; 4 tasks on *quantitative significance*; 2 tasks relating to *number composition*. A correct solution in each of the tasks earned 2 points, a partial solution 1 point, and a no/wrong answer 0 point. A single score was produced that included the total points from all 15 items. The grades range was 13–30, $\alpha = 0.83$.

7.2.2.2 The Illinois Test of Psycholinguistic Abilities: TPA

The TPA (Kirk et al. 1968) included 10 items that require a linguistic analogy. For example: "*I sit in the chair, I sleep in...*" (Correct answer: bed, wrong answer: chair, at night, at home. Correct solution was scored 1 point. Incorrect solution was scored 0 point. The grades-range is 0–10. Cronbach's alpha internal reliability was found to be high, $\alpha = 0.75$.

7.2.2.3 Mathematical Verbal Problem-Solving Test

The test included four routine problems similar to those practiced in class according to the official curriculum books, and two complex problems demanding sense making not trained in the class (see example in the Appendix). The verbal problems were administered on an individual basis. The duration of the test was about 20 min and was administered by the teacher to each child. A *correct* answer on each routine/ un routine task earned 2 points, an *incomplet*e answer was scored 1 point and *incorrect/no trial* was scored 0 point. The testing took place at three time points: T1 (before intervention), T2 (end of intervention) and T3 (2 months later).

7.2.2.4 Structured Observation to Assess Metacognitive and Meta-emotional SRL Skills

A structured observation was conducted during the child's individual practice aloud of the routine and non-routine problem solving with three trained assistants (one for each study group) blind to the aims of each group. Training lasted 2 h including explanation about problem solving timing process (before, during, after) and SRL (metacognition, meta-emotion) and its phases (planning, monitoring, evaluation), followed by practice with audio listening in kindergarten thinking aloud during the task solution, and SRL metacognitive and meta-emotional phases (planning, monitoring and control, and evaluation). The assistants were provided with examples and were asked to find additional spontaneous examples that were discussed in the group.

The observation was conducted at three time points: T1 (before intervention), T2 (end of intervention) and T3 (2 months later). At each testing time, the same trained assistant observed and audiotaped each individual student's solution. She recorded the SRL sentences focusing on metacognition and meta-emotion, according to the three SRL phases: planning, monitoring and control, and evaluation.

Statement Classification and Scoring Statements in each study group (MES, MS, CG) were classified as metacognitive or meta-emotional statement and by their appropriate SRL phase (planning, monitoring and control, and evaluation).

Table 7.1 Examples of metacognitive and meta-emotional regulation statements in each group[a] (MES, MS, CG) according to the SRL phases during a verbal problem

SRL phases	Metacognitive statements MES, MS, CG	Meta-emotional statements MES group
The problem: In the garden there are five more pink flowers than yellow flowers. There are four yellow flowers, how many pink flowers are in the garden?		
Planning-Before solution Understanding the problem	"Can you repeat the question?"—*MES* "It's hard, I will count with my fingers"—*MS* "It is difficult"—*CG*	"I'm sad I can't solve, I will try again with my clock"
Monitoring and control-During solution Re-selecting a strategy Self-assessment	"I know, I will count 4 here and add another 5"-MES, MS "I don't know"-CG	"I am pleased that I know the solution"
Reflection- After the solution Evaluation of the performance	"I checked the solution with the disks"-MES "I solved correctly"-MS "9 flowers"-CG	"I'm glad I was able to solve"

[a]Groups; *MES* Metacognitive Emotional Support, *MS* Metacognitive Support, *CG* Control Group

Scoring Each metacognitive/meta-emotional statement at each phase gained 1 point. A total summative score for each student's statements at each phase was calculated related to metacognition/meta-emotion.

For example: Child's statements classifications:

"*Can you repeat the statement*?" was identified as a *metacognitive* statement oriented to knowledge acquired *before* solving a task, as such it was classified to be part of the *planning* phase (MS group).

"It is hard for me but I will try again" was identified as a meta-*emotional* statement *during* the task solution, and classified to be part of the *monitoring and control* phase (MES group).

"I don't know...I have 4 and 5" was identified as a *metacognitive* statement *during* the task solution, and classified to be part of the *monitoring and control* phase (CG group).

"I am glad I finished the task" was identified as a *meta-emotional* statement *after* the task solution, and classified to be part of the *evaluation* phase (MES group).

More examples are presented in Table 7.1, referencing by group (MES, MS, CG). Inter-judgement reliability (91% agreement) was attained between observed judgments and tape-recorded audio analysis, calculated on 20% of the participants in each group.

7.2.3 The Intervention Programs: Teachers' Preparation

Three programs (MES, MS, CG) took place for 2 months. They were embedded in mathematical problem-solving activities, followed by the official goals in the math

Table 7.2 Structure of the two SRL programs MES (metacognitive and meta-emotional support) and MS (metacognitive support)

SRL	MES	MS
Components phases *Solution processes*	*Thinking and emotional clock* 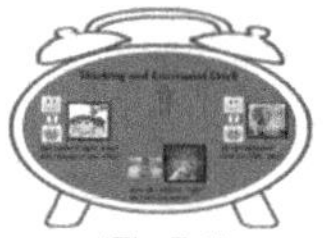 (Fig.7.1)	*Thinking clock* 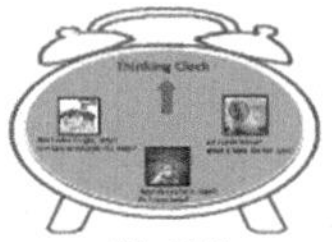 (Fig.7.2)
Planning- *Before* solution	Do I understand? How do I feel, why?	Do I understand? What is hard for me, why?
Monitoring **Controlling** *During* solution	How do I solve it, why? Do I need to relax? How?	How do I solve it, why? Do I need help? How?
Evaluation *After solution*	*Did I solve it right, why?* *Am I happy or sad, why?*	*Did I solve it right, why?* *Is it easy or hard for me, why?*

MES Metacognitive Emotional Support, *MS* Metacognitive Support, *CG* Control Group

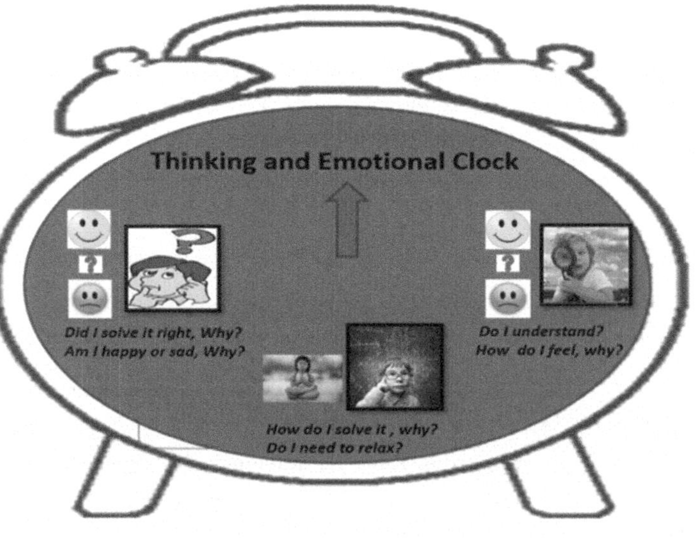

Fig. 7.1 "Thinking and Emotional Clock"-for the combined group (MES)

curriculum with "Interactive Storytelling" experiences challenged by questioning and discussions. Whereas the MES and MS were exposed to domain questions and SRL self-questions prompts according to the type of the program, supported by its "Thinking Clock" and symbolic icons (see Table 7.2; Figs. 7.1 and 7.2), the CG was exposed only to domain questions practice. Teachers in that group didn't know that they were serving as a control group. Each program (MES MS CG) was implemented by the preschool teacher who was exposed to a training session (2 h)

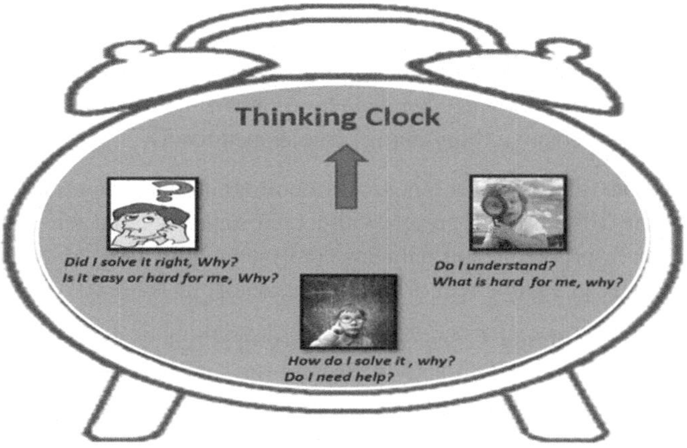

Fig. 7.2 "Thinking Clock"-for the metacognitive support group (MS)

under a research assistant's guidance that explained the rationale and structure of the program embedded with the structure of the "Interactive Storytelling" and its implementation with small groups of five children each time (elaboration in a forthcoming paragraph).

Teachers from the intervention groups were exposed to the SRL skills and self-question prompts embedded in a "Thinking Clock" according to the relevant intervention. The training was followed by discussion of preparing appropriate lesson plans with supported materials and posters to hang on the wall for each meeting. Two modeling sessions were conducted by the third researcher in each of the intervention groups. She visited the intervention groups and the CG group twice in each classroom to assess the fidelity of the activities to the planned intervention criteria as using SRL self-questioning and "Thinking Clocks" embedded in the "Interactive Storytelling", and provided feedback accordingly.

7.2.4 Structure of the Intervention Sessions in the Three Groups

A total of *eight* sessions in the second part of the year were held by the kindergarten teacher aided by ready-made scripts embedded in math tasks adapted to each group's rationale. The children's meetings took place in groups of five in a corner of the room, once a week. Each session lasted about 25 min for explanation and modeling followed by children's practice in daily authentic situations as games and math tasks. During that time other students were occupied by a research assistance.

7.2.4.1 Sessions Structure

Sessions 1–2 Goal presenting for each group (MES, MS, Control). Exposure to mathematical problem solving, guided by domain questions across solution processing with "Interactive Storytelling" (see Appendix A).

Sessions 3–5 The role of SRL components (metacognition and emotion) and phases as adapted to the MES and MS groups with its relevant clock and self-questions for coping with math problems and authentic daily situations (e.g., dilemmas raised while participating in a game with friends). See details in Table 7.2.

"Thinking and Emotional Clock"—MES Group Prior to the intervention program, the teacher conducted an activity around the topic of positive and negative emotions. She presented the children with four icons of emotions: angry, sad, happy and excited, and related a case/dilemma from the kindergarten, and then each child pointed to the emotion which aroused them. In order to strengthen familiarity with the icons, the icons were also presented on the board called *"Who's coming to the kindergarten?"*. The terms of thinking and emotions in the MES group were practiced and exemplified in the child's math solution processes (before, during, after) embedded with SRL phases (planning, monitoring and control, and evaluation). For example, before starting the solution, the MES kindergarten child was required to understand the task, to plan a strategy for the solution and to consider her/his emotions.

Throughout the three phases, the teacher modeled the use of the self-question prompts with the *"Thinking and Emotional Clock"* to stimulate children's thoughts and emotional awareness. Each phase included two questions, one directed to metacognition and the second to meta-emotion. See Table 7.2 for the six detailed questions. Finally, after getting to know the clock, the children built a personal clock with its icons and used it freely in daily situations, during a game or a contest between the children.

"Thinking Clock"—MS Group Prior to the intervention program, the teacher conducted an activity around the topic of thinking and its icon presentations. She presented a case/dilemma from the kindergarten and each child pointed to the solution it aroused them. In order to strengthen familiarity with the clock and its icons, it was presented on the board titled "*Who's coming to the kindergarten?*". The thinking clock with its six questions (2 questions in each phase) focused on metacognition (Table 7.2). The kindergarten teacher in the MS group explained the terms of the clock and the link between the child's solution processes (before, during, after) with SRL phases related to *metacognition awareness* without focus on emotion awareness. She modeled the use of the thinking clock with its metacognitive questions embedded in mathematical problem solving.

Similar to the MES group, after getting to know the clock in each group, the children built a personal clock and used it freely, during a game or a contest between the children to determine who would start the game.

Sessions 6–8 Integrating the clock (MES, MS) within the "Interactive Storytelling" problems. An application of each clock with its icons and self-questions (see Table 7.2, Figs. 7.1 and 7.2) was modeled and practiced in each group (MES, MS) while solving the "Tale of Five Balloons" (see Appendix A for the flow of "Interactive Storytelling" content questions), during which the preschool teacher stopped at predefined points and posed mathematical questions to the children which they had to answer: For example, "*How many balloons have exploded?*" "*Are there more or fewer balloons now?*" (After every balloon that had exploded). In case children had difficulty answering any of the questions, they were directed to the relevant clock questions and they proceeded in accordance with the SRL phases of the clock. During the sessions, the teacher implemented various story telling problems *but* asked fewer mathematical questions and encouraged children to raise their own questions and answer them with the relevant Clock support.

Control Group (CG) The teacher modeled and practiced the same mathematical problems with the "Interactive storytelling" and content questions with no SRL emphasis and implementation of the thinking and emotional clocks questions and their icons.

7.3 Results

7.3.1 Metacognitive and Meta-emotional Regulation. H1

One-way MANOVA analysis indicated no significant differences between the three study groups in the number of metacognitive and meta-emotional statements related to the three pre-intervention phases, $F(2,87) = 1.26, p = 0.290. \eta_p^2 = 0.03$. In order to examine the differences between the three groups (MES, ME, CG) by time (T1, T2, T3), two-way Mixed ANOVA analyses were conducted for each of the three phases (planning, monitoring control, evaluation) and for the metacognitive and meta-emotional regulation statements separately. The dependent variables were the number of metacognitive and meta-emotional statements for each of the three phases, and *group* (as the between subjects factor) and *time* (as the within subjects factor) were the independent variables (see Table 7.3).

7.3.2 Metacognitive Statements

7.3.2.1 Planning Statements

A significant Group*Time interaction was found. Bonferroni post hoc analyses in each study group separately revealed that while there was a significant increase (compared to T1) in the number of planning statements at the end of the intervention

Table 7.3 Mean (and *SD*) and *F* of the metacognitive and meta-emotional regulation statements by group and testing time in each SRL phase

SRL phases	Groups[a]	Pre-T1		Post-T2		Delayed-T3		$F(4172)$[b]	p	η_p^2
		M	*SD*	*M*	*SD*	*M*	*SD*			
Metacognitive statements										
Planning	MES	0.00	0.00	1.73	0.69	1.87	0.43			
	MS	0.00	0.00	1.33	0.55	1.37	0.72			
	CG	0.00	0.00	0.00	0.00	0.00	0.00	55.97***	0.000	0.57
Monitoring	MES	0.47	0.57	1.57	0.73	2.13	0.73			
	MS	0.47	0.51	1.50	0.63	1.50	0.78			
	CG	0.77	1.25	1.07	1.64	0.97	1.54	5.05***	0.001	0.11
Evaluation	MES	0.00	0.00	1.37	0.67	1.53	0.63			
	MS	0.00	0.00	1.10	0.61	1.23	0.90			
	CG	0.00	0.00	0.00	0.00	0.00	0.00	36.65***	0.000	0.46
Meta-emotional statements										
Planning	MES	0.00	0.00	1.67	0.76	1.50	0.57			
	MS	0.00	0.00	0.00	0.00	0.00	0.00			
	CG	0.00	0.00	0.00	0.00	0.00	0.00	78.50***	0.000	0.65
Monitoring	MES	0.00	0.00	1.67	0.99	1.37	0.67			
	MS	0.00	0.00	0.00	0.00	0.00	0.00			
	CG	0.00	0.00	0.00	0.00	0.00	0.00	53.79***	0.000	0.56
Evaluation	MES	0.00	0.00	1.40	0.67	1.47	0.78			
	MS	0.00	0.00	0.00	0.00	0.00	0.00			
	CG	0.00	0.00	0.00	0.00	0.00	0.00	57.33***	0.000	0.57

***$p < 0.001$; Range: 0–2
[a]Groups; *MES* Metacognitive Emotional Support, *MS* Metacognitive Support, *CG* Control Group
[b]Repeated measures (Group*Time)

(T2; $d = 2.51$ for the MES group; $d = 2.43$ for the MS group), and follow up 2 months later (T3; $d = 4.3$ for the MES group and $d = 1.9$ for the MS group), $p < 0.001$, there were no differences in the number of metacognitive statements (compared to T1) between the three measurement points for the control group.

7.3.2.2 Monitoring and Control Statements

A significant Group*Time interaction was found (see, Table 7.3). Bonferroni post hoc analyses revealed that there was a significant increase (compared to T1) in the number of monitoring and control statements at the end of the intervention favoring the MS group (T2; $d = 1.44$) compared to the MES group, (T2; $d = 1.30$). However, 2 months later the findings were *reversed*, so that the MES group manifested a greater increase (compared to T1) in metacognitive statements (T3; $d = 1.89$, $p < 0.001$) than the MS group (T3; $d = 1.35$). There were no differences in the number of statements between the three measurement times (compared to T1) for the control group.

7.3.2.3 Reflection/Evaluation Statements

A significant Group*Time interaction was found (Table 7.3). Bonferroni post hoc analyses revealed that while there was a significant increase in the number of reflection statements (compared to T1) at the end of the intervention for the two intervention groups (T2; $d = 2.04$ for the MES group; $d = 1.81$ for the MS group) as well as 2 months later (T3; $d = 2.44$ for the MES group; $d = 1.37$ for the MS group), $p < 0.001$, there were no differences in the number of statements between the three measurement times (compared to T1) in the control group.

7.3.3 Meta-emotional Statements

7.3.3.1 Planning Statements

A significant Group*Time interaction was found (see Table 7.3). Bonferroni post hoc analysis revealed that there was a significant increase in the number of emotional planning statements (compared to T1) at the end of the intervention for the MES group (T2; $d = 2.20$), and 2 months later (T3; $d = 2.62$), $p < 0.001$. However, there were no differences in the number of statements (compared to T1) between the three measurement times for the MS and CG groups (Table 7.2).

7.3.3.2 Monitoring and Control Statements

A significant Group*Time interaction was found. Bonferroni post hoc analysis revealed that there was a significant increase (compared to T1) in the number of emotional monitoring and control statements at the end of the intervention for the MES group (T2; $d = 1.68$), and 2 months later (T3; $d = 2.04$), $p < 0.001$. However, there were no differences in the number of emotional statements (compared to T1) in the MS and CG groups across the three measurement times.

7.3.3.3 Reflection/Evaluation Statements

A significant Group*Time interaction was found. Bonferroni post hoc analysis revealed that while there was a significant increase (compared to T1) in the number of the emotional reflection statements at the end of the intervention for the MES group (T2; $d = 2.07$), and 2 months later (T3; $d = 1.89$), $p < 0.001$, no differences were found in the number of statements (compared to T1) across the three times in the MS and CG groups.

7.3.4 Performance in Routine and Complex Problems. H2

One-way MANOVA (Groups*Types of problems) analyses indicated no significant differences between the three study groups in performance on the routine and complex problems before the intervention, $F(10,166) = 1.27, p = 0.254. \eta_p{}^2 = 0.07$.

7.3.4.1 Routine Problems

A follow-up two-way repeated ANOVA with performance on routine problems as dependent variable indicated a significant Group*Time interaction on the total score (see Table 7.4). Bonferroni post hoc analyses revealed a significant increase (compared to T1) of the routine tasks performance in the two intervention groups at the end of the intervention, favoring the MS group (T2; $d = 2.48$) compared to the MES group (T2; $d = 1.68$). However, a greater effect (compared to T1) was found for the MES group 2 months later (T3; $d = 1.4$) compared to the MS group ($d = 1$). There were no differences in performance on the routine problems between the three measurement times for the control group (compared to T1).

7.3.4.2 Complex Problems

A significant Group*Time interaction was found for performance on the complex tasks *(total score)*. Bonferroni post hoc analyses revealed a significant increase of performance on the complex problems for the MES group in T3 ($d = 1.29$), as compared to T1 and also compared to T2; ($d = 1.22$). However, there were no differences between the MS and CG groups on T2 and T3 compared to the starting gains (T1).

Table 7.4 Mean (and SD) and F of the performance on mathematical problem solving (routine, complex) by group and time

		Pre-T1		Post-T2		Delayed-T3				
Task type	Groups[a]	*M*	*SD*	*M*	*SD*	*M*	*SD*	*F*(4172)[b]	*p*	$\eta_p{}^2$
Routine	MES	1.22	0.28	1.69	0.15	1.90	0.19			
	MS	1.19	0.21	1.71	0.13	1.84	0.15			
	CG	1.21	0.26	1.22	0.57	1.07	0.69	16.67***	0.000	0.28
Complex	MES	1.13	0.35	1.07	0.25	1.80	0.41			
	MS	1.17	0.38	1.10	0.30	1.37	0.49			
	CG	1.20	0.41	1.17	0.70	1.10	0.48	10.18***	0.000	0.19

***$p < 0.001$; Range: 0–2 on a total score
[a]Groups; *MES* Metacognitive Emotional Support, *MS* Metacognitive Support, *CG* Control Group
[b]Repeated measures (Group*Time)

7.4 Discussion

The present study showed that the combination of metacognitive and meta-emotional support (MES) in kindergarten is instrumental for the exercise of metacognitive and emotional self-regulation and its maintenance over a 2-month period, as compared to a metacognitive support (MS) group and control group in the context of mathematical problem solving, activated with an "Interactive Storytelling" practice. We discuss the findings in relation to each of the hypotheses.

7.4.1 *Metacognitive and Meta-emotional Regulation in the Three Phases of SRL*

Metacognitive Regulation Hypothesis 1 predicted that the MES group would over time have more metacognitive regulation statements than the MS group, and both MES and MS groups would have more metacognitive statements than the CG. Our findings indicated that both intervention programs (MES, MS) significantly *increased* (compared to T1) children's verbal metacognitive statements along the three phases of SRL, as emerged at the end of the program (T2) and on T3 (follow up). In a comparison between the intervention groups, as expected, the highest metacognitive statements increase was found on T3 and favored the MES group, but on T2 this tendency was not attended. No differences were found between the intervention groups on the *planning* statements increase, and on the *monitoring* and *control* statements, in which the MS group outperformed the MES group. However, as regards the *evaluation* statements the combined MES group outperformed the MS group (as expected).

This discrepancy regarding H1 between the two groups on T2 can be explained by the fact that *both* groups were exposed to metacognitive self questioning training in the mathematical context empowered by *goal-oriented thinking (top-down* process) across the three phases (Mevarech and Kramarski 1997, 2014). Thus it had an immediate positive effect on both groups at the end of the program (T2) on the initial phases, planning monitoring and control that are less complicated than the evaluation regulation ability (Pintrich 2000; Zimmerman 2008), and also not on the *lasting effect* period while the program's scaffolds fad out. These two occasions were more favored in MES group with the help of the meta-emotional support (Tzohar-Rozen and Kramarski 2018; see elaboration in the next section). Finally, the control group did not show any increase in the use of metacognitive statements, thereby confirming Hypothesis 1 that the two intervention groups would score higher than the CG.

Meta-emotional Regulation Besides the metacognitive statements increase, as expected (H1), the MES group also showed an increase in meta-emotional statements at both T2 and T3 (compared to T1). These statements were distributed in all SRL phases (planning, monitoring and control, and evaluation), and often took the form of combined metacognitive and meta-emotional statements together in the same sentence (see Table 7.1). For example, in the evaluation phase a student stated: "*At first, I didn't understand, but you explained it to me again and I succeeded, so I'm really pleased*". In contrast, no meta-emotional statements were found in the MS and CG groups.

It seems that the "Thinking and Emotional Clock" with its self-question prompts succeeded in *concretizing* the two components (metacognition and emotions) of the circular model of SRL for young children. This raised children's "double attention" to their metacognitive goal-oriented thoughts (top-down processes) and emotional experiences (bottom-up processes) while solving verbal mathematical problems. These findings support previous claims that both types of regulation are necessary, but do not develop spontaneously. This seems to suggest, in particular, that learners should recognize their negative emotions and know how to deal with them (Gross 2013; Kramarski et al. 2010).

7.4.2 Performance on Verbal Routine and Complex Tasks

Hypothesis 2 predicted that MES would lead to higher performance on verbal mathematical tasks (routine or complex) compared to the MS group and CG.

Routine Verbal Tasks At the end of the intervention (T2), both the MS and MES groups increased their performance on routine tasks (compared to T1), but this time the MS group outperformed the MES group on routine problem-solving skills, contrary to the findings on the metacognitive and meta-emotional regulation. However, when testing for lasting effects, 2 months later (T3), the findings were reversed: a higher significant increase (compared to T1 and T2) was found in the *MES group* as compared to the MS group, that surpassed the control group which did not increase its problem-solving skills across the three measurement times despite the storytelling activator practice in mathematical problem solving.

The MS group's higher solution gains on T2 compared to the MES group in the routine tasks can be explained by the metacognitive self-questions power that matched to the solution phases directly and may lessen feelings of frustration and anxiety, thus increasing solution success (Kramarski et al. 2010; Mevarech and Kramarski 2014). In contrast, the use of the combined metacognitive and meta-emotional questions in MES group may be more overloaded for routine problem solution that may lessen success in solving tasks. Future studies will address this issue more deeply.

Complex Verbal Tasks In the case of the complex, sense-making task, only the MES group showed significant improvement in the two interval times (T2 and T3) compared to the MS and CG groups. Sense making requires high-order thinking that demands the ability to recruit previous knowledge and experience with routine tasks, and to use it along with an intuitive untrained open view of mathematical structures (NCTM 2000; OECD 2012).

It is plausible that integrating knowledge of non-routine tasks with intuitive approaches to math problem solving aroused feelings of frustration and anxiety (Kramarski et al. 2010; Pekrun et al. 2018). Thus, children who received the combined support, that included both metacognitive (top-down processes) and emotional guidance (bottom up experience awareness) raised their "transfer of attention" ability. That is, children switched attention between understanding the task and their emotional experiences that helped them to control their feelings, particularly during the follow up (T3). Consequently, they could be relaxed (see Table 7.2) and confident enough to reflect more carefully on the solution of the complex task, by considering all information and explaining their mathematical solution. This was not the case for the MS group, which received only metacognitive support, and the control group that did not receive any support.

The peak of performance on the complex tasks in the follow up testing period (T3) is in line with theories that SRL capacity takes time to develop and improve (Pintrich 2000; Zimmerman 2008). It supports research conclusions focused separately on each component alone, showing a larger impact of metacognitive effects in follow-up learning sessions than earlier measures of short-term effects (e.g., Bannert et al. 2015; Gidalevitch and Kramarski 2018).

The MES finding on metacognition, meta-emotion and mathematical complex problem solving at T3 supports previous conclusions with older students (grade 5), that combining both components may be loading at the first wave (T2), thus requiring more time to be familiar with emotional skills and its adaptability for personal use (Tzohar-Rozen and Kramarski 2013, 2018).

The combined benefit supports the added value of using the SRL aspects. The strategic of metacognition that help the long-term memorization and re-use of these learning skills to achieve deeper understanding (Bannert et al. 2015; Efklides 2011; Kuhn and Dean 2004). The affective aspect that "people when becoming aware of their affective state, use it as a cue along with other cues that come from the monitoring of task demands, features of cognitive processing and its outcomes" (Efklides et al. 2017, p. 70).

In conclusion, the beneficial effects of SRL metacognitive/meta-emotional training prompts among kindergarten children supports recent studies on kindergarten children improvement on self-regulation, math, and literacy after their participation in SRL program as presented by Duncan et al. (2018). Their findings suggest that self-regulation intervention leads to improved school readiness in children at higher risk for later school difficulties. Similarly, de Corte et al. (2000) found, among high school children, that an emotional regulation intervention significantly increased their ability to cope with the learning difficulties that arose in school studies.

7.4.3 Contribution of the Study, Limitations and Future Research

The study contributes evidence to the limited affective research findings about young children's SRL development (Efklides et al. 2017). The study showed that simultaneously using metacognitive and meta-emotional supports allows children to express and share their feelings, and thus to be emotionally available for more efficient and more effective use of cognitive skills acquired during problem-solving. This finding is in line with previous studies indicating that cultivation of metacognitive skills by itself is not sufficient to help students cope with difficulties faced in learning situations. Attention to learners' emotions and sense of self-efficacy should also be nurtured (Gross 2013; Mevarech and Kramarski 2014; Tzohar-Rozen and Kramarski 2018).

This study demonstrated that the explicit use of combined metacognitive and meta-emotional self-questioning support is essential for improving mathematical achievement (routine and complex tasks) among kindergarten children. This finding strengthens the conclusion that it is not enough to engage children with interactive environments such as "Storytelling" accompanied with content-related math questions and discourse as found in the control group.

This study has both theoretical and practical implications. Theoretically, it contributes to knowledge about the cognitive and emotional aspects of the SRL process and the impact of such components on preschool children's performance when dealing with verbal math problems. In terms of application, the design of the two intervention programs can serve as a practical basis for fostering mathematical education at the preschool level, in a self-regulated learning context.

This study is a response to recent pleas for interventions addressing the affective aspect of mathematics education (Schukajlow et al. 2017). Previous studies focused on older students (Mevarech and Kramarski 2014; Schukajlow et al. 2017), whereas this study was conducted among kindergarten children.

The study has some limitations. The intervention program conducted in this study included assessments of children from one district of the country. Fine-grained analysis should be done further, based on children's initial profiles as high/low achievers, emotional tendency, metacognitive tendency and its relatedness to problem solving gains at different task-complexity levels.

Further, the SRL analysis in this study was based on the frequency of children's verbal statements while solving the problem aloud. Future studies should incorporate deeper process analysis to understand the sequence of thinking processes by following mathematical metacognitive content between the teacher and the child (Azevedo 2014; Shilo and Kramarski 2019), also reinforced with complementary measures to assess behavioral gestures such as facial expressions. It is also recommended to follow up on the children that were exposed to such a program when they enter first grade, in order to examine the assimilation effect of the metacognitive and meta-emotional intervention in school while practicing math, and testing transferability to other domains such as reading comprehension.

Appendix A

A Tale of Five Balloons

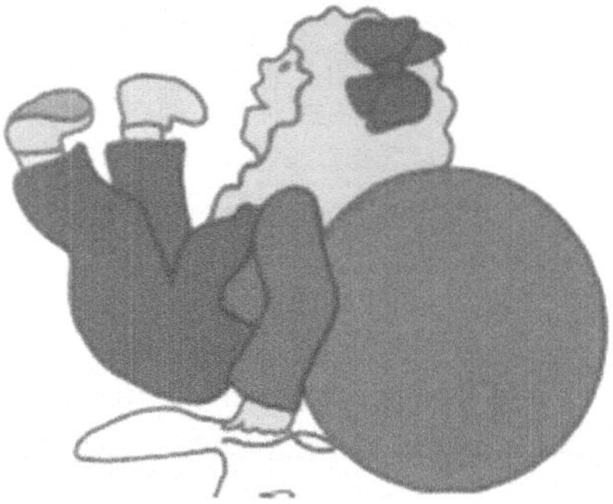

A story by Miriam Roth

Illustrated by Ora Ayal

Translated by Mya Feldman

Tale of five balloons

The story

Ruth's mother brought a gift: happiness... for each child a balloon

- Ruthie has a blue balloon
- Sara has a yellow balloon
- Rachel has a pink balloon
- David has a green balloon
- Uri has a purple balloon

The questions

How many balloons did Mom bring?

Are there enough for all children?

How many children were there? How many boys? How many girls?
And suddenly ... boom, what happened?
The balloon exploded, the balloon was torn
Please Uri don't be sorry
We'll get you another balloon
The questions
How many balloons were there?
How many have exploded?
Are there now more or less?
Continue the story...
Ask questions

Appendix B

Routine Problem

Noa has 5 pink dresses and 2 blue dresses. How many dresses does Noa have?

Structure: *The problem is clear, there is one answer. Students were trained in such tasks.*

Complex problem

Guy and Ofir play cards, if Guy loses one card, both of them will have an equal number of cards. What could be the number of cards for each? Can you find more options?

Structure: *No numeric data exists, there are several options. Most importantly, students were not trained on such a problem.*

References

Ahmed, W., van der Werf, G., Kuyper, H., & Minnaert, A. (2013). Emotions, self-regulated learning, and achievement in mathematics: A growth curve analysis. *Journal of Educational Psychology, 105*, 150–161. https://psycnet.apa.org/doi/10.1037/a0030160.

Azevedo, R. (2014). Issues in dealing with sequential and temporal characteristics of self- and socially-regulated learning. *Metacognition and Learning, 9*, 217–228. https://doi.org/10.1007/s11409-014-9123-1.

Bannert, M., Sonnenberg, C., Mengelkamp, C., & Pieger, E. (2015). Short- and long-term effects of students' self-directed metacognitive prompts on navigation behavior and learning performance. *Computers in Human Behavior, 52*, 293–306. https://doi.org/10.1016/j.chb.2015.05.038.

Boekaerts, M. (2007). Understanding students' affective processes in the classroom. In P. A. Schutz & R. Pekrun (Eds.), *Emotion in education* (pp. 37–56). San Diego: Elsevier.

Casey, B., Erkut, S., Ceder, I., & Young, J. M. (2008). Use of a storytelling context to improve girls' and boys' geometry skills in kindergarten. *Journal of Applied Developmental Psychology, 29*, 29–48. https://doi.org/10.1016/j.appdev.2007.10.005.

Cole, P. M., Martin, S. E., & Dennis, T. A. (2004). Emotion regulation as a scientific construct: Methodological challenges and directions for child development research. *Child Development, 75*, 317–333.

Davis, E. L., Levine, L. J., Lench, H. C., & Quas, J. A. (2010). Metacognitive emotion regulation: Children's awareness that changing thoughts and goals can alleviate negative emotions. *Emotions, 10*, 498–510. https://psycnet.apa.org/doi/10.1037/a0018428.

de Corte, E., Verschaffel, L., & Op't Eynde, P. (2000). Self-regulation: A characteristic and a goal of mathematics education. In M. Boekaerts, P. R. Pintrich, & M. Zeinder (Eds.), *Handbook of self-regulation* (pp. 687–726). San Diego: Elsevier.

Dignath, C., & Büttner, G. (2008). Components of fostering self-regulated learning among children: A meta-analysis on intervention studies at primary and secondary school level. *Metacognition and Learning, 3*, 231–264. https://doi.org/10.1007/s11409-008-9029-x.

Duncan, R. J., Schmitt, S. A., Burke, M., & McClelland, M. M. (2018). Combining a kindergarten readiness summer program with a self-regulation intervention improves school readiness. *Early Childhood Research Quarterly, 42*, 291–300. https://doi.org/10.1016/j.ecresq.2017.10.012.

Efklides, A. (2008). Metacognition: Defining its facets and levels of functioning in relation to self-regulation and co-regulation. *European Psychologist, 13*, 277–287. https://doi.org/10.1027/1016-9040.13.4.277.

Efklides, A. (2011). Interactions of metacognition with motivation and affect in self-regulated learning: The MASRL model. *Educational Psychologist, 46*, 6–25. https://doi.org/10.1080/00461520.2011.538645.

Efklides, A., Schwartz, B. L., & Brown, V. (2017). Motivation and affect in self-regulated learning: Does metacognition play a role? In D. H. Schunk & J. A. Greene (Eds.), *Handbook of self-regulation of learning and performance* (pp. 64–83). New York: Springer.

Eisenberg, N., & Spinrad, T. L. (2004). Emotion-related regulation: Sharpening the definition. *Child Development, 75*, 334–339. https://doi.org/10.1111/j.1467-8624.2004.00674.x.

Flavell, J. H. (1976). Metacognitive aspects of problem solving. In L. B. Resnick (Ed.), *The nature of intelligence* (pp. 231–236). Hillsdale: Erlbaum.

Flavell, J. H., Flavell, E. R., & Green, F. L. (2001). Development of children's understanding of connections between thinking and feeling. *Psychological Science, 12*, 430–432. https://doi.org/10.1111/2F1467-9280.00379.

Gidalevich, S., & Kramarski, B. (2017). Guidance for metacognitive judgements: A thinking-aloud analysis in math problem solving. *Hellenic Journal of Psychology, 14*, 88–113. Retrieved April 11, 2020 from https://pseve.org/wp-content/uploads/2018/03/Volume14_Issue2_Gidalevich.pdf

Gidalevich, S., & Kramarski, B. (2018). The value of fixed vs. faded self-regulatory scaffolds on fourth graders' mathematical problem solving. *Instructional Science, 47*, 39–68. https://doi.org/10.1007/s11251-018-9475-z.

Ginsburg, H. P., Lee, J. S., & Boyd, J. S. (2008). Mathematics education for young children: What it is and how to promote it. *Social Policy Report, 22*, 1–24. https://doi.org/10.1002/j.2379-3988.2008.tb00054.x.

Gross, J. J. (2013). Emotion regulation: Taking stock and moving forward. *Emotion, 13*, 359–365. https://psycnet.apa.org/doi/10.1037/a0032135.

Hanin, V., & Van Nieuwenhoven, C. (2018). Developing an expert and reflexive approach to problem-solving: The place of emotional knowledge and skills. *Psychology, 9*, 280–309. https://doi.org/10.4236/psych.2018.92018.

Kirk, S., McCarthy, J., & Kirk, W. (1968). *The Illinois test of psycholinguistic abilities* (Rev. Ed.). Urbana: University of Illinois Press.

Kramarski, B., Weiss, I., & Kololshi-Minsker, I. (2010). How can self-regulated learning support the problem solving of third-grade students with mathematics anxiety? *ZDM Mathematics Education, 42*, 179–193. https://doi.org/10.1007/s11858-009-0202-8.

Kuhn, D., & Dean, D. (2004). A bridge between cognitive psychology and educational practice. *Theory Into Practice, 43*, 268–273.

Mega, C., Ronconi, L., & De Beni, R. (2014). What makes a good student? How emotions, self-regulated learning and motivation contribute to academic achievement. *Journal of Educational Psychology, 106*, 121–131. https://psycnet.apa.org/doi/10.1037/a0033546.

Mevarech, Z. R. (1995). Metacognition, general ability, and mathematical understanding. *Early Education and Development, 6*, 155–168. https://doi.org/10.1207/s15566935eed0602_4.

Mevarech, Z. R., & Kramarski, B. (1997). IMPROVE: A multidimensional method for teaching mathematics in heterogeneous classroom. *American Educational Research Journal, 34*, 365–395. https://doi.org/10.3102/2F00028312034002365.

Mevarech, Z. R., & Kramarski, B. (2014). *Critical maths for innovative societies: The role of metacognitive pedagogies*. Paris: OECD.

Ministry of Education. (2010). *Mathematical curriculum in kindergarten*. Jerusalem: Department of Assessment and Measurements in Education. Retrieved April 11, 2020 from http://meyda.education.gov.il/files/Tochniyot_Limudim/KdamYesodi/Math1.pdf

National Council of Teachers of Mathematics [NCTM]. (2000). *Principles and standards for school mathematics*. Reston: NCTM.

Nelson, T. O., & Narens, L. (1994). Why investigate metacognition? In J. Metcalfe & A. P. Shimamura (Eds.), *Metacognition: Knowing about knowing* (pp. 1–25). Cambridge: MIT.

OECD. (2012). *PISA 2012. Assessment and analytical framework: Mathematics, reading, science, problem solving and financial literacy*. Paris: OECD Publication.

Organization for Economic Co-operation and Development [OECD]. (2000). Measuring students' knowledge and skills: A new framework for assessment. Paris: OECD. Retrieved April 11, 2020 from https://www.oecd.org/education/school/programmeforinternationalstudentassessment pisa/33693997.pdf

Pekrun, R., Goetz, T., Titz, W., & Perry, R. P. (2002). Academic emotions in students' self-regulated learning and achievement: A program of qualitative and quantitative research. *Educational Psychologist, 37*, 91–105. https://doi.org/10.1207/S15326985EP3702_4.

Pekrun, R., Muis, K. R., Frenzel, A. C., & Goetz, T. (2018). *Emotions at school*. New York: Routledge.

Pintrich, P. R. (2000). The role of goal orientation in self-regulated learning. In M. Boekaerts, P. R. Pintrich, & M. Zeidner (Eds.), *Handbook of self-regulation* (pp. 451–502). San Diego: Academic Press.

Pons, F., Harris, P. L., & de Rosnay, M. (2004). Emotion comprehension between 3 and 11 years: Developmental periods and hierarchical organization. *European Journal of Developmental Psychology, 1*, 127–152. https://www.tandfonline.com/doi/ref/10.1080/17405620344000022.

Schoenfeld, A. H. (1992). Learning to think mathematically: Problem solving, metacognition, and sense making in mathematics. In D. A. Grouws (Ed.), *Handbook of research on mathematics teaching and learning* (pp. 165–197). New York: Macmillan.

Schraw, G. (1998). Promoting general metacognitive awareness. *Instructional Science, 26*, 113–125. https://doi.org/10.1023/A:1003044231033.

Schraw, G., Crippen, K. J., & Hartley, K. (2006). Promoting self-regulation in science education: Metacognition as part of a broader perspective on learning. *Research in Science Education, 36*, 111–139. https://doi.org/10.1007/s11165-005-3917-8.

Schukajlow, S., Rakoczy, K., & Pekrun, R. (2017). Emotions and motivation in mathematics education: Theoretical considerations and empirical contributions. *ZDM: Mathematics Education, 49*, 307–322. https://doi.org/10.1007/s11858-017-0864-6.

Schunk, D. H., & Zimmerman, B. J. (Eds.). (2008). *Motivation and self-regulated learning: Theory, research, and applications*. New York: Erlbaum.

Shilo, A., & Kramarski, B. (2019). Mathematical-metacognitive discourse: How can it be developed among teachers and their students? Empirical evidence from a videotaped lesson and two case studies. *ZDM, Mathematics Education, 51*, 625–640. https://doi.org/10.1007/s11251-018-9475-z.

Tzohar-Rozen, M., & Kramarski, B. (2013). How does an affective self-regulation program promote mathematical literacy in young students? *Hellenic Journal of Psychology, 10*,

211–234. Retrieved April 11, 2020 from https://pseve.org/wp-content/uploads/2018/03/Volume10_Issue3_Tzohar-Rozen.pdf

Tzohar-Rozen, M., & Kramarski, B. (2018, April 13). *An holistic self-regulation model to enhance meta-cognition and meta-affect: A mixed methods study*. New York: Paper presented at the AERA conference.

Whitebread, D., & Coltman, P. (2010). Aspects of pedagogy supporting metacognition and self-regulation in mathematical learning of young children: Evidence from an observational study. *ZDM, Mathematics Education, 42*, 163–178. https://doi.org/10.1007/s11858-009-0233.

Zimmerman, B. J. (2008). Investigating self-regulation and motivation: Historical background, methodological developments, and future prospects. *American Educational Research Journal, 45*, 166–183. https://doi.org/10.3102/2F0002831207312909.

Chapter 8
Using Feedback to Support Children When Monitoring and Controlling Their Learning

Mariëtte H. van Loon and Claudia M. Roebers

Abstract Children's monitoring of learning is often inaccurate, and subsequent control of learning ineffective, making research on potential effects of feedback on metacognition very relevant. This chapter gives an overview of research on effects of feedback on metacognition in kindergarten and elementary school. We first introduce how feedback may affect learning and metacognition, by using Efklides' models on metacognition and self-regulated learning. Further, because children's ability to process feedback seems to depend on their cognitive and metacognitive development, we discuss how the content of the feedback message could be developmentally appropriate, such that it matches children's cognitive development. We then address research findings on effects of teachers' feedback, internal task feedback, and peer feedback on children's metacognition. Finally, the chapter describes open questions and directions for future research.

Keywords Metacognition · Monitoring · Control · Feedback · Development · Education

8.1 Children's Metacognition and Self-Regulated Learning

Nowadays, children grow up in a more and more complex world, a world that expects them to learn through multiple media, digital and analog, and to achieve increasingly demanding learning goals. In fact, today more than ever before, learning means more than just acquiring knowledge; it requires strategic application of knowledge and skills to meet demands under, as yet, complex and unknown circumstances. This is why education not only aims to focus children on the learning content, but also on 'learning-to-learn'. In other words, and ideally, children need to become self-regulated learners.

M. H. van Loon (✉) · C. M. Roebers
Department of Developmental Psychology, University of Bern, Bern, Switzerland
e-mail: mariette.vanloon@psy.unibe.ch

D. Moraitou, P. Metallidou (eds.), *Trends and Prospects in Metacognition Research across the Life Span*, https://doi.org/10.1007/978-3-030-51673-4_8

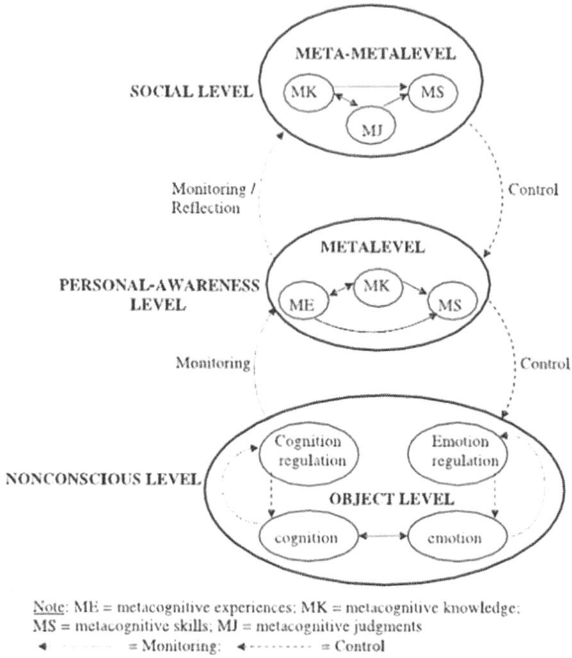

Fig. 8.1 Efklides' (2008) extended model of metacognition

Both experts in the field of self-regulated learning but also teachers agree that a core competence within self-regulated learning concerns metacognition. Nelson and Narens (1990) describe a model of metacognition, consisting of an object level (one's current state of knowledge and learning of the task at hand) and a metalevel (where thinking about the object level and adapting the object level take place through monitoring and control). To accurately monitor learning, individuals have to recognize how their metacognitive experiences, such as feelings of knowing, familiarity, ease of remembering, and varying degrees of certainty and uncertainty are related to their actual learning progress. Ideally, an individual has a set of adaptive metacognitive skills and strategies to effectively control their learning. This could concern monitoring-based allocation of study time, re-study selections, or withdrawal of incorrect answers.

The extended model of metacognition by Efklides (2008), depicted as Fig. 8.1, is based on the model of metacognition by Nelson and Narens (1990), and gives insights into the interplay between the object level and metalevel. Moreover, as can be seen in Fig. 8.1, the social level of metacognition affects the metalevel. In the present chapter, we will specifically focus on this extension of the original Nelson and Narens model, as it provides an ideal theoretical framework to investigate why and how teachers' co-monitoring and co-regulation of children's learning takes place. Efklides' model thereby conceptualizes that based on subjective judgments about a particular child's learning process and outcomes, teachers co-regulate children's learning. When guiding and steering children's learning, teachers give feedback to inform children about their performance, whether work on a task is going well or not, and how to proceed (Hattie and Timperley 2007). Thus, based on this model, the development of self-regulated learning skills in children also depends on the social level where feedback is—systematically or unsystematically—provided. Children have to actively interpret such feedback in relation to their own metacognition, their intrinsic goals, and also externally established tasks or educational goals (Butler and Winne 1995).

To support effective learning in and beyond the school context, children need support to learn how to monitor and control their learning. Teachers, and other interacting partners such as parents or peers, are an important source of support: They co-regulate learning by designing learning tasks and by giving feedback (Dignath and Büttner 2018; Vygotsky 1978). When aiming to investigate effects of feedback on children's metacognition, it is important to understand how metacognitive skills develop in childhood, as the effectiveness of feedback will largely depend on the degree to which metacognitive skills are developed. Since feedback affects children's metacognition, expanding our knowledge of effects of feedback on metacognitive experiences and metacognitive skills is crucial.

In this chapter, we specifically address effects of feedback on metacognition in kindergarten and elementary school. We first introduce how feedback may affect learning and metacognition, and discuss development of metacognition. We then address research on effects of feedback on children's metacognition; we distinguish between effects of teachers' feedback, internal task feedback, and peer feedback. Finally, we describe some questions for future research.

8.2 Effects of Feedback on Learning and Metacognition in School

Feedback informs students about how their present state of learning and performance relates to goals and standards (Nicol and Macfarlane-Dick 2006). When analyzing the content of feedback, this can be categorized on a continuum ranging from evaluative to descriptive (Skipper and Douglas 2015). Evaluative feedback expresses judgments about children's learning progress and performance according to norms, and this feedback can either be positive (confirming correct behavior and performance) or negative (pointing to errors). At the far end of the continuum, evaluative feedback focuses on correcting work or behavior. Further, evaluative feedback can go beyond disciplinary correction and be more neutral, by specifying what is wrong and addressing something to-be-learned. At the descriptive end of the continuum, feedback is rather focused on improvement and this relates more to competences. Such feedback can take many forms, such as giving hints and additional information, asking questions, providing extra study materials, and explaining correct answers (Shute 2008).

Research on the effects of feedback is done using very different methodological approaches, ranging from naturalistic classroom observations to experimental research comparing multiple feedback messages. For example, Skipper and Douglas (2015) investigated the content of feedback in the first years of elementary school. They showed that both evaluative and descriptive feedback is used by teachers in the classroom, across all curriculum subject areas. Classroom observation research by Eriksson et al. (2017) showed that evaluative feedback aimed at steering children by pointing out correct and incorrect performance was most frequently used by teachers. That is, when giving feedback, teachers often communicate that performance is assessed in accordance to norms (such as a correct or desirable answer, strategy, or behavior). They also observed that teachers regularly made use of descriptive feedback, aimed at promoting children's exploration discussions, and strategy use.

Both, theoretically and empirically, feedback is a significant factor in student learning. According to Hattie and Timperley (2007), feedback is one of the most powerful influences on learning and achievement, and meta-analyses by Black and Wiliam (1998) and Kluger and DeNisi (1996) found substantial effects of feedback on learning and school achievement across content areas, knowledge and skill types, as well as for different levels of education. However, the bulk of research on effects of feedback on learning investigates how feedback (flowing from the social level of metacognition) modifies children's object level (that is, their cognition and task performance). To benefit from feedback, learners must (a) know what good performance is, (b) have insights into how their current performance relates to good performance, and (c) know how to close the gap between current and good performance (Nicol and Macfarlane-Dick 2006; Sadler 1989). Importantly, in order to compare actual performance with performance goals, and to take action to close the gap, children must possess self-monitoring skills and they should be able to use these to control learning.

As visible in the extended model of metacognition by Efklides (Fig. 8.1), the social level of metacognition does not directly connect to a child's object level, but to the metalevel instead. That is, from this theoretical perspective, feedback and co-regulation of learning does not directly affect learning and cognition at the object level, but it does so indirectly, through the processes involved at the metalevel of metacognition. In other words, and from the theoretical perspective taken here, children may become aware through feedback that they are not studying the right way or that they are not yet understanding the learning content, and this may then lead them to control their learning and alter the content of the object level. This means that—ideally—teachers should thus use feedback to strengthen the self-monitoring skills of their students, so that students become able to better control their learning. However, although numerous studies investigate effects of feedback on cognition and performance, most of this research does not recognize and address whether and how feedback affects the metalevel of metacognition, that is, children's monitoring of metacognitive experiences and control of learning through application of metacognitive skills.

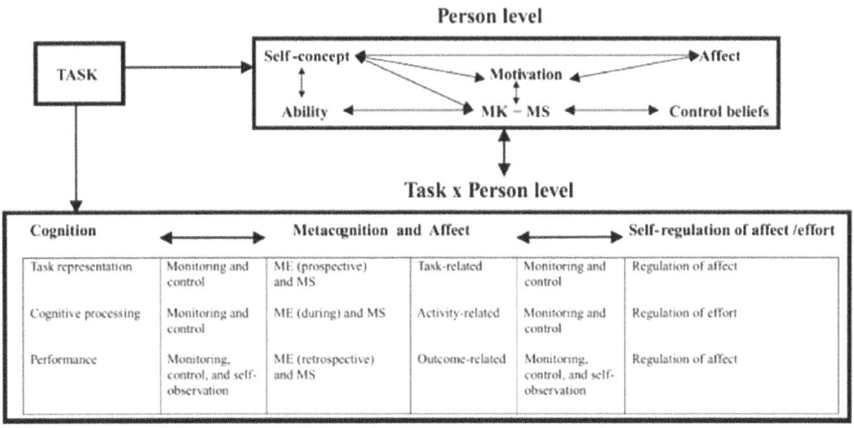

Fig. 8.2 The MASRL model (Efklides 2011)

To understand effects of feedback on metacognition in a broader self-regulated learning context, the metacognitive and affective model of self-regulated learning (MASRL model) by Efklides (2011), as shown in Fig. 8.2, can be helpful. This model explains how feedback can affect metacognition and learning when a person is working on a task. As shown in Fig. 8.2, this MASRL model comprises the task, general person characteristics, and the interaction between the person and the task. Person characteristics consist of cognitive and metacognitive components, but also motivational and affective components play an important role. When receiving feedback on learning, characteristics of the task and the person level interact. In this chapter, we describe research addressing this interaction, by investigating effects of feedback on monitoring (in the form of metacognitive experiences) and control (i.e., metacognitive skills). Thus, the main focus of this chapter is on effects of feedback on children's metacognition, which relates to the metacognitive component of the MASRL model.

8.3 Development of Metacognition and Children's Use of Feedback

8.3.1 Metacognitive Development During the Early Years of Schooling

During kindergarten and in elementary school, pronounced development takes place in children's ability to engage in metacognition and to use their metacognitive experiences and skills to guide self-regulated learning. In the pre-school and kindergarten years, one of children's most striking characteristics is their overoptimistic view of themselves; they believe that if they only try hard enough, they can succeed in almost all tasks (Lipko-Speed 2013; Lipowski et al. 2013). However, even though children are overly optimistic, their ability to self-monitor, the frequency of self-monitoring activities, and the ability to act based on monitoring outcomes develop gradually between the third and seventh year of life (Bryce and Whitebread 2012; Ghetti et al. 2013; Schneider and Löffler 2016). Using simple perceptual tasks, several studies showed that preschool children are in principle able to monitor their performance (Balcomb and Gerken 2008; Coughlin et al. 2015). For instance, Coughlin et al. (2015) asked 3-year-old children to complete a perceptual identification task and to indicate how confident they were that their responses were correct. Children were less confident about incorrect than correct responses. Further, children were more likely to seek help when they indicated that they were uncertain and this strategic help-seeking behavior improved task performance. At the same time, however, about 40–50% of children's confidence judgements and help-seeking decisions were inaccurate.

In the kindergarten years, also other facets of metacognition undergo developmental improvements. From the age of four onwards, children slowly learn to distinguish partial knowledge from full knowledge (Kim et al. 2016; Rohwer et al. 2012). That is, the ability to discriminate between gradations of (un)certainty begins to emerge (Flavell 2000). Further, children's sensitivity to task difficulty develops; children become less confident about performance for difficult than for easy task items (Geurten et al. 2015; Paulus et al. 2014). However, even though rudimentary signs of self-monitoring skills emerge and are detectable in the pre-school and kindergarten years, children's discrimination between correct and incorrect performance is far from perfect, and remains extensively overconfident (Destan and Roebers 2015; Rohwer et al. 2012; Destan et al. 2017).

During the early elementary school years, children gradually become less overconfident (Lipko et al. 2009; Roebers 2014) and improve their discrimination between correct and incorrect responses (Hembacher and Ghetti 2014). Particularly, children become better aware of errors (Destan et al. 2014), and between 5 and 6 years of age, they become sensitive to the fact that errors can occur because responses may be based on guessing rather than actual knowledge (Rohwer et al. 2012). However, these emerging skills are fragile; children's ability to monitor and control learning largely depends on the type of task. That is, children's ability to monitor more complex memory-related performance seems to improve even more slowly (Roebers 2014). With use of a task for which children had to learn Japanese symbols (*Kanji*) with their meaning, Destan et al. (2014) showed that 5- and 6-year-old children could differentiate between correct and incorrect performance at a recognition test, and that monitoring affected control, such that children spent more time studying hard than easy items, and were more likely to withdraw incorrect rather than correct responses to improve their test answers. Again however, despite these signs of emerging skills, inaccurate (overoptimistic) monitoring and inefficient control decisions were frequent.

Further development in monitoring and control is visible in the elementary and the secondary school years (Schneider and Löffler 2016). When using simple learning materials (e.g., when learning vocabulary or correcting spelling errors), monitoring skills appear to be effectively developed by the age of eight (Roebers and Spiess 2017). However, for more complex learning tasks that require conceptual understanding and comprehension of cause-and-effect relations, skills to monitor learning seem to develop only between the age of 10 and 12 (De Bruin et al. 2011). Importantly, during the course of elementary school, the beneficial effect of accurate monitoring on control of learning becomes more pronounced (Metcalfe and Finn 2008; Roebers 2017), rending metacognitive skills into the center of self-regulated learning activities. From the age of ten onwards, children seem to become increasingly able to strategically focus attention on, and allocate study time to difficult or not-yet-learned items (Dufresne and Kobasigawa 1989). This relationship between monitoring and control continues to grow at least until late adolescence (Crone and Steinbeis 2017; Metcalfe and Finn 2013).

8.3.2 Why Does Metacognition Develop?

Through brain maturation and through repeated experiences with tasks, instructions, co-regulation, and feedback, children continuously learn to better monitor and control learning (Efklides and Tsiora 2002; Roebers et al. 2019). Based on behavioral data, research on this issue proposes two main, not mutually exclusive explanations for children's development of metacognition. Firstly, when children grow older, they are less biased by self-protective factors. Young children base their self-monitoring on their desire for good performance, and their monitoring judgments indicate their wishes for correct performance, even when actual performance is incorrect (i.e., they exhibit a wishful thinking bias, Schneider 1998; Shin et al. 2007; Stipek 1984). Further, young children strongly believe in effort as a means to be successful, and disregard their actual ability and the difficulty of the tasks to complete (Destan et al. 2017; Nicholls 1978; Stipek 1984). This is for instance demonstrated by their tendency to think that they will receive credit points for incorrect task responses (Destan et al. 2017). Reliance on self-protection is assumed to keep the motivation to learn high and thus to be adaptive, especially early in development. During the course of elementary school, children become less prone to conflating effort with ability (Kurtz-Costes et al. 2005). This reduced sensitivity to self-protective biases and improvement in taking actual performance into account seems—at least in part—to explain developmental progression in metacognitive skills.

A further explanation for children's improved monitoring accuracy is the fine-tuning of their ability to use valid experiential cues as a basis for their metacognitive judgments. Cues such as study time, experienced ease of studying, the ease with which information comes to mind when making a retrieval attempt (retrieval fluency, accessibility), and one's ability to apply studied information in a novel context can all be valid indicators of actual understanding and performance (Koriat 1997; Roebers et al. 2019; Van Loon et al. 2013). Throughout elementary school, children detect valid cues and can distinguish them increasingly well from invalid cues (e.g., font size), and become more skilled to strategically use valid instead of invalid cues while monitoring (Van Loon et al. 2017a, b; Koriat et al. 2009). For instance, although kindergarten children seem somewhat sensitive to experiences of task difficulty (Geurten et al. 2015; Destan et al. 2017), children's use of task difficulty cues improves extensively during elementary school (Paulus et al. 2014). Moreover, from the age of ten onwards, children begin to strategically base judgments on cues that are related to their study and retrieval experiences (Van Loon et al. 2017a, b). Yet, children's monitoring and control of their increasingly demanding learning, remains often inaccurate, making research on potential effects of feedback very relevant.

8.3.3 Ensuring Developmentally Appropriate Feedback

Because inaccurate metacognition has disadvantages for children's learning in the educational context (Destan and Roebers 2015; Rinne and Mazzocco 2014; Zhang and Whitebread 2017), feedback should support them to improve their monitoring and control. Feedback has been described as an important factor for enhancing metacognition (Efklides 2006), and children as young as kindergartners seem to be sensitive to feedback on performance and use this to adapt their monitoring judgments (Muis et al. 2015; Destan et al. 2017; Van Loon and Roebers, under review). Particularly in the early years of schooling, children are very dependent on external feedback, as development is still in the early stages. Therefore, younger and inexperienced children may benefit from direct and detailed feedback from their teachers. In contrast, older and more experienced children, with further developed metacognitive skills, may already take more control over their own learning, and teachers may offer feedback when children seek for it (Collins et al. 1988).

Based on the insights into children's development of metacognition, assumptions can be made about how the content of the feedback message could match children's developmental stage. From the age of four onwards, it seems likely that feedback could help kindergartners to increasingly consider task difficulty. From the age of five onwards, feedback addressing the difference between guessing and knowing is likely to be understood. Moreover, at this age, simple, evaluative feedback, informing how performance compares to standards, may be helpful to improve metacognition. Kindergarten children seem well able to base their metacognitive judgments (and specifically their error recognition) on feedback addressing performance when solving reasoning tasks (Van Loon and Roebers, under review) as well as memory tasks (Destan et al. 2017). When children begin to differentiate ability from effort, performance feedback can have even stronger effects on the self-regulated learning process (Schunk 1984). In the later years of elementary school, approximately from age ten onwards, descriptive feedback to guide children to focus on their learning competences and on cues related to their learning progress (e.g., the ease of learning, ease of retrieval, and one's ability to apply the learned information) is likely to be helpful. Moreover, after the age of 10, feedback could guide children on how to use their monitoring to make strategic study decisions.

8.3.4 Working Memory Capacity Affects Feedback Processing

Importantly, to ensure that children optimally benefit from feedback, children's information processing capacity should be taken into account. When working on a task, attending to external feedback competes for additional working memory resources (Schooler and Anderson 1990). That is, children need to flexibly shift attention from ongoing task activities to the content of the feedback, so they can update their task understanding and their insights into the progress they are making. There are large individual differences in working memory between children at any age, and working memory capacity has a substantial effect on school achievement (Alloway and Alloway 2010). Working memory capacity is limited (even more so for kindergartners and young elementary school children as for adults), and therefore, feedback processing may be very challenging (Gathercole et al. 2006; Strasser and Del Rio 2014). Effects of working memory capacity on feedback processing has been demonstrated by Fyfe et al. (2015), who provided young elementary school children (6–9-year-olds) with feedback on their strategy use and task outcomes during completion of problem-solving tasks. Working memory capacity was positively related to their ability to improve performance after receiving feedback. Moreover, Van Loon and Roebers (under review) showed that kindergartners' working memory capacity also predicted the extent to which they were able to make use of feedback to improve their monitoring accuracy. From these studies can be concluded that feedback is most helpful when it is sufficiently simple, so that it can be processed easily without bringing too much cognitive load (Shute 2008).

8.4 Effective Feedback to Improve Children's Monitoring and Control

To benefit from feedback, this needs to give children a true picture of their performance. Even though it is important that feedback points out successes, children seem well able to also deal with negative feedback on errors (Dweck 1999). Research comparing effects of positive and negative feedback on children's reasoning abilities showed that negative feedback concerning erroneous task performance yielded the greatest learning benefits (Ball et al. 2010; Muldoon et al. 2007). In addition to improving performance, pointing out errors can benefit monitoring accuracy for children as young as kindergartners (Van Loon and Roebers, under review). Importantly, to help children to discriminate between errors and correct performance, feedback seems most effective when it addresses item-specific performance. Aggregate feedback on learning seems less helpful because it does not inform the individual about how well they did for particular items (Pashler et al. 2005). The assumption that such general feedback about overall task performance may not be used as well as item-specific feedback is strengthened by studies in which kindergartners who memorized items repeatedly received aggregate feedback about the number of correctly remembered items. Children remained overconfident and did not take the feedback into consideration when predicting their performance for subsequent tasks (Lipko et al. 2009, 2012; Lipko-Speed 2013; Schneider 1998).

Moreover, feedback timing appears to influence feedback effects. Immediate feedback that is given during, or immediately after children work on the assigned tasks seems more preferable than delayed feedback, particularly when completing complex tasks (Kulik and Kulik 1988; Webb et al. 1997). Delayed feedback after task completion only seems to be effective when completing relatively simple tasks that do not present too many cognitive demands.

8.4.1 Effects of Teacher Feedback

In the school context, it is most often the teacher who passes on feedback messages to children, by telling them about correct performance and errors, and about strengths and weaknesses in their work. According to Hattie and Timperley (2007), feedback has most potential when students are informed about their learning process, and paths towards meeting tasks goals, rather than only addressing learning outcomes. That is, feedback may be most helpful when it supports children to explore the way towards correct solutions, rather than having a focus on whether performance is correct or incorrect. For children, as young as kindergartners, feedback aiming to support children's task exploration, rather than direct feedback on children's learning actions, leads to most improvements in learning and transfer (Weisberg et al. 2016). When supporting explorative learning, teachers give feedback in line with the principles of child-centered teaching (Lerkkanen et al. 2016). Rather than focusing children's attention on learning outcomes, such feedback aims to support children's learning through discovery of the task (Bonawitz et al. 2011). This way, children are helped to focus on task dimensions of interest, in order to reach the goals and standards. When using such an indirect, child-centered feedback approach, teachers could, for instance, highlight learning goals, or encourage children to question. Another way to guide children to explore reasons for why they are doing well or making mistakes is by giving them feedback and asking them to self-explain the feedback. When 6–7-year-old children completed a problem-solving task, giving feedback about performance alongside asking to self-explain why performance was correct or incorrect had most benefits on learning (Cheshire et al. 2005).

However, although these studies indicate that child-centered feedback practice can improve learning performance and transfer, to our knowledge, only one study connects teacher feedback to children's monitoring and control of learning. Van Loon et al. (under review) showed that child-centered feedback practice might improve performance as well as metacognition. With a classroom observation study, it was investigated how 21 teachers' classroom instructions and feedback affected 8 and 10-year-old elementary school children's metacognitive monitoring (in terms of confidence judgments), and their control of learning (measured with restudy selections). Although all teachers used teacher-directed and child-centered feedback styles, teacher-directed feedback was more common, such that teachers most often explicitly told children what to work on and how to use strategies. However, in the classes in which child-centered feedback was given more often, not only task performance, but also metacognition benefitted. That is, giving child-centered feedback (i.e., using feedback to guide children to explore and experience the task themselves) was related to more accurate monitoring and more adaptive restudy selections. Moreover, although the advantage of child-centered feedback was shown for both grades, effects were more pronounced for older children; this may indicate that they were more skilled to take control over their own learning, and therefore, they may have profited even more.

8.4.2 Designing Tasks with Feedback Opportunities to Improve Monitoring and Control

To support metacognition with a child-centered and individualized approach, teachers could create tasks that give students frequent opportunities to acquire internal task feedback. A few studies with elementary school children showed that asking them to complete so-called generation tasks after learning seems to be a useful way to support improvement of monitoring and subsequent control. With generation tasks, children try to apply the studied information. By doing this, they generate internal task feedback about their understanding of the learned content. Van Loon et al. (2017a, b) showed that from age 10 onwards, children are able to strategically base their monitoring judgments on cues derived from their generation task experiences. Research by Van Loon et al. (2013) investigated effects of delayed sentence generation instructions on 9–12-year-olds metacognition when studying complex idiomatic phrases. After learning the idioms and their meanings, they were asked to make novel sentences in which they applied the studied idioms. Children who generated sentences were better able to self-monitor and control their learning (by selecting idioms for restudy) than children who did not generate sentences. That is, through these generative activities, they acquired internal task feedback which helped them to judge what they understood well, and what had not yet been learned well and thus needed further study.

Further, from the age of 10 onwards, generation of keywords and summaries can be another useful tool for children to generate their own feedback and thus to acquire insights into whether they understood and are able to apply studied textual information (De Bruin et al. 2011). It is important to note, though, that such self-generated feedback only seems to have a beneficial effect on monitoring and control when generation tasks are done after a delay, rather than during or immediately after study. This effect of the timing of generation is shown when comparing studies by De Bruin et al. (2011) and Engelen et al. (2018). Both studies used the same type of materials and tested the same age group (12-year-olds): Children had to study complex texts containing information about details as well as causality. Then they were asked to self-generate task feedback by either writing down keywords or making summaries about the studied texts. In the study by De Bruin et al. (2011), the generation tasks were completed delayed, and these tasks improved metacognitive monitoring (as indicated by the relation between subjective judgments of learning and objective test performance per text) and control (as measured with the effectiveness of restudy selections). However, in the study by Engelen et al. (2018), children generated keywords or summaries immediately after reading, and no improvement of monitoring and control was shown. Presumably, only after a delay, children self-test their comprehension and application skills with these generation tasks. This way, they self-generate feedback to acquire metacognitive experiences indicating to what extent they really remember and understand the learned information. When they complete such tasks during or immediately after study, they are not yet testing these skills, but instead, they can rely more on the accessibility of learned details in working memory (Thiede et al. 2005).

Another way to give children systematic opportunities to use feedback for improving their monitoring and control is by asking them to self-test their understanding, and then provide them with feedback in the form of expected standards (i.e., showing what correct performance consists of). For kindergartners, inspecting computer feedback indicating whether responses were correct or incorrect improved judgments about performance on a memory task (Destan et al. 2017). For second graders, such feedback after self-testing had even more beneficial effects on their ability to monitor performance than for kindergartners, again pointing out the importance of developmentally appropriate feedback. For older elementary school children, feedback standards can also support them to monitor the quality of open-ended test responses. Van Loon and Roebers (2017) asked 10–12-year-old children to study difficult concepts, to take a self-test, to judge the quality of their performance and to make restudy selections. Then, they presented them with feedback standards and asked children again to judge their test performance and to select items for restudy. The feedback standards had strong benefits on children's monitoring accuracy and their subsequent control decisions. However, this kind of feedback will only be useful to improve metacognition when it gives sufficient detail about the ideas that the children should have mentioned in their self-test responses (Lipko et al. 2009; Miller and Geraci 2011). This way, children can become aware of the discrepancies between their actual performance and the learning goals, and feedback can then be a helpful tool to support recognition and correction of errors (Hattie and Timperley 2007; Mory 2004).

However, although inspection of feedback standards improved monitoring and control for elementary school children (Van Loon and Roebers 2017), even after receiving feedback, children often expected that they would receive more credit points for their responses than they would objectively receive. This suggests that children were not always detecting errors when using feedback, indicating that in some cases feedback is ignored, rejected, or even re-interpreted such that it fits committed errors (Mory 2004).

8.4.3 Studies on Peer Feedback

There are indications that metacognition may benefit even more when children engage in collaborative scoring activities together with their peers, rather than in self-scoring activities only. One valuable approach to support students' monitoring and control is to give children opportunities to provide feedback on each other's work. Children who have just learned something may be able to explain this to their peers in a comprehensive language. And by giving peer feedback, children may develop the skills to make accurate judgments, and these skills may be transferred when they are in turn asked to monitor and control their own learning (Okita 2014).

A study by Destan et al. (2017) asked kindergartners' and second grade elementary school children to judge memory task performance of themselves and of an unknown peer. To support children to judge the correctness of their answers on a recognition test with four alternatives, they were shown which of the alternatives was the correct response, and whether they had chosen this correct alternative. That is, the task was completed on a computer, and on the screen, they saw a black rectangle around the given response, and a green rectangle around the correct response. If the given response and the correct response did not match, this indicated that an error was made. Surprisingly, even after getting such unambiguous feedback, children in both age groups were still overconfident when judging the quality of their responses. However, when making judgments for peers, children were more accurate in their discrimination between correct and incorrect responses. Presumably, because monitoring judgments are—at least in part—based on self-serving and self-protective biases, when monitoring performance of peers, more objective reasoning about performance quality may occur (Efklides 2008; Koriat and Ackerman 2010; Thomas and Jacoby 2013). This seems to explain why children are better able to use feedback about response correctness when judging peers.

For older elementary school children (age 9–13), a study by Van Loon and Van de Pol (2019) investigated whether children are also able to make use of feedback when judging their peers' performance to open-ended questions. Particularly on open-ended tests, commission errors (i.e., entirely incorrect responses) are hard to detect and correct. Children studied difficult concepts, took a test, and then they were provided with feedback standards which described the ideal correct responses would consist of. With use of these standards, children then scored their own and their peers' test responses. Findings showed that children better recognized others' errors than their own mistakes, indicating that they were more eager to catch their peers' than their own errors. However, even though the accuracy of self-score judgments was better for peers' errors than for own mistakes, the accuracy of self-score judgments for correct responses was lower for peers than for oneself. That is, children were stricter when scoring responses of their peers, which led to underestimation of peer performance when responses were partially or fully correct.

Findings suggesting that children are able to use feedback standards indicate that performance feedback does not always need to be provided by teachers. When aiming to target correct recognition and correction of errors, designing collaborative learning and feedback activities during which children have to score each other's answers may be promising. When using online tutoring systems, making use of peer feedback could potentially be helpful to give children insight into how well they are progressing on tasks. Online tutoring systems can give detailed performance feedback when using multiple-choice questions and when learning memory materials (such as when learning second language vocabulary). When more complex learning materials are used and students have to show that they understood the gist, such systems are less effective in giving feedback. Peer feedback may be more useful with such kinds of more complex tasks. However, although peer-scoring activities are potentially useful to improve monitoring and control of learning, when using such activities, teachers have to keep in mind that children may sometimes be very strict concerning their peers' performance. Therefore, teachers should instruct children how to use scoring criteria, and closely monitor the quality of self and peer scoring.

8.5 Open Questions and Directions for Future Research

The abovementioned research shows that feedback can improve monitoring and control, and that effects of feedback may depend on the child's metacognitive development. It has to be noted, though, that research on effects of feedback on young children's metacognitive experiences and metacognitive skills is very limited. Therefore, future research should continue with efforts to clarify how feedback can be most efficient in supporting children with individualized, differential learning across development. We specifically consider three points important for future research: Addressing (a) the accuracy of teachers' monitoring and control of children's learning, (b) effects of metacognitive, rather than cognitive feedback and, (c) the complex interplay between metacognition and motivation.

8.5.1 Teachers' Metacognitive Accuracy

As shown in Fig. 8.1, teachers' perceptions (as well as perceptions of others who provide feedback) give input to co-regulation of, and feedback on children's learning processes (Salonen et al. 2005). To give adaptive and appropriate feedback, teachers should thus have accurate insight into students' changing needs. That is, not only children, but also teachers need to have accurate metacognition. However, the few studies addressing teachers' monitoring accuracy of elementary school children's learning seem to indicate that teachers often do not have insight into their students' metacognitive experiences. Although teachers are fairly accurate when making single judgments per student about their average performance and their grades (Südkamp et al. 2012), in these studies, teachers only provided one single judgment per child. To give effective feedback when guiding students how to proceed with tasks, teachers should be able to discriminate between occasions when work is going well, and occasions when students are not working well towards goals (Van de Pol et al. 2011). However, it seems challenging for teachers to make detailed and accurate estimations about children's learning progress.

There are only two studies investigating whether teachers can perceive differences between well-learned and less-learned materials on the side of the students, one study with elementary school children aged 10–13 (Engelen et al. 2018) and one study with adolescents (aged 14) in secondary school (Van de Pol et al. 2019). In these studies, children were reading texts, and findings show that teachers could not accurately judge the differences in their students' text-by-text test performance. Teachers do not seem to have insights into children's awareness of task difficulty, nor into the effort children put into learning (Salonen et al. 2005), that is, they may not have access to valid cues related to children's learning experiences and outcomes. Moreover, a study by Van Loon et al. (under review) shows that for teachers, it is more difficult to predict children's performance on unfamiliar tasks (learning Japanese symbols) than for more familiar tasks (studying texts). This strengthens the assumption that it is often challenging for teachers to acquire insight into cues that are predictive of children's actual learning.

Interestingly, Van de Pol et al. (2019) tried to improve teachers' insights into cues related to 14-year-old adolescents' text comprehension. They asked students to complete a generation task after reading texts, by making diagrams about causal events in the texts. This intervention improved students' monitoring. Then teachers were asked to inspect student diagrams, and, based on this, to decide for each student which texts needed further study. Inspecting the diagrams provided teachers with cues about students' intra-individual text comprehension, as indicated by the finding that they made more adaptive restudy selections for students for which diagrams were inspected than for students for which they did not see the diagrams. This research may be a promising first step towards the design of feedback interventions to not only trying to improve student metacognition, but also targeting teacher metacognition and the quality of individualized feedback. Taken together, there are many reasons to investigate how teachers can get more insight into students' metacognition and learning for different types of tasks.

8.5.2 Distinguishing Between Cognitive and Metacognitive Feedback

In the research described in this chapter, feedback addressed children's cognition, i.e., their performance and their progress towards task standards and learning goals. However, potentially, feedback addressing children's metacognition could also benefit monitoring and control, and probably even more so than feedback on cognition itself. Indeed, for adults, such metacognitive feedback has been shown to decrease overconfidence when predicting exam scores (Callender et al. 2016; Nietfeld et al. 2006). There are a few studies that give insight into whether metacognitive feedback may also be suitable for young children; however, findings of these studies are mixed and do not seem to show an ubiquitous benefit of metacognitive feedback over and beyond cognitive feedback.

Geurten and Meulemans (2017) asked children aged four to eight to memorize items and to evaluate their memory performance. Then, children received aggregate metacognitive feedback addressing to what extent the number of remembered task items matched their subjective judgment. Although this feedback led children to lower their judgments about performance on subsequent tasks, it did not improve monitoring accuracy. That is, children rather seemed to base the lowering of their judgments on an anchoring heuristic, without taking the task characteristics and their performance into account.

In a study by Van Loon and Roebers (under review), effects of item-specific cognitive feedback were compared with effects of metacognitive feedback. Kindergarten children (age five to six) completed analogical reasoning tasks, for which they had to match image pairs. After matching each pair, children made a monitoring judgment, with which they indicated whether they thought the match was correct or not. Then, some children received cognitive feedback, i.e., they were told whether their response was correct. Other children were assigned to a metacognitive feedback group; these children were informed whether their subjective judgments matched their objective performance (i.e., whether their monitoring judgments were correct or not). Children who received metacognitive feedback became better at recognizing their errors, but at the same time, they also became more cautious and more often judged their correct performance as incorrect. This may also indicate that they based judgments on an anchoring heuristic, and generally lowered these without taking their actual performance into account. Further, the metacognitive feedback group had lower task performance than the cognitive feedback group.

A kindergarten observation by Muñoz and Santa Cruz (2016) suggested that feedback aiming to stimulate metacognitive reflection on how tasks are carried out led to more planning, monitoring, and evaluation processes. However, also in this study, children's task performance did not improve as a result of metacognitive feedback. Possibly, for young children, it is too difficult to process the metacognitive feedback; dealing with information about performance and monitoring when at the same time paying attention to the task at hand may pose too many demands.

It is not yet clear from what age on metacognitive feedback will yield to positive effects; even for secondary school children, processing this type of feedback may be very demanding. Roll et al. (2011) investigated effects of metacognitive feedback on adolescents' help-seeking skills and on their performance when working on a computerized geometry learning task. After receiving metacognitive feedback, students took more time to read information, and their help-seeking for errors improved. However, also in this research, these changes in learning behavior did not lead to improved task performance. Considering the differences between research findings on effects of metacognitive feedback for adults and young learners, future research could further investigate how task conditions and developmental level can explain to what extent metacognitive feedback may benefit monitoring, control, and also ultimately learning outcomes.

8.5.3 Accounting for Interactions Between Metacognition and Motivation

Although metacognition plays an important role for self-regulated learning processes (Dunlosky and Rawson 2012), as can be derived from the MASRL model (Fig. 8.2), only aiming to improve metacognition does not seem sufficient to ensure effective learning. The motivational component of self-regulated learning predicts to what extent learners are willing to monitor their learning, to base their control on their monitoring, and to make use of feedback to reach learning goals. Learners' experiences of control, their feelings of competence, their beliefs about the value of reaching task goals, and their emotions provide the basis for appraisals of the learning task, metacognition, and feedback (Pekrun 2006; Ryan and Deci 2017). Efklides (2011) states that motivation to learn seems to be explained by learners' goal orientations (i.e., whether they learn for mastery or to show good performance), their expectancy-value beliefs, their self-concept, affect and emotions, and volition. Viewing feedback solely as a process through which monitoring and control of learning can be adapted ignores the way feedback also impacts motivation and affect. In addition to having effects on metacognition, feedback affects emotions (such as interest, joy, pride, curiosity, surprise and confusion), and motivational beliefs, which in turn influence what and how children work on tasks (Dweck 1999; Efklides 2016). Further, emotions and motivational beliefs can also affect the way children interpret feedback messages (e.g., an explanation why feedback on failures may not be used well to improve self-monitoring may be due to wishes to maintain perceptions of self-efficacy).

Although research on interactions between feedback, metacognition, and motivation is very limited for young children, there is no doubt that one's motivation to learn may affect one's interpretation of feedback and moderates how feedback affects metacognition and learning. Although negative feedback seems to decrease students' feelings of confidence and increase their experiences of difficulty (Efklides and Dina 2007), effects of feedback on metacognition may depend on motivational factors such as goal orientations and feelings of competence. A study by Dina and Efklides (2009) with 12–14-year-olds showed that students with performance avoidance goal orientations and low experiences of competence may not be open for feedback, because this can reveal that they are not performing well. Instead, students with high self-efficacy and performance goal orientations seem to be open for feedback, because this communicates to them that they are proceeding well towards goals. These students are then likely to use the feedback for control of learning, by effectively allocating and increasing learning effort.

8.6 To Conclude: How Can We Use Feedback to Improve Metacognition?

Clearly, future research investigating how to support teachers to give appropriate feedback is warranted. This research could pay attention to the feedback message and feedback content, and clarify how effects of feedback depend on the type of tasks, as well as developmental differences and individual differences in children's processing capacity. Despite the necessity to further examine these issues, the research findings summarized in this chapter integrate insights into risks and benefits of feedback and may bring suggestions about how to improve feedback practice in the educational setting.

Children's ability to process feedback seems to depend on their cognitive and metacognitive development. Feedback for young children seems mainly helpful when it draws their attention to ability and performance, whereas feedback for older children can also focus them on their learning experiences, and how these cues can be indicative of their progress towards task goals. Further, feedback seems only useful when it gives detailed information about how children are progressing on their tasks, so that children can learn to discriminate between subtasks for which progress is going well, and tasks for which they made mistakes or got stuck. Questioning, guiding, and asking children to explain reasons for correct performance and errors may help to engage in metacognition, and to transfer insights when working on novel tasks. After receiving feedback, children should be able to use the acquired insights as a basis for their control of learning, such as selection of learning strategies and actions. Feedback can only benefit learning, in the short and longer term, when children repeatedly get the opportunity to make use of it to improve self-regulation.

Teachers have a high workload, and finding the time to give individualized, child-appropriate feedback that meets actual learning requirements may often be challenging. It is therefore valuable to consider who provides the feedback, in relation to its effectiveness in supporting metacognition. Collaborative peer-learning and peer-feedback activities seem promising for children as young as kindergartners, since children are better able to recognize others' than their own mistakes. From mid-elementary school onwards, children also seem well able to distinguish between different gradations of response quality. Further, for older elementary school children, teachers can design tasks such that children can get internal task feedback. Teachers may, for instance, tell children to self-test their learning, and then give children feedback standards to compare their responses with, so they can monitor to what extent they reached learning goals. Further, children could complete generation tasks after studying, to acquire internal task feedback about whether and to what extent they are able to apply the studied information.

To conclude, the Efklides' models on metacognition and self-regulated learning provides an excellent framework for investigating mechanisms of self-regulated learning as well as for exploring how aspects of the social context impact metacognitive skills. In this chapter, we have focused on effects of feedback on children's metacognitive skills. We have discussed several lines of research, and distinguished between externally provided and internally generated feedback. Effects of feedback have been shown to be substantial, underscoring that the extension of the original Nelson and Narens' model (1990) on metacognition proposed by Efklides (2008) has been useful. We are positive that it will further influence research efforts by allowing a differentiated view on the social context in which metacognitive processes take place. The empirical evidence clearly suggests that metacognition is not only bound to its object or task level but has to be understood and investigated within larger contexts. At the same time, the Efklides' models are not primarily developmental; that is, they are not conceptualized for theoretically framing metacognitive development *per se*. Yet, from our view, they bear important developmental aspects that may be helpful to stimulate future research. As we have outlined, children's cue utilization stems from metacognitive experiences, that is, different cues related to the social or task context inform monitoring and subsequent control. Moreover, in this chapter we have strongly emphasized the critical aspect of taking individual differences in learners' skills into account. In the course of children's development, metacognitive monitoring and control skills improve and consequently, feedback provided in the social context needs to match these changing skills. In this specific respect, research is still in its early stages, but we are convinced that Efklides' impact on the field of metacognitive development and educational practices will be long lasting.

References

Alloway, T. P., & Alloway, R. G. (2010). Investigating the predictive roles of working memory and IQ in academic attainment. *Journal of Experimental Child Psychology, 106*, 20–29.

Balcomb, F. K., & Gerken, L. (2008). Three-year-old children can access their own memory to guide responses on a visual matching task. *Developmental Science, 11*, 750–760.

Ball, L. J., Hoyle, A. M., & Towse, A. S. (2010). The facilitatory effect of negative feedback on the emergence of analogical reasoning abilities. *British Journal of Developmental Psychology, 28*, 583–602.

Black, P., & Wiliam, D. (1998). Assessment and classroom learning. *Assessment in Education: Principles, Policy and Practice, 5*, 7–74.

Bonawitz, E., Shafto, P., Gweon, H., Goodman, N. D., Spelke, E., & Schulz, L. (2011). The double-edged sword of pedagogy: Instruction limits spontaneous exploration and discovery. *Cognition, 120*, 322–330.

Bryce, D., & Whitebread, D. (2012). The development of metacognitive skills: Evidence from observational analysis of young children's behavior during problem-solving. *Metacognition and Learning, 7*, 197–217.

Butler, D. L., & Winne, P. H. (1995). Feedback and self-regulated learning: A theoretical synthesis. *Review of Educational Research, 65*, 245–281.

Callender, A. A., Franco-Watkins, A. M., & Roberts, A. S. (2016). Improving metacognition in the classroom through instruction, training, and feedback. *Metacognition and Learning, 11*, 215–235.

Cheshire, A., Ball, L. J., & Lewis, C. N. (2005). Self-explanation, feedback and the development of analogical reasoning skills: Microgenetic evidence for a metacognitive processing account. In B. G. Bara, L. W. Barsalou, & M. Bucciarellli (Eds.), *Proceedings of the twenty-seventh annual conference of the cognitive science society* (pp. 435–441). Mahwah: Lawrence Erlbaum Associates.

Collins, A., Brown, J. S., & Newman, S. E. (1988). Cognitive apprenticeship: Teaching the craft of reading, writing and mathematics. *Thinking: The Journal of Philosophy for Children, 8*, 2–10.

Coughlin, C., Hembacher, E., Lyons, K. E., & Ghetti, S. (2015). Introspection on uncertainty and judicious help-seeking during the preschool years. *Developmental Science, 18*, 957–971.

Crone, E. A., & Steinbeis, N. (2017). Neural perspectives on cognitive control development during childhood and adolescence. *Trends in Cognitive Sciences, 21*, 205–215.

De Bruin, A. B. H., Thiede, K. W., Camp, G., & Redford, J. (2011). Generating keywords improves metacomprehension and self-regulation in elementary and middle school children. *Journal of Experimental Child Psychology, 109*, 294–310.

Destan, N., & Roebers, C. M. (2015). What are the metacognitive costs of young children's overconfidence? *Metacognition and Learning, 10*, 347–374.

Destan, N., Hembacher, E., Ghetti, S., & Roebers, C. M. (2014). Early metacognitive abilities: The interplay of monitoring and control processes in 5- to 7-year-old children. *Journal of Experimental Child Psychology, 126*, 213–228.

Destan, N., Spiess, M. A., De Bruin, A., Van Loon, M., & Roebers, C. M. (2017). 6-and 8-year-olds' performance evaluations: Do they differ between self and unknown others? *Metacognition and Learning, 12*, 315–336.

Dignath, C., & Büttner, G. (2018). Teachers' direct and indirect promotion of self-regulated learning in primary and secondary school mathematics classes–insights from video-based classroom observations and teacher interviews. *Metacognition and Learning, 13*, 127–157.

Dina, F., & Efklides, A. (2009). Student profiles of achievement goals, goal instructions and external feedback: Their effect on mathematical task performance and affect. *European Journal of Education and Psychology, 2*, 235–262.

Dufresne, A., & Kobasigawa, A. (1989). Children's spontaneous allocation of study time: Differential and sufficient aspects. *Journal of Experimental Child Psychology, 47*, 274–296.

Dunlosky, J., & Rawson, K. A. (2012). Overconfidence produces underachievement: Inaccurate self evaluations undermine students' learning and retention. *Learning and Instruction, 22*, 271–280.

Dweck, C. S. (1999). Caution-praise can be dangerous. *American Educator, 23*, 4–9.

Efklides, A. (2006). Metacognitive experiences: The missing link in the self-regulated learning process. *Educational Psychology Review, 18*, 287–291.

Efklides, A. (2008). Metacognition: Defining its facets and levels of functioning in relation to self-regulation and co-regulation. *European Psychologist, 13*, 277–287.

Efklides, A. (2011). Interactions of metacognition with motivation and affect in self-regulated learning: The MASRL model. *Educational Psychologist, 46*, 6–25.

Efklides, A. (2016). Metamemory and affect. In J. Dunlosky & S. U. K. Tauber (Eds.), *The Oxford handbook of metamemory* (pp. 245–168). Oxford: Oxford University Press.
Efklides, A., & Dina, F. (2007). Is mastery orientation always beneficial for learning. In F. Salili & R. Hoosain (Eds.), *Culture, motivation and learning: A multicultural perspective* (pp. 131–168). Charlotte: Information Age Publishing.
Efklides, A., & Tsiora, A. (2002). Metacognitive experiences, self-concept, and self-regulation. *Psychologia, 45*, 222–236.
Engelen, J. A. A., Camp, G., Van de Pol, J., & De Bruin, A. B. H. (2018). Teachers' monitoring of students' text comprehension: Can students' keywords and summaries improve teachers' judgment accuracy? *Metacognition and Learning, 13*, 287–307.
Eriksson, E., Björklund Boistrup, L., & Thornberg, R. (2017). A categorisation of teacher feedback in the classroom: A field study on feedback based on routine classroom assessment in primary school. *Research Papers in Education, 32*, 316–332.
Flavell, J. H. (2000). Development of children's knowledge about the mental world. *International Journal of Behavioral Development, 24*, 15–23.
Fyfe, E. R., DeCaro, M. S., & Rittle-Johnson, B. (2015). When feedback is cognitively-demanding: The importance of working memory capacity. *Instructional Science, 43*, 73–91.
Gathercole, S. E., Lamont, E., & Alloway, T. P. (2006). Working memory in the classroom. *Working Memory and Education, 21*, 219–240.
Geurten, M., & Meulemans, T. (2017). The effect of feedback on children's metacognitive judgments: A heuristic account. *Journal of Cognitive Psychology, 29*, 184–201.
Geurten, M., Willems, S., & Meulemans, T. (2015). Beyond the experience: Detection of metamemorial regularities. *Consciousness and Cognition, 33*, 16–23.
Ghetti, S., Hembacher, E., & Coughlin, C. A. (2013). Feeling uncertain and acting on it during the preschool years: A metacognitive approach. *Child Development Perspectives, 7*, 160–165.
Hattie, J., & Timperley, H. (2007). The power of feedback. *Review of Educational Research, 77*, 81–112.
Hembacher, E., & Ghetti, S. (2014). Don't look at my answer: Subjective uncertainty underlies preschoolers' exclusion of their least accurate memories. *Psychological Science, 25*, 1768–1776.
Kim, S., Paulus, M., Sodian, B., & Proust, J. (2016). Young children's sensitivity to their own ignorance in informing others. *PloS One, 11*, 1–15.
Kluger, A. N., & DeNisi, A. (1996). The effects of feedback interventions on performance: A historical review, a meta-analysis, and a preliminary feedback intervention theory. *Psychological Bulletin, 119*, 254–284.
Koriat, A. (1997). Monitoring one's own knowledge during study: A cue-utilization approach to judgments of learning. *Journal of Experimental Psychology-General, 126*, 349–370.
Koriat, A., & Ackerman, R. (2010). Choice latency as a cue for children's subjective confidence in the correctness of their answers. *Developmental Science, 13*, 441–453.
Koriat, A., Ackerman, R., Lockl, K., & Schneider, W. (2009). The memorizing effort heuristic in judgments of learning: A developmental perspective. *Journal of Experimental Child Psychology, 102*, 265–279.
Kulik, J. A., & Kulik, C.-L. C. (1988). Timing of feedback and verbal learning. *Review of Educational Research, 58*, 79–97.
Kurtz-Costes, B., McCall, R. J., Kinlaw, C. R., Wiesen, C. A., & Joyner, M. H. (2005). What does it mean to be smart? The development of children's beliefs about intelligence in Germany and the United States. *Journal of Applied Developmental Psychology, 26*, 217–233.
Lerkkanen, M.-K., Kiuru, N., Pakarinen, E., Poikkeus, A.-M., Rasku-Puttonen, H., Siekkinen, M., & Nurmi, J.-E. (2016). Child-centered versus teacher-directed teaching practices: Associations with the development of academic skills in the first grade at school. *Early Childhood Research Quarterly, 36*, 145–156.

Lipko, A. R., Dunlosky, J., & Merriman, W. E. (2009). Persistent overconfidence despite practice: The role of task experience in preschoolers' recall predictions. *Journal of Experimental Child Psychology, 103*, 152–166.
Lipko, A. R., Dunlosky, J., Lipowski, S. L., & Merriman, W. E. (2012). Young children are not underconfident with practice: The benefit of ignoring a fallible memory heuristic. *Journal of Cognition and Development, 13*, 174–188.
Lipko-Speed, A. R. (2013). Can young children be more accurate predictors of their recall performance? *Journal of Experimental Child Psychology, 114*, 357–363.
Lipowski, S. L., Merriman, W. E., & Dunlosky, J. (2013). Preschoolers can make highly accurate judgments of learning. *Developmental Psychology, 49*, 1505–1516.
Metcalfe, J., & Finn, B. (2008). Evidence that judgments of learning are causally related to study choice. *Psychonomic Bulletin and Review, 15*, 174–179.
Metcalfe, J., & Finn, B. (2013). Metacognition and control of study choice in children. *Metacognition Learning, 8*, 19–46.
Miller, T. M., & Geraci, L. (2011). Training metacognition in the classroom: The influence of incentives and feedback on exam predictions. *Metacognition and Learning, 6*, 303–314.
Mory, E. H. (2004). Feedback research revisited. In M. J. Spector, D. M. Merrill, J. Van Merriënboer, & M. P. Driscoll (Eds.), *Handbook of research on educational communications and technology* (Vol. 2, pp. 745–783). New York: Taylor & Francis Group.
Muis, K. R., Ranellucci, J., Trevors, G., & Duffy, M. C. (2015). The effects of technology-mediated immediate feedback on kindergarten students' attitudes, emotions, engagement and learning outcomes during literacy skills development. *Learning and Instruction, 38*, 1–13.
Muldoon, K. P., Lewis, C., & Berridge, D. (2007). Predictors of early numeracy: Is there a place for mistakes when learning about number? *British Journal of Developmental Psychology, 25*, 543–558.
Muñoz, L., & Santa Cruz, J. (2016). The preschool classroom as a context for cognitive development: Type of teacher feedback and children's metacognitive control. *Electronic Journal of Research in Educational Psychology, 14*, 23–44.
Nelson, T. O., & Narens, L. (1990). Metamemory: A theoretical framework and new findings. *Psychology of Learning and Motivation, 26*, 125–141.
Nicholls, J. G. (1978). The development of the concepts of effort and ability, perception of academic attainment, and the understanding that difficult tasks require more ability. *Child Development, 49*, 800–814.
Nicol, D. J., & Macfarlane-Dick, D. (2006). Formative assessment and self-regulated learning: A model and seven principles of good feedback practice. *Studies in Higher Education, 31*, 199–218.
Nietfeld, J. L., Cao, L., & Osborne, J. W. (2006). The effect of distributed monitoring exercises and feedback on performance, monitoring accuracy, and self-efficacy. *Metacognition and Learning, 1*, 159–179.
Okita, S. Y. (2014). Learning from the folly of others: Learning to self-correct by monitoring the reasoning of virtual characters in a computer-supported mathematics learning environment. *Computers and Education, 71*, 257–278.
Pashler, H., Cepeda, N. J., Wixted, J. T., & Rohrer, D. (2005). When does feedback facilitate learning of words? *Journal of Experimental Psychology: Learning, Memory, and Cognition, 31*, 3–8.
Paulus, M., Tsalas, N., Proust, J., & Sodian, B. (2014). Metacognitive monitoring of oneself and others: Developmental changes during childhood and adolescence. *Journal of Experimental Child Psychology, 122*, 153–165.
Pekrun, R. (2006). The control-value theory of achievement emotions: Assumptions, corollaries, and implications for educational research and practice. *Educational Psychology Review, 18*, 315–341.
Rinne, L. F., & Mazzocco, M. M. M. (2014). Knowing right from wrong in mental arithmetic judgments: Calibration of confidence predicts the development of accuracy. *PloS One, 9*, 1–11.

Roebers, C. M. (2014). Children's deliberate memory development: The contribution of strategies and metacognitive processes. In P. J. Bauer & R. Fivush (Eds.), *The Wiley handbook on the development of Children's memory* (Vol. I/II, pp. 865–894). Chichester: John Wiley & Sons, Ltd.

Roebers, C. M. (2017). Executive function and metacognition: Towards a unifying framework of cognitive self-regulation. *Developmental Review, 45*, 31–51.

Roebers, C. M., & Spiess, M. (2017). The development of metacognitive monitoring and control in second graders: A short-term longitudinal study. *Journal of Cognition and Development, 18*, 110–128.

Roebers, C. M., Mayer, T., Bayard, N., Steiner, M., & Van Loon, M. H. (2019). The role of children's metacognitive experiences for cue utilization and monitoring accuracy: A longitudinal study. *Developmental Psychology, 55*, 2077–2089.

Rohwer, M., Kloo, D., & Perner, J. (2012). Escape from metaignorance: How children develop an understanding of their own lack of knowledge. *Child Development, 83*, 1869–1883.

Roll, I., Aleven, V., McLaren, B. M., & Koedinger, K. R. (2011). Improving students' help-seeking skills using metacognitive feedback in an intelligent tutoring system. *Learning and Instruction, 21*, 267–280.

Ryan, R. M., & Deci, E. L. (2017). *Self-determination theory. Basic psychological needs in motivation, development and wellness*. New York: The Guilford Press.

Sadler, D. R. (1989). Formative assessment and the design of instructional systems. *Instructional Science, 18*, 119–144.

Salonen, P., Vauras, M., & Efklides, A. (2005). Social interaction-what can it tell us about metacognition and coregulation in learning? *European Psychologist, 10*, 199–208.

Schneider, W. (1998). Performance prediction in young children: Effects of skill, metacognition and wishful thinking. *Developmental Science, 1*, 291–297.

Schneider, W., & Löffler, E. (2016). The development of metacognitive knowledge in children and adolescents. In J. Dunlosky & S. U. K. Tauber (Eds.), *The Oxford handbook of metamemory* (pp. 191–517). Oxford: Oxford University Press.

Schooler, L. J., & Anderson, J. R. (1990). The disruptive potential of immediate feedback. *Paper presented at the Proceedings of the Twelfth Annual Conference of the Cognitive Science Society*, Carnegie-Mellon University.

Schunk, D. H. (1984). Sequential attributional feedback and children's achievement behaviors. *Journal of Educational Psychology, 76*, 1159–1169.

Shin, H., Bjorklund, D. F., & Beck, E. F. (2007). The adaptive nature of children's overestimation in a strategic memory task. *Cognitive Development, 22*, 197–212.

Shute, V. J. (2008). Focus on formative feedback. *Review of Educational Research, 78*, 153–189.

Skipper, Y., & Douglas, K. (2015). The influence of teacher feedback on children's perceptions of student-teacher relationships. *British Journal of Educational Psychology, 85*, 276–288.

Stipek, D. J. (1984). Young children's performance expectations: Logical analysis or wishful thinking. *Advances in Motivation and Achievement, 3*, 33–56.

Strasser, K., & Del Río, F. (2014). The role of comprehension monitoring, theory of mind, and vocabulary depth in predicting story comprehension and recall of kindergarten children. *Reading Research Quarterly, 49*, 169–187.

Südkamp, A., Kaiser, J., & Möller, J. (2012). Accuracy of teachers' judgments of students' academic achievement: A meta-analysis. *Journal of Educational Psychology, 104*, 743–762.

Thiede, K. W., Dunlosky, J., Griffin, T. D., & Wiley, J. (2005). Understanding the delayed-keyword effect on metacomprehension accuracy. *Journal of Experimental Psychology: Learning, Memory and Cognition, 31*, 1267–1280.

Thomas, R. C., & Jacoby, L. L. (2013). Diminishing adult egocentrism when estimating what others know. *Journal of Experimental Psychology: Learning, Memory, and Cognition, 39*, 473–486.

Van de Pol, J., Volman, M., & Beishuizen, J. (2011). Patterns of contingent teaching in teacher–student interaction. *Learning and Instruction, 21*, 46–57.

Van de Pol, J., De Bruin, A., Van Loon, M. H., & Van Gog, T. (2019). Students' and teachers' monitoring and regulation of students' text comprehension: Effects of comprehension cue availability. *Contemporary Educational Psychology, 56*, 236–249.
Van Loon, M. H., & Roebers, C. M. (2017). Effects of feedback on self-evaluations and self-regulation in elementary school. *Applied Cognitive Psychology, 31*, 508–519.
Van Loon, M. H., & Roebers, C. M. (under review). Using Feedback to Improve Monitoring Accuracy in Kindergarten Children.
Van Loon, M. H., & Van de Pol, J. (2019). Judging own and peer performance when using feedback in elementary school. *Learning and Individual Differences, 74*, 101754. https://doi.org/10.1016/j.lindif.2019.101754.
Van Loon, M. H., De Bruin, A. B. H., Van Gog, T., & Van Merriënboer, J. J. G. (2013). The effect of delayed-JOLs and sentence generation on children's monitoring accuracy and regulation of idiom study. *Metacognition and Learning, 8*, 173–191.
Van Loon, M., De Bruin, A., Leppink, J., & Roebers, C. (2017a). Why are children overconfident? Developmental differences in the implementation of accessibility cues when judging concept learning. *Journal of Experimental Child Psychology, 158*, 77–94.
Van Loon, M. H., Destan, N., Spiess, M. A., de Bruin, A., & Roebers, C. M. (2017b). Developmental progression in performance evaluations: Effects of children's cue-utilization and self-protection. *Learning and Instruction, 51*, 47–60.
Vygotsky, L. S. (1978). Interaction between learning and development. In M. Gauvain & M. Cole (Eds.), *Readings on the development of children* (pp. 34–40). New York: Scientific American Books.
Webb, J. M., Pridemore, D. R., Stock, W. A., Kulhavy, R. W., & Henning, J. E. (1997). Remembering responses and cognitive estimates of knowing: The effects of instructions, retrieval sequences, and feedback. *Contemporary Educational Psychology, 22*, 147–164.
Weisberg, D. S., Hirsh-Pasek, K., Golinkoff, R. M., Kittredge, A. K., & Klahr, D. (2016). Guided play: Principles and practices. *Current Directions in Psychological Science, 25*, 177–182.
Zhang, H., & Whitebread, D. (2017). Linking parental scaffolding with self-regulated learning in Chinese kindergarten children. *Learning and Instruction, 49*, 121–130.

Chapter 9
The Role of Parents and Teachers in Fostering Children's Self-regulated Learning Skills

Irini Dermitzaki and Eleni Kallia

Abstract Recent research offers new insights on the role of parents and teachers in the development of children's self-regulated learning (SRL) skills. Parental behaviors that support children's early learning efforts, such as parental contingent support and autonomy encouragement, are associated with the development of children's SRL skills. When children enter school, teachers are expected to foster students' learning and SRL skills, but this is often not the case. Teacher professional development programs aiming at promoting teacher self-regulation of their own learning and teaching as well as student SRL show promising results but also highlight the constraints of transferring such knowledge in teaching practices in the classroom. The implications of research findings for the cultivation of student SRL by parents and teachers are discussed from the point of view of theoretical and methodological shifts needed.

Keywords Self-regulated learning skills · Parental contingency · Children's autonomy support · Instruction of SRL

9.1 Introduction

Over the last three decades, a substantial body of research supported that self-regulation is a fundamental process in learning and academic performance. Several studies provided documentation that students' active engagement in the learning process, such as setting meaningful goals and learning plans, selecting appropriate strategies, monitoring their learning, and reflecting on cognitive outcomes, is positively related to improved academic performance and higher motivation levels (Boekaerts 1997; Efklides 2011; Schunk and Greene 2018; Zimmerman 2000). A central assumption within the SRL literature is that students' skills and strategies are

I. Dermitzaki (✉) · E. Kallia
Department of Early Childhood Education, University of Thessaly, Volos, Greece
e-mail: idermitzaki@uth.gr

D. Moraitou, P. Metallidou (eds.), *Trends and Prospects in Metacognition Research across the Life Span*, https://doi.org/10.1007/978-3-030-51673-4_9

core components of SRL and can play a critical role in academic performance (Alexander 2018; Pressley and Harris 2008). Skills, such as planning the learning process, self-monitoring, and self-evaluation after a cognitive endeavor, are key processes and behaviors oriented to control cognition in order to attain a learning goal (Efklides 2008; Zimmerman 2002). Alexander et al. (1998) postulated that skills and strategies share common characteristics but they are distinct constructs differing in automaticity and intentionality. Strategies regard conscious, intentional and effortful processing that facilitate the acquisition, understanding, or later transfer of new knowledge and skills (Alexander et al. 1998; Weinstein et al. 2000). Henceforth, we use jointly the terms skills and strategies because SRL presupposes both skills and strategies and, in addition, in most of the existent studies these two terms are used interchangeably (Alexander 2018).

The development of skills and strategies in children is affected by both individual and contextual/situational factors. For example, the development of children's nervous and sensory systems, their cognitive abilities, the general and specific knowledge they possess, their beliefs and values systems, and motivation, are all personal factors that can influence the development of children's learning skills (Littlefield-Cook and Cook 2009). Besides personal traits, learning largely takes place within social situations. Early childhood learning experiences within the family context, along with early school experiences, play a very important role in developing students' learning skills and strategies. For instance, parental child-rearing style, the frequency and quality of self-regulation that the environment requests from the child, the kind of support provided to the child's learning efforts by both parents and teachers are assumed to influence the development of students' SRL skills (Bernier et al. 2010; Bronson 2000; Dignath and Büttner 2018; Efklides and Misailidi 2019; Kistner et al. 2010; Paris and Paris 2001; Perry and VandeKamp 2000).

One of the basic tenets of SRL theory is that strategy use in learning can be trained (Boekaerts 1997; Perry and VandeKamp 2000; Zimmerman 2002). A social-cognitive perspective on academic self-regulation is nested in many assumptions of the present paper (Zimmerman 2000). It is claimed that capable individuals from the child's social environment provide various forms of support to children's self-regulatory development and strategy use, such as implicit and explicit social models to emulate, direct instruction, scaffolding, guidance and facilitation, feedback, encouragement, and rewards (Martinez-Pons 2002). In the following units, contemporary evidence on the contribution of parents and teachers in the development of students' SRL is presented with the aim of highlighting relevant theory and research lines. Moreover, possible paths for future research are proposed and implications for parental and teaching practices are discussed.

9.2 Parental Contribution to the Development of Children's SRL

Although self-regulation of learning is not always evident in younger ages, its foundations are set early in the child's life. In the family context, children are expected to gradually acquire the competences to self-regulate their behavior, cognition, emotions, and motivation (Bronson 2000). There are important indications that parents initially contribute with various ways to their children's developing abilities to self-regulate. For example, infants' social interactions with their caregivers provide them information on emotional states, allow them linking emotions with overt behaviors, and provide chances to encounter experiences of emotion regulation driven by parents, as parents often use emotion-regulation strategies to regulate infant distress (Efklides and Misailidi 2019).

As children grow older, they are encouraged to take responsibility and develop independence within diverse contexts according to their age and abilities. The family emotional climate and environmental cognitive stimulations communicate, directly and indirectly, practices related to self-regulation within social and cognitive contexts. These early parent-child interactions can be the starting point for children to explore the environment, to acquire knowledge, and to develop autonomy and responsibility, competences that are particularly important for effectively controlling behavior and gradually regulating learning efforts (Bronson 2000; Efklides and Misailidi 2019; Neitzel and Stright 2003; Pino-Pasternak and Whitebread 2010; Robinson et al. 2009). Early co-regulation of learning between competent persons and children gradually transforms into self-regulation through internalization processes (Erdman and Hertel 2019).

The frequency and quality of parent-child interactions over time related to learning situations are claimed to influence children's executive functions and cognitive flexibility (Hammond et al. 2012; Zeytinoglu et al. 2019), attention regulation and effortful control (Kochanska et al. 2000; Robinson et al. 2009), self-regulated learning skills and performance (Bronson 2000; Hill and Tyson 2009; Neitzel and Stright 2003; Pino-Pasternak and Whitebread 2010; Zhang and Whitebread 2017) and students' motivation (Gonzalez-DeHass et al. 2005). Children's developing skills and learning outcomes are significantly boosted by parents' support and assistance, particularly when children encounter problems beyond their capabilities (Neitzel and Stright 2003). The different aspects of parental support related to children's self-regulation skills are presented in the following paragraphs.

9.2.1 Aspects of Parental Support

One of the aspects of parental support appearing frequently in literature is cognitive support. It refers to parental assistance offered to the children (e.g., instructions, cues, hints, prompts) so that they understand and handle the cognitive demands of the task. Cognitive support can take various forms such as how to analyze and combine information, to find out the key features of task instructions, to elaborate and organize material, to remember information, etc. (Kallia and Dermitzaki 2017; Leerkes et al. 2011; Neitzel and Stright 2003, 2004; Zhang and Whitebread 2017). Furthermore, parental support of the child's metacognitive skills, as a part of cognitive support, it refers to any kind of assistance that activates the child's metacognition, e.g., the ability to organize and plan the steps towards a solution, to select and follow solution strategies, to self-monitor and self-regulate during learning, and to evaluate the learning outcomes.

Emotional support refers to the emotional and motivational climate that characterizes the parent-child interaction during learning, and the adult's efforts to attract and retain the child's interest, motivation, and engagement with the task. Parents' encouragement, praise, warm voice tone, responsiveness, sensitivity, and positive affect are indicative of emotional support (e.g., Efklides and Misailidi 2019; Kallia and Dermitzaki 2017; Leerkes et al. 2011; Neitzel and Stright 2003).

Promotion of the child's autonomy during learning is another dimension of parental support. Transfer of responsibility and autonomy support refers to the degree to which the parent encourages the child's gradual autonomy, independent learning, and active involvement during problem solving and it is associated with children's developing competence in self-regulation (Grolnick et al. 2002; Neitzel and Stright 2003, 2004; Zhang and Whitebread 2017).

Finally, a dimension of parental support that is claimed to play an instrumental role in children's developing skills is parental contingent support, namely, parental adjustment of the level and quality of support provided according to children's understanding. That is, parents increase of their instructions and reduction of the cognitive demand when children encounter difficulties, and conversely, parents provide less support and increase the cognitive demand when children succeed (Pino-Pasternak 2014; Wood and Middleton 1975; Zhang and Whitebread 2017).

Although parents play an instrumental role in children's developing competence to control and regulate internal processes and behaviors, few studies so far have thoroughly examined the associations between multiple dimensions of parental support and children's various academic and SRL skills (e.g., Kallia and Dermitzaki 2017; Neitzel and Stright 2003; Pino-Pasternak et al. 2010; Zhang and Whitebread 2017). In the following unit, current evidence is reviewed in order to outline the above relations.

9.2.2 Parental Support of Learning and Children's SRL Skills

Based on the evidence so far, it seems that different facets of parental support might be differentially associated with different learning skills in students. More specifically, Zhang and Whitebread (2017) reported that mothers' cognitive support of their children's learning efforts was significantly associated with young children's use of cognitive strategies and their metacognitive skills. Further, parental cognitive support of children's learning efforts, was connected with students' perceptual skills (Hubbs-Tait et al. 2002), behavior control strategies, and their cognitive outcomes (Leerkes et al. 2011; Mulvaney et al. 2006). A recent study by Sun and Tang (2019) explored the relations between maternal scaffolding during joint problem solving and Chinese preschool children's self-regulation. The findings of the study indicated that children's self-regulation and executive functions (attention, inhibitory control, shifting response) were positively predicted by maternal elaborative cognitive assistance and positive feedback.

Associations between maternal scaffolding and executive functions in 3- and 4-year old were also reported by Lowe et al. (2014). In line with this study, a recent meta-analysis reported significant associations between different aspects of parental support, such as cognitive behaviors (e.g., cognitive stimulation, scaffolding, autonomy support), and 0–8 years-old children's executive functions (inhibition, shifting and working memory) (Valcan et al. 2018). The researchers concluded that parental cognitive behaviors are especially influential during early childhood for children's executive functions. As regards metacognitive processes, the provision of metacognitive information from mothers to children, as well as the way they provide instructions (e.g., review of the steps, regulation of the difficulty of the project), predicted children's metacognitive talk, monitoring, and help seeking in the classroom (Neitzel and Stright 2003). On the contrary, low level of cognitive support (e.g., modelling, manual help, target-specific words related to the task) has been associated with lower levels of children's attention skills, engagement, and persistence (e.g., Hustedt and Raver 2002) while the provision of parental teaching strategies (e.g., higher use of target words related to the task) related to children's engagement to the task (Fender et al. 2010). Moreover, maternal directive instructions negatively predicted children's autonomous behaviors after controlling for maternal education and parenting beliefs (Stright et al. 2009).

Regarding the children's emotional support during learning, Leerkes et al. (2011) reported that maternal emotional support (i.e., encouragement, praise, interest) and the quality of home learning environment were predictors of children's pre-academic skills (i.e., language skills, behavior control strategies, early work habits) in 3 and 4 years of age. Valcan et al. (2018) in their meta-analysis reported a stable association between positive parental behaviors (e.g., support, involvement, sensitivity, praise), and negative parental behaviors (e.g., intrusiveness, control, hostility, negative affect) with executive functions (inhibition, shifting and working memory) across ages 0–8 years. Zhang and Whitbread (2017) reported that maternal emotional support during problem solving was associated with preschool children's actual cognitive, metacognitive, and motivational strategic behaviors during problem solving.

Moreover, parental emotional support has been found to foster students' self-monitoring and metacognitive talk in the classroom (Stright et al. 2001). In addition, maternal emotional support and transfer of responsibility were related to children's behavior control in school (Neitzel and Stright 2003) while maternal sensitivity was related to children's self-control skills, such as delay of gratification (Razza and Raymond 2013). Parents' emotion expression and coaching of children's emotional skills help children to self-regulate emotions in social contexts (Efklides and Misailidi 2019). Motivational aspects of children's learning have been also found to be associated with parental emotional support. For example, the emotional support provided by parents was positively correlated with children's effort and task persistence (Mokrova et al. 2012; Neitzel and Stright 2003).

Significant links were detected so far between another aspect of parental support, i.e., autonomy support, and children's cognitive and metacognitive skills in learning. For example, Kallia and Dermitzaki (2017) reported that maternal practices for autonomy support were positively related to children's actual use of cognitive strategies, planning skills, and monitoring skills during problem-solving in two different cognitive domains, namely language and visual-spatial tasks. In addition, in the latter domain, maternal autonomy support was positively associated with children's actual motivational strategic behaviors, i.e., persistence, concentration, and autonomous activity. Moreover, Bernier et al. (2010) claimed that autonomy support was the strongest predictor of children's executive function skills. Past studies have also shown that children encouraged by their mothers to engage actively in the learning process usually demonstrate improved executive function, better performance as well as better social and school adaptation skills (Grolnick et al. 2002; Joussemet et al. 2005). Furthermore, researchers maintained that parental autonomy support was positively associated with students' motivational skills, such as engagement, effort, and autonomous motivation (Vasquez et al. 2016).

On the contrary, parental overcontrol, that is, parents who either provide the answers themselves or heavily guide their children's actions exceeding children's needs, or when parents undertake themselves the completion of a learning project, has been linked to maladaptive students' academic and psychological outcomes. For example, maternal overcontrol was negatively associated with preschoolers' actual cognitive strategy use, planning and monitoring skills when solving visual-spatial tasks–but not with reference to language tasks (Kallia and Dermitzaki 2017). Research on helicopter parenting, i.e., low levels of promotion of independent behavior, excessive control, physical and social contact, revealed that perceived helicopter parenting positively predicted students' procrastination practices and that the latter negatively predicted students' SRL (i.e., performance monitoring, goal setting, pursuing goal) (Hong et al. 2015). Excessive parental control and pressure were also negatively associated with students' academic performance (Karbach et al. 2013; Silinskas et al. 2015).

Parental contingent support of children's learning efforts has received scant attention so far in literature. A recent study by Zhang and Whitebread (2017) revealed that, among the facets of the parental support examined, contingent support was the only independent predictor of young children's actual strategic behavior during learning and of their task performance. Moreover, parental contingent support has been associated with children's executive functions (Devine et al. 2016; Hammond et al. 2012), children's regulation of cognition, metacognitive knowledge, motivation, language skills, and academic competence (e.g., Mattanah et al.

2005; Mermelshtine and Barnes 2016; Pino-Pasternak and Whitebread 2010; Pino-Pasternak et al. 2010).

In conclusion, the associations between different parental supportive practices of children's learning efforts and children's SRL skills need further investigation. Only a few studies examined the associations between multiple dimensions of parental support and children's various SRL skills (e.g., Kallia and Dermitzaki 2017; Neitzel and Stright 2003; Pino-Pasternak et al. 2010; Zhang and Whitebread 2017). The evidence presented in this section indicates that children in their effort to master a task and become independent learners need both cognitive stimulating environments and emotionally supportive parents (Valcan et al. 2018). In addition, promotion of children's autonomy during problem solving and parental contingency, i.e., adjustment of support provided according to children's understanding, appear to be favorable conditions for optimal self-regulation skills in children. Early childhood seems to be a critical period during which parental support is especially influential for children's developing skills for self-regulation. These early interactions between parents and children can play an instrumental role in children's understanding and regulation of cognition, affect, and behavior. Although the evidence presented thus far makes clear the parental practices that support SRL, it is unclear why parents adopt a particular way in their supportive behaviors.

9.2.3 Factors Associated with Parental Support of Learning

There is evidence that parents' supportive behaviors and parent-child interactions during learning are related to parent- and to child-specific factors as well as to situational/contextual factors. To mention some of these influencing factors, parental self-efficacy, that is, parents' beliefs about their capability to deal with parenting duties, or effectively handle situations arising from child-rearing and parenting, is a factor that appears to be associated with the quality of parent-child interaction (Hess et al. 2004). Higher levels of parental self-efficacy are associated with positive parenting behaviors, such as encouragement, involvement, discussion, consistent parenting behaviors and monitoring, which in turn lead to better school performance, positive adjustment and socio-emotional competence in children (Dumka et al. 2010; Glatz and Buchanan 2015). Parental educational level is another factor that seems to be associated with characteristics of parental support. It has been found that higher educational level is associated with higher levels of contingent support, which in turn predicts higher levels of children's strategic behaviors and task performance (Zhang and Whitebread 2017). However, there is not conclusive evidence regarding the role of such parent-related factors in children's learning skills and further research is needed.

The child's temperament and parent's perception of it is another factor linked to the quality of parent-child interactions in learning. Specifically, parents' reactions and behavior patterns towards the child seem to vary depending on the extent to which the child's temperament and behaviors match parental expectations. For example, Stright et al. (2008) reported that children's perceived temperament moderated the associations between maternal parenting styles during early childhood and children's first-grade academic competence, social skills, and relationships with teachers and peers. Relations between parenting and first-grade outcomes were stronger for difficult in temperament than for less difficult infants. Furthermore, parents' positive behaviors towards the child (e.g., warmth, responsiveness) are positively linked to children's effortful control and self-regulation (e.g., Colman et al. 2006; Karreman et al. 2008). Specifically, children's effortful control was positively associated with positive parenting, such as setting of boundaries, responsiveness, and boosting the child's autonomy (Lengua et al. 2007; Slobodskaya et al. 2019). However, there are bidirectional relations between children's temperament and parental response (e.g., Eisenberg et al. 1999; Lengua 2006). When children are more adaptable, calm and social, it is more likely for their parents to show warm attitude and responsiveness in contrast to irritable or socially withdrawn children (Kochanska et al. 2000). And vice versa, parents' warm attitude can reduce children's negative emotions while a distant stance can increase them.

An example of a contextual factor that appears to be involved in the kind of parental support offered to the child is the nature of the cognitive task, that is, the cognitive domain of the task-to-be-solved that may affect the relations between parental support and children's learning skills. For instance, in a study by Kallia and Dermitzaki (2017) several significant relations between maternal boosting of children's autonomy and preschoolers' SRL skills were detected with reference to visual-spatial tasks but not with reference to language tasks that mothers and children jointly solved. Further research is needed in order to enlighten whether parental support during learning is affected by the nature of the cognitive tasks and to deeper understand the associations between parental support of learning and children's learning skills depending on the nature of the task.

Summing up, in the present unit, the contribution of parental support to children's developing abilities to regulate their learning efforts was highlighted along with indicative factors assumed to affect the above relations. Growing evidence shows that different aspects of parental support of children's learning, especially parental contingent support and promotion of children's autonomy, might differentially affect children's various SRL skills. These parent-child interactions can initiate self-regulatory development and lead to the independent exercise of academic skills and competences that are particularly important for effectively controlling behavior and gradually regulating learning efforts. Later, when children enter school, teachers can play an instrumental role in the development of students' skills and abilities to self-regulate learning in the classroom. This issue is discussed in the following units.

9.3 The Role of Teachers in Promoting SRL Strategies in the Classroom

Knowing and effectively applying various types of strategies for SRL is associated with cognitive and affective gains in students and with improved academic performance (Dent and Koenka 2016; Efklides 2008; Schunk and Greene 2018). However, self-regulation skills such as goal setting, progress monitoring, and reflection (see Zimmerman 2000) are not spontaneously used by students in the classroom (de Bruin and van Merriënboer 2017). This calls for teaching practices that can support the development and application of such skills. Teachers are expected to help students learn how to learn and to self-regulate their learning and this should be a central and explicit goal within education (Moos and Ringdal 2012; Paris and Paris 2001).

Instruction of self-regulation strategies for increasing students' active involvement and improved achievement needs to be explicitly and strategically integrated within the teaching and learning process in the classroom. This goal can be achieved by providing students with learning strategies and supportive learning environments. Adjustments teachers make to the learning environment and their teaching practices might have positive effects on skills such as self-monitoring, heightened awareness of the quality of their performance, and increased commitment to school learning (Anderman et al. 2011; Perry and VandeKamp 2000; Perry et al. 2002). Research evidence on teachers' practices that promote students' SRL in the classroom, their effectiveness and related teacher factors is highlighted in the following paragraphs. Teacher training programs for improving the development of students' SRL skills are also delineated.

9.3.1 Instruction of SRL Strategies in the Classroom

A great bulk of evidence regarding the instruction of SRL strategies in the classroom comes from both teachers' beliefs and perceptions about the fostering of SRL in their students and from classroom observations. Teachers' perceptions are investigated through questionnaires or/and teachers' interviews about instruction of SRL in the classroom. For example, Chatzistamatiou et al. (2014) investigated elementary school teachers' perceptions of how frequently they foster students' SRL strategies in mathematics learning. From the different groups of strategies examined, the strategies for encouraging students' metacognitive and reflection skills were the less frequently activated according to teachers' reports. Overall, it was found that teachers' reports were rather over-optimistic with regards to SRL strategy instruction in the classroom, as the high mean scores of their answers denoted. In line with the above findings, Dignath and Büttner (2018) found that, with reference to mathematics, primary and secondary school teachers reported they instructed mainly cognitive strategies and less often motivation strategies, whereas little instruction of metacognitive strategies was mentioned. In addition, the same study provided data from classroom observations and from interviews on teachers' knowledge of SRL. Dignath and Büttner (2018) reported that neither observation nor teachers' interviews were associated with teachers' perceptions of the frequency of their strategy teaching in the classroom.

Similar findings had been previously reported by Kane et al. (2002) with reference to university teachers. Several unsupported claims about teaching SRL practices were found. Furthermore, Spruce and Bol (2015) assessed teachers' reports of promoting SRL in the classroom and, additionally, observed them in the classroom. Overall, they found that there were gaps between what teachers reported and their actual practice of SRL. The researchers conducted interviews by asking teachers questions on the application of SRL in the classroom. They found differences in teachers' answers depending on the phase of SRL cycle process (Zimmerman 2000). For example, regarding planning strategies, some teachers were able to provide examples of application of such strategies, but "...yet little explicit connections were made between the actions taken and how these helped students regulate their learning" (Spruce and Bol 2015, p. 261). The teachers had difficulties in explaining how these actions were applied in the classroom and how they helped students' SRL. Regarding monitoring processes many teachers "struggled to articulate what they did to encourage their students to monitor learning" (p. 263). Explicit connections between teachers' presentation of monitoring strategies, an explanation of why these are employed and how these might help students to regulate their learning were missing. In conclusion, teachers' individual reports are not always well grounded and they may not correspond to their actual instructional practices in the classroom context.

Apart from teachers' self-reports, to what extent teachers do actually teach students how to learn in everyday instruction in the classroom? It is postulated that few teachers do actually prepare pupils to learn on their own and steer the learning process (Boekaerts 1997; Zimmerman 2002). Indeed, data from observation studies conducted in the classroom show that teachers spend only little of their instruction time on strategy teaching, and, especially, on explicit strategy teaching. For example, Hamman et al. (2000) showed that middle school teachers devoted a small amount of their instructional activity to coaching students in learning both in math/science and in English/social studies. Hamman et al. (2000) also reported that students' reported strategy use was positively related to teachers' observed coaching of learning.

On the other hand, there is observational data testifying that teachers do spend time on strategy instruction in mathematics (Kistner et al. 2010). However, in the same study it was pointed out that a great amount of strategy teaching took place in an implicit way, whereas explicit strategy teaching was rare. It was explicit strategy instruction by the math teachers though, and not implicit instruction, that was positively related to students' learning gains. Moreover, Kistner et al. (2010) showed that teachers mostly instruct cognitive strategies, and not so often motivational or metacognitive strategies, and that they differ widely among them in how often they instruct these strategies. Finally, the researchers concluded that mathematics teachers hardly create a learning environment that fosters SRL. In line with the above study, Dignath and Büttner (2018), based on observational data, found that primary and secondary school teachers spent little time explicitly teaching SRL strategies, and when they did, they taught mainly cognitive strategies whereas motivational and metacognitive strategies were less often taught. Moreover, secondary education teachers exhibited a highly teacher-directed style of teaching, in comparison to the primary school teachers, that did not allow students to have an active role in their learning.

It is interesting to note, however, that not only teachers' reports but also their actual practices were differentiated depending on Zimmerman's (2000) phase of the SRL cyclic process (Spruce and Bol 2015). Specifically, the instructional practices to encourage monitoring of learning in various school subjects (grades 3–8), such as attention focusing or checking progress towards learning goals, were common. However, teachers demonstrated few activities for encouraging planning and goal setting at the initiation of task processing or subsequent evaluation after task completion. None of the observed teachers, after task completion, made direct connections to student effort and outcome.

In conclusion, regarding teaching practices that promote students' SRL, although data from teachers' reports are rather optimistic, observations in the classroom show that teachers do not actually devote sufficient time to directly instruct SRL in the classroom. Explicit teaching of SRL is not frequent nor is teaching of SRL efficiently embedded in everyday instruction. When teachers instruct strategies, these are mainly cognitive strategies. It can be concluded that teachers may not explicitly incorporate direct promotion of students' SRL in the classroom without training how to do it (Spruce and Bol 2015). It is worth to better understand the factors that might affect teachers' instruction of SRL in the classroom.

9.3.2 Teachers' Beliefs and Knowledge of SRL

Recently, it has been argued that teachers' beliefs and values about teaching and learning expand or limit SRL promotion in the classroom and, consequently, student use of SRL strategies (Lawson et al. 2019). Further, teachers' epistemological beliefs about learning and teaching, their knowledge about the promotion of SRL, and the value they attribute to fostering SRL in students have been found to affect teachers' instructional practices (Moos and Ringdal 2012). Overall, when teachers have positive beliefs toward SRL they are inclined to promote it in school (Lombaerts et al. 2009; Yan 2018).

Regarding teachers' knowledge of SRL, Waeytens et al. (2002) found that teachers hold different views regarding the notion "learning to learn" and that these different viewpoints were related to their approach to learning and their own teaching behaviors. Similarly, teachers were not familiar with the conceptualization of and rationale underlying SRL and did not have the necessary knowledge in relation to it. Moreover, Spruce and Bol (2015) reported that teachers' knowledge how to describe SRL to their students was low and diverse. Specifically, teachers demonstrated greater knowledge of monitoring processes during a learning event than for planning or evaluating. Although teachers recognized the value of reflection and evaluation, many of the participants in the above study were unable to describe self-evaluation of a learning outcome and few demonstrated knowledge how to help students reflect on their learning outcomes. Furthermore, teachers did not mention lack of training as a reason for low SRL integration into their classrooms. They may be unaware of the gaps in their SRL-related knowledge and, therefore, do not recognize the need for professional development in this area.

Spruce and Bol (2015) concluded that teachers' beliefs and knowledge about SRL and their observed classroom practices were not consistently aligned. Chatzistamatiou and Dermitzaki (2013), on the other hand, found that elementary school teachers considered self-regulation in mathematics as important both for their teaching and students' learning. In the same study, teachers' reports about ways to foster students' SRL reflected the three cyclical phases of SRL, as suggested by Zimmerman (2000). That is, three categories of strategies for promoting SRL in the classroom emerged: strategies for promoting students' planning and forethought skills, metacognitive and reflection skills, and solution evaluation skills.

In a recent study, Yan (2018) showed that teacher beliefs about SRL affected their SRL instructional practices. Dignath and Büttner (2018) conducted interviews with eight secondary school teachers on their knowledge of SRL strategies and their actual use in the classroom. They found that teachers lacked knowledge about metacognition as a main component of SRL and, at the same time, were reluctant to promote it. Teachers considered cognitive and motivational strategies to be more important for learning than metacognitive strategies. Indeed, observational data in the same study confirmed that teachers taught mainly cognitive strategies. In a previous study, Dignath-van Ewijk (2016) showed that teachers' beliefs about fostering SRL in the classroom, their knowledge about ways to promote SRL, and their self-efficacy toward the promotion of SRL significantly predicted teachers' reports on the promotion of SRL in the classroom.

Lawson et al. (2019) recently examined a range of teachers' beliefs about learning and SRL strategies. Their aim was to investigate the potential negative impact such beliefs may have on fostering students' SRL. The researchers underscored that even if teachers believe that SRL is important for teaching and learning, frequently they do not think it is necessary to make it explicit in the classroom. This is might be related to an implicit belief may teachers hold, namely, that SRL does not constitute a content domain that is different or independent from subject-specific knowledge and skills and, hence, the instructor does not need to dispose deep and complex knowledge of it. Lawson et al. (2019) conjectured that such beliefs might limit the promotion of SRL by teachers. In the same vein, even if teachers believe that SRL is useful, sometimes they do not view it as practical for their students. For example, Spruce and Bol (2015) found that teachers believed that their middle-school students may not be ready to self-regulate. Also, teachers may be unsure about how much and what kinds of guidance young children need to become masters of their own learning (Perry and VandeKamp 2000).

To conclude, the need to strengthen teachers' beliefs and knowledge about SRL is associated with their willingness and their instructional practices to promote SRL in the classroom. In many cases, change in such belief systems is needed, but inducing change might be a slow process (Lawson et al. 2019).

9.3.3 Teacher Self-Efficacy, Value Beliefs and Individual Differences Factors Related to SRL Instructional Practices

Beyond teachers' beliefs and knowledge about SRL, other individual factors might impact the instruction of SRL. One such factor is self-efficacy for teaching. Teachers are often concerned about their capability to turn students into self-regulated learners (Boekaerts 1997). Specifically, teaching self-efficacy beliefs are significantly associated with teacher self-regulation and use of instructional strategies (Capa-Aydin et al. 2009; De Smul et al. 2018; Ghonsooly and Ghanizadeh 2011). High self-efficacy beliefs about teaching lead to higher motivation, greater effort, resilience and persistence of the teacher, which usually result in improved instruction. Positive teaching self-efficacy beliefs are associated with greater levels of teacher planning and organization, with more time spent on student learning and with greater support of students in the pursuit of their goals (Zimmerman 2000). Furthermore, there is evidence suggesting that teachers' value beliefs are associated with their use of self-regulation instructional strategies. For example, there are links between pre-service teachers' value for learning strategy instruction and their own degree of strategy use and self-regulation (Hamman 1998) and between task value and reported self-regulation strategies (Arsal 2010). Chatzistamatiou et al. (2014) also found that teaching self-efficacy, the value teachers attribute to mathematics as a cognitive domain, and their emotional commitment to their profession were directly and positively associated with teachers' reports of fostering SRL strategies in the classroom. In addition, the above factors predicted the strategies teachers reported using for regulating their own teaching of mathematics.

Further, other teacher characteristics such as teaching experience and gender may also be associated with SRL-related instructional practices. For instance, experienced teachers employ their own and students' metacognitive processes for SRL more than novice teachers do. The latter focus on covering content knowledge and on time management (Artzt and Armour-Thomas 2001; Stewart et al. 2007). Comparisons between expert and novice teachers also show that there are differences between them in the planning and implementation of instruction and in their reflection regarding what happens in the classroom (Zohar 2004). Regarding gender differences, there is evidence showing that female teachers are more likely to employ more individualized student-centered instructional strategies and to encourage cooperation in the classroom in comparison to males (Retelsdorf et al. 2010). Yan (2018) showed that female teachers reported higher levels of SRL-related instructional practices than males. Similarly, Chatzistamatiou and Dermitzaki (2013) found that female teachers differed from their male colleagues in the type of strategies they report using in mathematics teaching. Females reported using more frequently strategies for planning their mathematics instruction and for evaluating the attainment of teaching goals. However, such findings are not always consistent as there are studies that report no differences in instructional practices between the two genders (e.g., Opdenakker and Van Damme, 2006).

Briefly, teachers' motivational and individual differences factors may affect promotion of students' SRL skills in the classroom, although more research is needed to shed further light on these associations. However, even when teachers believe in the importance of SRL, hold positive teaching efficacy beliefs and value a cognitive domain, the question is whether they have themselves the necessary skills in order to regulate learning and teaching. Effective instruction of SRL is grounded on the instructor's skills to self-regulate.

9.3.4 Teachers' Skills for Self-Regulation of Learning and Instruction. Relations with Promoting SRL in the Classroom

In order to facilitate students' learning, teachers need to actively direct, regulate, and reflect on their own cognition, motivation and instructional practices (Hartman 2001; Paris and Paris 2001). Classroom instruction needs among others clear teaching aims, a plan and methods on how to achieve these aims, teaching strategies, monitoring of the implementation of the instruction plan, control and regulation of the teaching processes, evaluation of teaching effectiveness and reflection on it. Moreover, classroom instruction requires teachers who are willing to examine different perspectives and seek support when instructional challenges arise. That is, for effective teaching it is important to regulate instructional processes (Paris and Paris 2001; Stoeger and Ziegler 2011).

There are not many studies investigating what teachers do in order to regulate their own learning and instruction and how this is associated with promotion of SRL in the classroom. Teachers report some use of SRL strategies in relation to their own learning, "...though not all are able to explain what those strategies are" (Spruce and Bol 2015, p. 260). Spruce and Bol (2015) reported that several teachers were unable to describe what they knew about goal setting and monitoring of their own learning. In another study, with reference to mathematics teaching, elementary school teachers claimed that they use more frequently strategies for planning and preparing the lesson compared to other subject domains and for evaluating whether the teaching goals have been accomplished (Chatzistamatiou et al. 2014). According to teachers' reports, they activated less frequently strategies for monitoring their instruction and for reflecting on it. However, teachers' perceptions of their own skills to strategically regulate their instruction seem to be conceptually distinct from their perceptions of the instructional strategies that support students' efforts to self-regulate their learning (e.g., see Chatzistamatiou and Dermitzaki 2013).

Concerning the relations between teachers' self-regulation of instruction and practices that promote students' SRL, elementary school teachers who reported frequent employment of strategies for regulating mathematics instruction also reported frequent use of strategies for promoting students' SRL in mathematics (Chatzistamatiou et al. 2014). Furthermore, when teachers receive training regarding their own skills, such as metacognitive skills, they become better prepared to support their students' SRL in the classroom (Kramarski and Michalsky 2009; Zohar 2004). Therefore, strengthening teachers' own skills to self-regulate learning and instruction seems to be a promising path to promoting students' SRL in the classroom (Butler et al. 2004; Peters-Burton and Botov 2017). Other options for improving instructional practices of SRL in the classroom are highlighted below.

9.3.5 Improving Teachers' Knowledge and Practice of SRL in the Classroom

As already mentioned, teachers' understanding and practicing of SRL in the classroom is not optimal, and this calls for interventions that can improve and facilitate transfer to classroom instruction. There is evidence that professional development programs can be effective in improving teachers' capability to teach SRL to their students (Moos and Ringdal 2012) under certain conditions.

Some past studies focused on teachers' training in explicitly instructing SRL in the classroom with diverse findings. Veenman et al. (1999) trained secondary school teachers to explicitly instruct SRL strategies. The SRL training program had little effect on classroom practices. It is likely that embedding explicit instruction of SRL strategies in teaching is time consuming and the outcomes may not be immediately visible. Moreover, as the authors pointed out, SRL is not common practice in Dutch secondary schools, and this might be a possible interpretation for these outcomes.

Perry and VandeKamp (2000) built a community of primary school teachers and students who worked together to design tasks and structure interactions between them to maximize opportunities for students to exercise metacognition, increase intrinsic motivation, and develop strategic action. Teachers consistently involved students in open-ended activities, choosing what to learn, modifying tasks to reach an optimal level of challenge, and evaluating their own and others' learning processes. Furthermore, teachers were highly skilled at providing explicit instruction of SRL and extensive scaffolding that is required for young children to build knowledge about the cognitive tools that affect learning. In these classrooms, students were observed to be engaged in independent, academically effective forms of learning. In another study, Hilden and Pressley (2007) engaged primary school teachers in SRL-based reading instruction training over 1 year. At the end of the program, teachers demonstrated capacity to implement SRL-based instruction in the classroom, yet they had not achieved full efficiency in SRL-based instruction.

Perels et al. (2009) trained kindergarten teachers in order to be able to foster self-regulation in their preschool students. The teachers learned both self-regulatory strategies for their own learning, in order to be able to act as a role model for their students, and strategies for supporting the SRL of preschoolers. The results showed that the self-regulation of the kindergarten teachers and the SRL of preschoolers improved significantly, although not on all aspects expected. Kramarski and Michalsky (2009) investigated preservice teachers' professional growth in SRL learning environments. They found that preservice teachers in the supported SRL conditions outperformed their unsupported peers on all professional growth measures.

More recently, Festas et al. (2015) trained middle school teachers through a professional development program in order to teach the Self-Regulated Strategy Development (SRSD) program for essay writing to their students. The instructed students showed greater gains than the comparison students immediately after instruction of the SRSD program and at a follow up 2 months later. In another intervention study, Dermitzaki and Kriekouki (2017) trained elementary school teachers to implement themselves a program aiming at fostering students' SRL strategies in reading comprehension. Teachers effectively taught cognitive skills in order to support students' text comprehension and were successful in engaging and inspiring their students to actively participate into the training program. However, it was noted that, even after training, teachers lacked the adoption of a consistent "learning to learn" approach embedded in the classroom. The authors concluded that further teachers' training and long-term support is needed in order to effectively promote students' metacognitive skills and an autonomous, student-regulated learning. Teachers' difficulties to connect SRL instruction with everyday classroom practice and with subject-specific content instruction have been noticed in the past (Zohar 2004).

Regarding interventions for improving teachers' self-regulation of their teaching, Butler et al. (2004) engaged teachers in interactive discussions within collaborative groups that helped them learn how to reflectively guide their own (teaching) activities. The aim was teachers to self-regulate their teaching based on a clear view of (instructional) goals, and to critically monitor outcomes to re-/co-construct knowledge about effective teaching processes. Peters-Burton and Botov (2017), during a professional development program for elementary school teachers, examined, by means of microanalysis, the self-regulatory learning cycles that teachers experienced while engaged in inquiry learning. The researchers found that, as professional development progressed, teachers improved their goal setting and self-monitoring skills, and their learning tactics. Xu and Ko (2019) examined whether teachers' knowledge of how to promote students' SRL would improve within a professional development program. It was reported that over a period of 6 months most teachers improved their knowledge of SRL-based instruction and, especially, their repertoire of strategies regarding how to create a high-SR classroom.

Teacher professional development programs are a viable means for cultivating SRL instruction in the classroom. However, teacher personal epistemologies and systems of beliefs, and teacher related motivational and individual differences factors need to be taken into consideration when planning a teacher training program (Moos and Ringdal 2012). So far, empirical evidence highlights the need for continued professional development of teachers in SRL strategies and their application in the classroom.

To summarize the present unit, explicit instruction of SRL is not frequently observed in authentic classroom environments. Teachers' knowledge, beliefs, values, their skills for self-regulating own learning and instruction and promoting those of their students, interact with SRL promotion in the classroom. Professional development programs and interventions in SRL instruction provide promising results. However, more research is needed to delimit the conditions that can render such programs successful at a large scale and embed them in classroom instruction.

9.4 General Conclusions and Implications for Research and Practice

As children grow, they are expected to gradually acquire competences to self-regulate their behavior and learning processes. The central claim of the present paper is that parents and teachers play a key role in children's developing skills to self-regulate their learning efforts. Regarding the role of parents in fostering children's SRL skills, it has been shown that stimulating cognitively children's learning efforts within an emotionally and motivationally supportive environment is associated with gains in children's developing executive functions, behavior control, cognitive, metacognitive, and motivational skills during learning. For example, aspects of parental support, such as contingent support and encouraging the child's independent learning and gradual autonomy are essential for SRL skills to grow as well as for school performance and social and school adaptation. Research in this area should further investigate how different aspects of parental support of learning differentially impact children's various groups of SRL skills and the role of contextual factors, such as school practices, in the above relations. This is important because SRL lies at the junction of parental and school practices as well as child characteristics. This calls for complex research designs that make use of multiple informants and multiple research methods tapping different aspects of SRL.

Regarding teachers' role in fostering students' SRL skills, it has been shown that when explicit and meaningful instruction of learning strategies takes place in the classroom, important cognitive, motivational and performance gains for students are evidenced. Teachers may act as role model for SRL by making explicit the strategies they use to self-regulate their own learning and teaching or include explicit instruction of SRL skills in their lessons. Teachers may also engage students in discussions about SRL strategies in a meaningful learning context.

Teacher professional development programs for promotion of student SRL can be effective but there is a need to adapt the SRL strategies trained to the characteristics of different knowledge domains and subject matter taught in the classroom. That is, SRL should be viewed as both domain-free and domain-specific skills. Such an approach could conciliate teacher need to promote content knowledge and skills with the use of cognitive and regulatory strategies that are specific to that content. Such an approach to SRL instruction in school requires both a theoretical shift in the conceptualization of SRL and a paradigm shift in teacher professional development programs. For example, such programs could address the needs of teachers of specific subject matter and content knowledge, the differences in pedagogical knowledge and belief or value systems among teachers, the matching of student characteristics with the SRL demands of the specific knowledge domains, the provision of opportunities for teacher active learning of SRL skills and embedding SRL in their teaching practices, as well as provision of feedback on their teaching performance while learning (see Harris et al. 2015). Future interventions focusing on teacher professional development should also support teachers' reflection on, evaluation of, and revision of teaching practices to construct new conceptual knowledge (Butler et al. 2004) but also beliefs and attitudes regarding teaching and learning in the classroom.

References

Alexander, P. A. (2018). Commentary looking down the road: Future directions for research on depth and regulation of strategic processing. *British Journal of Educational Psychology, 88*, 152–166.

Alexander, P. A., Graham, S., & Harris, K. (1998). A perspective on strategy research: Progress and prospects. *Educational Psychology Review, 10*, 129–154.

Anderman, L. H., Andrzejewski, C. E., & Allen, J. (2011). How do teachers support students' motivation and learning in their classrooms? *Teachers College Record, 113*, 969–1003.

Arsal, Z. (2010). The effects of diaries on self-regulation strategies of pre-service science teachers. *International Journal of Environmental and Science Education, 5*, 85–103.

Artzt, A., & Armour-Thomas, E. (2001). Mathematics teaching as problem solving: A framework for studying teacher metacognition underlying instructional practice in mathematics. In H. J. Hartman (Ed.), *Metacognition in learning and instruction* (pp. 127–148). The Netherlands: Kluwer Academic Publishers.

Bernier, A., Carlson, S. M., & Whipple, N. (2010). From external regulation to self-regulation: Early parenting precursors of young children's executive functioning. *Child Development, 81*, 326–339.

Boekaerts, M. (1997). Self-regulated learning: A new concept embraced by researchers, policy makers, educators, teachers, and students. *Learning and Instruction, 7*, 161–186.

Bronson, M. (2000). *Self-regulation in early childhood: Nature and nurture*. New York: Guilford Press.

Butler, D., Lauscher, H., Jarvis-Selinger, S., & Beckingham, B. (2004). Collaboration and self-regulation in teachers' professional development. *Teaching and Teacher Education, 20*, 435–455.

Capa-Aydin, Y., Sungur, S., & Uzuntiryaki, E. (2009). Teacher self-regulation: Examining a multidimensional construct. *Educational Psychology, 29*, 345–356.

Chatzistamatiou, M., & Dermitzaki, I. (2013). Teaching mathematics with self-regulation and for self-regulation: Teachers' reports. *Hellenic Journal of Psychology, 10*, 253–274.
Chatzistamatiou, M., Dermitzaki, I., & Bagiatis, V. (2014). Self-regulatory teaching in mathematics: Relations to teachers' motivation, affect and professional commitment. *European Journal of Psychology of Education, 29*, 295–310.
Colman, R. A., Hardy, S. A., Albert, M., Raffaelli, M., & Crockett, L. (2006). Early predictors of self-regulation in middle childhood. *Infant and Child Development, 15*, 421–437.
de Bruin, A. B. H., & van Merriënboer, J. J. G. (2017). Bridging cognitive load and self-regulated learning research: A complementary approach to contemporary issues in educational research. *Learning and Instruction, 51*, 1–9.
De Smul, M., Heirweg, S., Van Keer, H., Devos, G., & Vandevelde, S. (2018). How competent do teachers feel instructing self-regulated learning strategies? Development and validation of the teacher self-efficacy scale to implement self-regulated learning. *Teaching and Teacher Education, 71*, 214–225.
Dent, A. L., & Koenka, A. C. (2016). The relation between self-regulated learning and academic achievement across childhood and adolescence: A meta-analysis. *Educational Psychology Review, 28*, 425–474.
Dermitzaki, I., & Kriekouki, M. (2017). Implementing a teacher education program on fostering students' self-regulated learning. In D.-M. Kakana & P. Manoli (Eds.), *Digital proceedings from the 3rd international symposium on new issues on teacher education-ISNITE 2015* (pp. 302–309). Volos: University of Thessaly Press.
Devine, R., Bignardi, G., & Hughes, C. (2016). Executive function mediates the relations between parental behaviors and children's early academic ability. *Frontiers in Psychology, 7*, 1902.
Dignath, C., & Büttner, G. (2018). Teachers' direct and indirect promotion of self-regulated learning in primary and secondary school mathematics classes–insights from video-based classroom observations and teacher interviews. *Metacognition and Learning, 13*, 127–157.
Dignath-van Ewijk, C. (2016). Which components of teacher competence determine whether teachers enhance self-regulated learning? Predicting teachers' self-reported promotion of self-regulated learning by means of teacher beliefs, knowledge, and self-efficacy. *Frontline Learning Research, 4*, 83–105.
Dumka, L. E., Gonzales, N. A., Wheeler, L. A., & Millsap, R. E. (2010). Parenting self-efficacy and parenting practices over time in Mexican American families. *Journal of Family Psychology, 24*, 522–531.
Efklides, A. (2008). Metacognition: Defining its facets and levels of functioning in relation to self-regulation and co-regulation. *European Psychologist, 13*, 277–287.
Efklides, A. (2011). Interactions of metacognition with motivation and affect in self-regulated learning: The MASRL model. *Educational Psychologist, 46*, 1–20.
Efklides, A., & Misailidi, P. (2019). Emotional self-regulation in the early years: The role of cognition, metacognition and social interaction. In D. Whitebread, K. Kumpulainen, M. McClelland, V. Grau, & A. Pasternak (Eds.), *The sage handbook of developmental psychology and early childhood education* (pp. 502–516). London: Sage Publications.
Eisenberg, N., Fabes, R. A., Shepard, S. A., Guthrie, I. K., Murphy, B. C., & Reiser, M. (1999). Parental reactions to children's negative emotions: Longitudinal relations to quality of children's social functioning. *Child Development, 70*, 513–534.
Erdmann, K. A., & Hertel, S. (2019). Self-regulation and co-regulation in early childhood. Development, assessment and supporting factors. *Metacognition and Learning, 14*, 229–238.
Fender, J. G., Richert, R. A., Robb, M. B., & Wartella, E. (2010). Parent teaching focus and toddlers' learning from an infant DVD. *Infant and Child Development, 19*, 613–627.
Festas, I., Oliveira, A. L., Rebelo, J. A., Damião, M. H., Harris, K., & Graham, S. (2015). Professional development in self-regulated strategy development: Effects on the writing performance of eighth grade Portuguese students. *Contemporary Educational Psychology, 40*, 17–27.
Ghonsooly, B., & Ghanizadeh, A. (2011). Self-efficacy and self-regulation and their relationship: A study of Iranian EFL teachers. *Language Learning Journal, 41*, 1–17.

Glatz, T., & Buchanan, C. M. (2015). Over-time associations among parental self-efficacy, promotive parenting practices, and adolescents' externalizing behaviors. *Journal of Family Psychology, 29*, 427–437.
Gonzalez-DeHass, A. R., Willems, P. P., & Holbein, M. F. D. (2005). Examining the relationship between parental involvement and student motivation. *Educational Psychology Review, 17*, 99–123.
Grolnick, W. S., Gurland, S. T., De Courcey, W., & Jacob, K. (2002). Antecedents and consequences of mothers' autonomy support: An experimental investigation. *Developmental Psychology, 38*, 143–155.
Hamman, D. (1998). Preservice teachers' value for learning-strategy instruction. *The Journal of Experimental Education, 66*, 209–221.
Hamman, D., Berthelot, J., Saia, J., & Crowley, E. (2000). Teachers' coaching of learning and its relation to students' strategic learning. *Journal of Educational Psychology, 92*, 342–348.
Hammond, S. I., Müller, U., Carpendale, J. I., Bibok, M. B., & Liebermann-Finestone, D. P. (2012). The effects of parental scaffolding on preschoolers' executive function. *Developmental Psychology, 48*, 271–281.
Harris, K. R., Graham, S., & Adkins, M. (2015). Practice-based professional development of self-regulated strategy development for tier 2 at-risk writers in second grade. *Contemporary Educational Psychology, 40*, 5–16.
Hartman, J. H. (2001). Teaching metacognitively. In H. J. Hartman (Ed.), *Metacognition in learning and instruction* (pp. 149–172). The Netherlands: Kluwer Academic Publishers.
Hess, C. R., Teti, D. M., & Hussey-Gardner, B. (2004). Self-efficacy and parenting of high-risk infants: The moderating role of parent knowledge of infant development. *Journal of Applied Developmental Psychology, 25*, 423–437.
Hilden, K. R., & Pressley, M. (2007). Self-regulation through transactional strategies instruction. *Reading and Writing Quarterly, 23*, 51–75.
Hill, N. E., & Tyson, D. F. (2009). Parental involvement in middle school: A meta-analytic assessment of the strategies that promote achievement. *Developmental Psychology, 45*, 740–763.
Hong, J. C., Hwang, M. Y., Kuo, Y. C., & Hsu, W. Y. (2015). Parental monitoring and helicopter parenting relevant to vocational student's procrastination and self-regulated learning. *Learning and Individual Differences, 42*, 139–146.
Hubbs-Tait, L., Culp, A. M., Culp, R. E., & Miller, C. E. (2002). Relation of maternal cognitive stimulation, emotional support, and intrusive behavior during head start to children's kindergarten cognitive abilities. *Child Development, 73*, 110–131.
Hustedt, J. T., & Raver, C. C. (2002). Scaffolding in low-income mother-child dyads: Relations with joint attention and dyadic reciprocity. *International Journal of Behavioral Development, 26*, 113–119.
Joussemet, M., Koestner, R., Lekes, N., & Landry, R. (2005). A longitudinal study of the relationship of maternal autonomy support to children's adjustment and achievement in school. *Journal of Personality, 73*, 1215–1236.
Kallia, E., & Dermitzaki, I. (2017). Assessing maternal practices that support children's self-regulated learning. *Hellenic Journal of Psychology, 14*, 83–112.
Kane, R., Sandetto, S., & Heath, C. (2002). Telling half the story: A critical review of research on the teaching beliefs and practices of university academics. *Review of Educational Research, 72*, 177–228.
Karbach, J., Gottschling, J., Spengler, M., Hegewald, K., & Spinath, F. M. (2013). Parental involvement and general cognitive ability as predictors of domain-specific academic achievement in early adolescence. *Learning and Instruction, 23*, 43–51.
Karreman, A., Van Tuijl, C., Van Aken, M. A., & Deković, M. (2008). Parenting, coparenting, and effortful control in preschoolers. *Journal of Family Psychology, 22*, 30–40.

Kistner, S., Rakoczy, K., Otto, B., Dignath-van Ewijk, D., Büttner, G., & Klieme, E. (2010). Promotion of self-regulated learning in classrooms: Investigating frequency, quality, and consequences for student performance. *Metacognition and Learning, 5*, 157–171.

Kochanska, G., Murray, K. T., & Harlan, E. T. (2000). Effortful control in early childhood continuity and change: Antecedents, and implications for social development. *Developmental Psychology, 36*, 220–232.

Kramarski, B., & Michalsky, T. (2009). Investigating preservice teachers' professional growth in self-regulated learning environments. *Journal of Educational Psychology, 101*, 161–175.

Lawson, M. J., Vosniadou, S., Van Deur, P., Wyra, M., & Jeffries, D. (2019). Teachers' and students' belief systems about the self-regulation of learning. *Educational Psychology Review, 31*, 223–251.

Leerkes, E. M., Blankson, A. N., O'Brien, M., Calkins, S. D., & Marcovitch, S. (2011). The relation of maternal emotional and cognitive support during problem solving to pre-academic skills in preschoolers. *Infant and Child Development, 20*, 353–370.

Lengua, L. J. (2006). Growth in temperament and parenting as predictors of adjustment during children's transition to adolescence. *Developmental Psychology, 42*, 819–832.

Lengua, L. J., Honorado, E., & Bush, N. R. (2007). Contextual risk and parenting as predictors of effortful control and social competence in preschool children. *Journal of Applied Developmental Psychology, 28*, 40–55.

Littlefield-Cook, J. L., & Cook, G. (2009). *Child development. Principles and perspectives* (2nd ed.). Boston: Pearson Education.

Lombaerts, K., Engels, N., & van Braak, J. (2009). Determinants of teachers' recognitions of self-regulated learning practices in elementary education. *Journal of Educational Research, 102*, 163–173.

Lowe, J., Erickson, S. J., MacLean, P., Duvall, S. W., Ohls, R. K., & Duncan, A. F. (2014). Associations between maternal scaffolding and executive functioning in 3 and 4 year olds born very low birth weight and normal birth weight. *Early Human Development, 90*, 587–593.

Martinez-Pons, M. (2002). Parental influences on children's academic self-regulatory development. *Theory Into Practice, 41*, 126–131.

Mattanah, J. F., Pratt, M. W., Cowan, P. A., & Cowan, C. P. (2005). Authoritative parenting, parental scaffolding of long-division mathematics, and children's academic competence in fourth grade. *Journal of Applied Developmental Psychology, 26*, 85–106.

Mermelshtine, R., & Barnes, J. (2016). Maternal responsive–didactic caregiving in play interactions with 10-month-olds and cognitive development at 18 months. *Infant and Child Development, 25*, 296–316.

Mokrova, I. L., O'Brien, M., Calkins, S. D., Leerkes, E. M., & Marcovitch, S. (2012). Links between family social status and preschoolers' persistence: The role of maternal values and quality of parenting. *Infant and Child Development, 21*, 617–633.

Moos, D. C., & Ringdal, A. (2012). Self-regulated learning in the classroom: A literature review on the teacher's role. *Education Research International, 2012*, 1–15.

Mulvaney, M. K., McCartney, K., Bub, K. L., & Marshall, N. L. (2006). Determinants of dyadic scaffolding and cognitive outcomes in first graders. *Parenting: Science and Practice, 6*, 297–320.

Neitzel, C., & Stright, A. D. (2003). Mothers' scaffolding of children's problem solving: Establishing a foundation of academic self-regulatory competence. *Journal of Family Psychology, 17*, 147–159.

Neitzel, C., & Stright, A. D. (2004). Parenting behaviours during child problem solving: The roles of child temperament, mother education and personality, and the problem-solving context. *International Journal of Behavioral Development, 28*, 166–179.

Opdenakker, M. C., & Van Damme, J. (2006). Teacher characteristics and teaching styles as effectiveness enhancing factors of classroom practice. *Teaching and Teacher Education, 22*, 1–21.

Paris, S. G., & Paris, A. H. (2001). Classroom applications of research on self-regulated learning. *Educational Psychologist, 36*, 89–101.
Perels, F., Merget-Kullmann, M., Wende, M., Schmitz, B., & Buchbinder, C. (2009). Improving self-regulated learning of preschool children: Evaluation of training for kindergarten teachers. *British Journal of Educational Psychology, 79*, 311–327.
Perry, N. E., & VandeKamp, K. O. (2000). Creating classroom contexts that support young children's development of self-regulated learning. *International Journal of Educational Research, 33*, 821–843.
Perry, N. E., VandeKamp, K. O., Mercer, L. K., & Nordby, C. J. (2002). Investigating teacher-student interactions that foster self-regulated learning. *Educational Psychologist, 37*, 5–15.
Peters-Burton, E. E., & Botov, I. S. (2017). Self-regulated learning micro-analysis as a tool to inform professional development delivery in real time. *Metacognition and Learning, 12*, 45–78.
Pino-Pasternak, D. (2014). Applying an observational lens to identify parental behaviours associated with children's homework motivation. *British Journal of Educational Psychology, 84*, 352–375.
Pino-Pasternak, D., & Whitebread, D. (2010). The role of parenting in children's self-regulated learning. *Educational Research Review, 5*, 220–242.
Pino-Pasternak, D., Whitebread, D., & Tolmie, A. (2010). A multidimensional analysis of parent–child interactions during academic tasks and their relationships with children's self-regulated learning. *Cognition and Instruction, 28*, 219–272.
Pressley, M., & Harris, K. R. (2008). Cognitive strategies instruction: From basic research to classroom instruction. *The Journal of Education, 189*, 77–94.
Razza, R. A., & Raymond, K. (2013). Associations among maternal behavior, delay of gratification, and school readiness across the early childhood years. *Social Development, 22*, 180–196.
Retelsdorf, J., Butler, R., Streblow, L., & Schiefele, U. (2010). Teachers' goal orientations for teaching: Associations with instructional practices, interest in teaching, and burnout. *Learning and Instruction, 20*, 30–46.
Robinson, J. B., Burns, B. M., & Davis, D. W. (2009). Maternal scaffolding and attention regulation in children living in poverty. *Journal of Applied Developmental Psychology, 30*, 82–91.
Schunk, D. A., & Greene, J. A. (Eds.). (2018). *Handbook of self-regulation of learning and performance* (2nd ed.). New York: Routledge.
Silinskas, G., Kiuru, N., Aunola, K., Lerkkanen, M. K., & Nurmi, J. E. (2015). The developmental dynamics of children's academic performance and mothers' homework-related affect and practices. *Developmental Psychology, 51*, 419–433.
Slobodskaya, H. R., Petrenko, E. N., Loginova, S. V., Kornienko, O. S., & Kozlova, E. A. (2019). Relations of child effortful control to personality, well-being and parenting. *International Journal of Psychology, 1–10*, 144–153. https://doi.org/10.1002/ijop.12568.
Spruce, R., & Bol, L. (2015). Teacher beliefs, knowledge, and practice of self-regulated learning. *Metacognition and Learning, 10*, 245–277.
Stewart, P. W., Cooper, S. S., & Moulding, L. R. (2007). Metacognitive developments in professional educators. *The Researcher, 21*, 32–40.
Stoeger, H., & Ziegler, A. (2011). Self-regulatory training through elementary-school students' homework completion. In B. J. Zimmerman & D. H. Schunk (Eds.), *Handbook of self-regulation of learning and performance* (pp. 87–101). New York: Routledge.
Stright, A. D., Neitzel, C., Sears, K. G., & Hoke-Sinex, L. (2001). Instruction begins in the home: Relations between parental instruction and children's self-regulation in the classroom. *Journal of Educational Psychology, 93*, 456–466.
Stright, A. D., Gallagher, K. C., & Kelley, K. (2008). Infant temperament moderates relations between maternal parenting in early childhood and children's adjustment in first grade. *Child Development, 79*, 186–200.
Stright, A. D., Herr, M. Y., & Neitzel, C. (2009). Maternal scaffolding of children's problem solving and children's adjustment in kindergarten: Hmong families in the United States. *Journal of Educational Psychology, 101*, 207–218.

Sun, J., & Tang, Y. (2019). Maternal scaffolding strategies and early development of self-regulation in Chinese preschoolers. *Early Child Development and Care, 189*, 1525–1537.
Valcan, D. S., Davis, H., & Pino-Pasternak, D. (2018). Parental behaviours predicting early childhood executive functions: A meta-analysis. *Educational Psychology Review, 30*, 607–649.
Vasquez, A. C., Patall, E. A., Fong, C. J., Corrigan, A. S., & Pine, L. (2016). Parent autonomy support, academic achievement, and psychosocial functioning: A meta-analysis of research. *Educational Psychology Review, 28*, 605–644.
Veenman, S., Beems, D., Gerrits, S., & Op de Weegh, G. (1999). Implementation effects of a training program for self-regulated learning. *Journal of Research and Development in Education, 32*, 148–159.
Waeytens, K., Lens, W., & Vandenberghe, R. (2002). "Learning to learn": Teachers' conceptions of their supporting role. *Learning and Instruction, 12*, 305–322.
Weinstein, C. E., Husman, J., & Dierking, D. R. (2000). Self-regulation interventions with a focus on learning strategies. In M. Boekaerts, P. R. Pintrich, & M. Zeidner (Eds.), *Handbook of self-regulation* (pp. 727–747). San Diego: Academic.
Wood, D., & Middleton, D. (1975). A study of assisted problem-solving. *British Journal of Psychology, 66*, 181–191.
Xu, H., & Ko, P. Y. (2019). Enhancing teachers' knowledge of how to promote self-regulated learning in primary school students: A case study in Hong Kong. *Teaching and Teacher Education, 80*, 106–114.
Yan, Z. (2018). How teachers' beliefs and demographic variables impact on self-regulated learning instruction. *Educational Studies, 44*, 564–577.
Zeytinoglu, S., Calkins, S. D., & Leerkes, E. M. (2019). Maternal emotional support but not cognitive support during problem-solving predicts increases in cognitive flexibility in early childhood. *International Journal of Behavioral Development, 43*, 12–23.
Zhang, H., & Whitebread, D. (2017). Linking parental scaffolding with self-regulated learning in Chinese kindergarten children. *Learning and Instruction, 49*, 121–130.
Zimmerman, B. J. (2000). Attaining self-regulation: A social-cognitive perspective. In M. Boekaerts, P. R. Pintrich, & M. Zeidner (Eds.), *Handbook of self-regulation* (pp. 13–39). San Diego: Academic.
Zimmerman, B. J. (2002). Becoming a self-regulated learner: An overview. *Theory Into Practice, 41*, 64–70.
Zohar, A. (2004). *Higher order thinking in science classrooms: Students' learning and teachers' professional development*. Dordrecht: Kluwer Academic Publishers.

Part III
Metacognition and Affect in Life-Span Development

Chapter 10
Understanding Cognitive Mental States and Emotions in Early Childhood: Dissociation and Interconnectedness

Plousia Misailidi

Abstract This chapter focuses on the development of children's abilities to understand cognitive mental states and emotions in early childhood. Are these abilities dissociable or interconnected components of the young child's theory of mind (ToM)? We approach this question by reviewing the findings of recent developmental and neuropsychological studies. The developmental evidence supports both the dissociation and the interconnectedness of the two abilities. Similarly, the neuropsychological data indicate that common and independent neural substrates are involved in the processing of cognitive and emotional mental states. It is concluded that the two abilities should be regarded as components of a "nearly decomposable" ToM system that develops dynamically during the early years of life.

Keywords Children · Cognitive mental states · Dissociation · Emotions · Interconnectedness · Theory of mind

10.1 Introduction

Children's theory of mind (ToM) has dominated developmental research for the last 35 years. ToM studies investigate children's ability to attribute mental states—such as beliefs, intentions, emotion and knowledge—to oneself and to other people (Premack and Woodruff 1978). This research has documented that ToM emerges early in life and is key to a child's understanding of the social world (for reviews see Sabbagh and Bowman 2018 and Wellman 2011, 2014). ToM enables children to understand and predict other people's behaviour and successfully navigate in their social environment. Once a child develops a ToM, "the assumption is that this understanding guides all social action and interaction" (Wellman 1993, p. 10).

P. Misailidi (✉)
Department of Primary Education, University of Ioannina, Ioannina, Greece
e-mail: pmisaili@uoi.gr

D. Moraitou, P. Metallidou (eds.), *Trends and Prospects in Metacognition Research across the Life Span*, https://doi.org/10.1007/978-3-030-51673-4_10

Research examining the development of ToM in early childhood has traditionally focused on children's ability to understand what other people believe and know and specifically on their growing awareness of others' false beliefs (Wellman et al. 2001). However, ToM extends beyond the ability to understand cognitive mental states. It also involves the ability to make inferences about other people's (and one's own) emotions, and to appreciate that others can have both palpable and concealed emotional experiences (Lane et al. 2010; Pons et al. 2004).

The aim of this chapter is to provide a review of studies on the development of children's abilities to understand cognitive mental states and emotions during the first years of life. The overarching question that guides this review is: to what extent can these abilities be considered dissociable or interconnected components of the young child's ToM? After a brief presentation of competing views about the unitary vs. componential nature of ToM, the main part of this review concentrates on the presentation of studies investigating the major milestones of young children's abilities to understand cognitive mental states and emotions. This research indicates that the two abilities develop along independent trajectories in the early years of life.[1] Then, some recent developmental work is discussed documenting interrelations between the two abilities. Next, neuroimaging studies are presented which add new data into the picture, supporting that the neural systems associated with children's understanding of cognitive mental states and emotions are subserved by independent and common neural systems. Finally, the implications of these findings for the architecture (/structure) of ToM and for research investigating the links between ToM and metacognition are discussed.

10.2 Theory of Mind: Unitary or Componential?

A theoretical challenge in the field of ToM is the lack of agreement about the structure of this ability: is ToM a unitary system for making inferences about others' mental states or a collection of individual, more specialized, abilities or components? For many years the dominant approach posited that ToM is a unitary inferential system, in many ways analogous to scientific theories (Gopnik and Wellman 1994). However, as Naito (2004) has put forward, the notion that ToM is unitary has hampered efforts to explore the exact nature of the individual mental-state abilities that comprise ToM.

More recently, a shift in the traditional ToM approach has taken place. Researchers have put forward that ToM is "a suite of distinct capacities" (Boyer and Barrett 2005, p. 106) or components (Schaafsma et al. 2015; Tager-Flusberg and Sullivan 2000), each one dedicated to carrying out a specific function in the prediction and explanation of action. Componential models (see Tsoi 2016 for a

[1]This chapter does not review clinical data on children's abilities to understand cognitive mental states and emotions. Instead, its aim is to provide a review of studies that have focused on the typical development of these abilities in early childhood.

review) emphasize distinctions between different ToM components, such as an intuitive and a reflective ToM (Astington and Hughes 2013), an implicit and an explicit ToM (Apperly and Butterfill 2009; Dienes and Perner 1999), an early- and a late-developing ToM (Saxe et al. 2004) and so forth. Here, the essential distinction that is considered is that between cognitive and emotional (or affective) ToM[2] (Dvash and Shamay-Tsoory 2014; Shamay-Tsoory and Aharon-Peretz 2007; Smith et al. 2003). These are often characterized as the "cold" and "hot" aspects of ToM (Brothers and Ring 1992).

Are inferences about "cold" cognitive mental states different from inferences about "hot" emotional states? First, although both abilities are expressions of the mind's capacity to form "higher-order representations with lower-order representations embedded within them" (i.e., metarepresentations, Wilson 2000, p. 411), in the former the lower-order representations are epistemic states (e.g., beliefs, knowledge, thinking) whereas in the latter the lower-order representations are emotions (e.g., happiness, sadness, guilt, shame). Second, for some researchers inferences about cognitive mental states and inferences about emotions rely on different types of information cues: on the one hand, emotion inferences rely primarily on decoding immediately available observable stimuli (i.e., facial cues); on the other hand cognitive mental state inferences depend mainly on contextual cues (e.g., background scenery) (Sabbagh 2004; Sabbagh and Bowman 2018). However, more recent accounts postulate that neither type of cue "wins out" or dominates inferences about cognitive mental states or emotions respectively (e.g., Mitchell and Phillips 2015; see also Ong et al. 2015). Inferring others' cognitive mental states and emotions depend similarly on the integration of different types of observable and contextual cues. In fact, combining multiple and sometimes competing cues, such as facial expressions and information about the context, is necessary in order to make inferences about the two classes of mental states (Ong et al. 2015).

10.3 Evidence for Dissociation: Independent Developmental Trajectories

A number of studies have investigated the development of young children's abilities to understand cognitive mental states and emotions in early childhood. These studies have reported evidence indicating that the two abilities follow distinct

[2]While reviewing the available literature, it became clear that the term emotional (or affective) ToM has more than one interpretations. Some researchers adopt a broad meaning of the term by describing emotional ToM not only as a person's understanding of emotions but also as her or his "empathic appreciation" of these mental states ("...knowledge and empathic understanding of their emotional states and feelings", Shamay-Tsoory and Aharon-Peretz 2007, p. 3055). This definition is not adopted here. Instead, the term emotional ToM is used narrowly to specifically denote children's ability to make inferences about others' (and their own) emotional states (see also Efklides and Misailidi 2019).

developmental trajectories. We first provide a review of research on young children's understanding of cognitive mental states, starting from their ability to explicitly (and implicitly) attribute false beliefs to their ability to make sophisticated inferences about other people's thinking. We then turn to a review of studies on young children's ability to understand others' emotions, beginning with a discussion of recent work revealing an early-emerging understanding of the links between other people's goals and emotions to research documenting an abstract appreciation of the links between beliefs and emotions and the distinction between real and apparent emotions.

10.3.1 Understanding Cognitive Mental States

The milestone that has attracted the greatest attention from researchers studying children's understanding of cognitive mental states is the development of their ability to understand beliefs. Typically, this ability is measured with false belief tasks, which assess children's capacity to understand that other people (as well as themselves) might have beliefs that do not coincide with external reality. In a classic version of this task (Wimmer and Perner 1983), children are presented with a story about a character who hides an object in a specific place and then exits the scene. While the character is away, a second character moves the object from its original place to a different location. Children are then asked to predict where the first character will seek out the object. Children aged 4 years or older correctly predict that the character will look for the object in the first location, indicating that they have developed an adult-like ability to attribute false beliefs to others. In contrast, 3-year-olds are unable to take into account the character's false belief and consistently respond that the first character will look for the object where they themselves know that it really is located.

This 3- to 4-year-old shift in children's thinking about false belief is one of the most consistently replicated and robust findings. A meta-analytic investigation of 178 false belief studies has shown that, despite task modifications, children transition from giving reality-based responses to answering correctly the false belief question between the ages of 3 to 4 years (Wellman et al. 2001). Other meta-analytic studies have shown that this shift is relatively stable across cultures (Liu et al. 2008). A number of researchers have suggested that this shift indicates a qualitative conceptual change: the point at which children are able to successfully pass classic false belief tasks is the point at which they are able to understand that the world is represented in the mind and that our mental representations of the world—even the incorrect ones—guide our everyday behaviour (Astington 2003; Perner 1991).

Although the majority of studies on children's understanding of false belief have concentrated on preschoolers, more recently researchers have begun advocating that knowledge of belief begins at 15 months of age (Onishi and Baillargeon 2005) or younger (Luo and Baillargeon 2007; Surian et al. 2007). Using non-verbal false belief tasks (e.g., tasks that measure violation of expectation looking times, anticipatory looking patterns), these researchers have shown that infants have an implicit understanding of false belief. Nevertheless, this conclusion has been debated by other investigators who have put forward that infants' good performance on such tasks is the result of other abilities (e.g., application of behaviour rules, Perner and Ruffman 2005; lower level associations, Ruffman 2014) and does not reflect a genuine understanding of belief. Furthermore, other evidence indicates that the abilities measured by the non-verbal and the verbal false belief tasks are dissociated (Schneider et al. 2014).

Children's understanding of cognitive mental states expands during the preschool period. For example, at about the same time they begin to pass verbal false-belief tasks, children also demonstrate a capacity to distinguish between appearance and reality. In a standard appearance-reality task, children are shown a deceptive object (e.g., a sponge that is painted to look like a brick) and, without knowledge of the deception, they are asked what the object looks like. Immediately afterwards, the real identity of the object is revealed to children and two questions are asked: "What does it look like?" and "What is it really?". Four- and 5-year-olds respond correctly that the object is really a sponge but it looks like a brick. In contrast, the 3-year-olds, fail to differentiate between the object's appearance and reality and respond either that the object looks like a brick and is a brick ("phenomenalism error") or that it looks like a sponge and is a sponge ("realism error") (Flavell et al. 1986; Moll and Tomasello 2012, Experiment 2). These results indicate that from about the age of 4 years, children develop the ability to hold dual representations of a deceptive object's apparent and real identity. Moreover, children's performance on appearance-reality tasks typically correlates with their performance on standard false belief tasks (Carlson and Moses 2001; Gopnik and Astington 1988), which indicates that they both are indexes of an understanding of the representational nature of cognitive mental states (Wellman 2014).

By the time children develop the ability to pass false belief and appearance-reality tasks, they are also able to understand the non-physical (mental) status of thoughts—such as the thought of a grape–, and to distinguish them from their physical counterparts–a grape inside a person's stomach (Estes 1998; Watson et al. 1998). They also understand the "seeing-leads-to-knowing principle", that is, they judge that a person who had visual access inside a box will know what its contents are, but a person who simply touched or lifted the box, without looking inside, will not know (Pratt and Bryant 1990).

Understanding of cognitive mental states continues to develop in important respects beyond the preschool years. At the age of 6 or 7 years, children develop the ability to understand thinking as an internal mental activity (e.g., Flavell et al. 1997, 2000). For example, in contrast to preschoolers, who do not understand that thinking is embedded in a continuous stream of consciousness (James 1890), 6- to 7-year-olds acknowledge that a woman who sits quietly in a chair, having a thoughtful pose, has some thoughts in her mind—that is, that the mind is continuously engaged in thinking (Flavell et al. 1993, 1995, 1998). After age 7, children also develop an understanding of cognitive cueing (Flavell et al. 1998). They gradually recognize that one thought automatically triggers another related thought and that these thoughts can sometimes be unwanted and intrusive and they are difficult to get rid of (Flavell et al. 1995). These abilities have been interpreted as evidence that older children have developed an understanding of the mind "as a homunculus or processing device that is constantly active" (Harris 2006, p. 833).

10.3.2 Understanding Emotions

Compared to the large number of studies examining the development of children's ability to understand false beliefs and other cognitive mental states, considerably fewer studies have investigated young children's mentalistic understanding of emotions in the first years of life (Harris 2008). Infants younger than 10 months of age can detect the positive vs. negative affective valence of facial expressions of emotion (Vaillant-Molina et al. 2013) and they use the emotions expressed in the faces of their caregivers' as signposts on how to behave when they are confronted with an ambiguous situation (Striano and Rochat 2000; Vaish and Striano 2004). This has been interpreted as evidence that infants know that the caregiver's emotional expression signals her or his emotional stance towards a particular object or situation (Repacholi 1998; see also Harris 2006).

Other researchers disagree that the infant's ability to discriminate emotions in the faces of others is a sign of a mentalistic understanding of emotions. They propose, instead, that children's understanding of emotional mental states begins to develop when they are able to use the emotion expressed in a person's face to predict how that person will act (Reschke et al. 2017). A number of studies have investigated the relation between emotional expressions and goal-directed actions (Phillips et al. 2002; Skerry and Spelke 2014). For example, Phillips et al. (2002) reported that by the age of 14 months infants use the combined information about a person's emotional expression and direction of gaze to predict that person's actions. More recently, Skerry and Spelke (2014) showed that even at the age of 10 months infants are able to predict that an agent who has attained its goal will express a positive emotion rather than a negative emotion. Ten-month-olds in their study looked longer at the agent who expressed a negative emotion when it followed an attained goal than when it followed a goal that was not attained.

By the age of 2 to 3 years, children's understanding of emotional mental states expands to include a more sophisticated understanding of their causes. For example, 2-year-olds use emotion terms in a way indicating that they appreciate the links between the emotions and the situations or events that cause them (e.g., "Grandma mad. I wrote on wall"; "Me fall down. Me cry"; Bretherton et al. 1986, p. 534). When they reach the age of 3 years, children also begin to appreciate that external situations can elicit specific emotional states (Borke 1972; Harris et al. 1987). For example, 3-year-olds are able to predict the happiness a child feels at receiving a beautiful gift or the sadness that precipitates the loss of a cherished toy. Nevertheless, at this age, children are unable yet to understand that it is not the objective features of a situation but the mental states of the person appraising the situation which trigger the emotion (Harris et al. 2014). An appreciation of the role that cognitive mental states play in the elicitation of emotion is a later achievement.

In a pioneering investigation of young children's understanding of beliefs as causes of emotions, Harris et al. (1989) presented 4- to 6-year-old children with a series of stories, each featuring an animal character, a monkey named Mickey, who liked to play tricks on others. In one of the stories, the monkey played a nasty trick on an elephant, named Ellie, whose desire was to drink coke and nothing else. Mickey replaced the contents of a coke can with milk and offered it to Ellie. Children were asked to predict how Ellie would feel when she saw the coke can and how she would feel when she tasted its real contents. The results showed that the majority of the 4-year-olds failed to take into consideration Ellie's false belief and predicted that she would feel sad both on seeing the coke can and after tasting it. In contrast, 6-year-olds answered correctly that Ellie would feel happiness before opening the can and sadness afterwards. These results have been replicated in subsequent studies (e.g., de Rosnay et al. 2004; Harris et al. 1989; Pons et al. 2004), while more recent research has shown that the same findings hold when children are questioned about their own false beliefs as causes of emotions (Bender et al. 2011).

By 6 years, children also develop the ability to distinguish between genuine and dissembled emotions. Six-year-olds begin to understand that some social situations require dissembling one's real emotion. For example, when given a disappointing gift it is appropriate to display happiness rather than sadness. Thus, they begin to understand that the outward expression (appearance) can be dissembled and, thus, it will not correspond to the emotion felt subjectively (reality) (Gross and Harris 1988; Misailidi 2006). Six-year-old children are also able to (a) understand the different motives (prosocial, self-protective) for emotional dissemblance (Gosselin et al. 2002; Naito and Seki 2009) and (b) acknowledge the misleading effect that an individual's dissembled emotion can have upon the minds of others (Gross and Harris 1988).

To summarize, the studies that have been reviewed so far provide evidence that significant changes occur during the first years of life in children's abilities to understand cognitive mental states and emotions. Crucially, this research has shown that the two abilities develop asynchronously in early childhood. Children's understanding of emotion seems to develop more precociously and sometimes less precociously than understanding of cognitive mental states. For example, the development of an implicit understanding of emotions in infancy (i.e., the prediction of emotions on the basis of goals) develops much earlier than the implicit understanding of false beliefs. On the other hand, the distinction of real and apparent emotions, develops much later than children's understanding of the appearance-reality distinction. Overall, these results suggest that the two ToM abilities follow distinct developmental trajectories. This evidence provides substance to the claim that a predominant dissociation exists between children's understanding of cognitive mental states and emotions during early childhood. In the next section, we turn to research examining associations between young children's abilities to understand the two classes of mental states in early childhood.

10.4 Evidence for Interconnections: Association Between Children's Understanding of Cognitive Mental States and Emotions

The literature examining associations between children's ability to understand cognitive mental states and emotions in early childhood is limited and has produced inconsistent findings. Early studies concluded that the two abilities are "distinct aspects" of the young child's ToM (Cutting and Dunn 1999, p. 861) and any associations between them should be attributed to the influence of shared socio-demographic factors (Cutting and Dunn 1999; Dunn 1995; Dunn et al. 1991). For example, in a study by Cutting and Dunn (1999) the two abilities were found to be unrelated, when the effects of age, verbal ability and family background were statistically controlled. In that study, however, children's understanding of emotion was measured with emotion-labeling and causes-of-emotion tasks (two emotional ToM abilities that develop early), whereas cognitive mental state understanding was measured with false belief tasks (a cognitive ToM ability that emerges later in development and has higher processing demands). This limitation in the measures used to assess the two ToM abilities may be the reason for the lack of significant association.

In more recent studies, children's understanding of cognitive mental states and emotions have been found to be positively associated (e.g., Bender et al. 2011; Harwood and Farrar 2006; Ornaghi et al. 2016; Weimer et al. 2012). For example, Harwood and Farrar (2006) administered children aged 3–5 years a battery of false belief tasks and a task assessing their ability to predict others' emotions. After controlling for age and verbal ability, they found that children's understanding of false beliefs was positively correlated to their ability to predict another individual's emotion when it was different (i.e. conflicting) from their own emotion, but not when it was congruent with their own emotion. In another study, Weimer et al. (2012) examined the relation between 4.5- and 6.5-year-old children's false belief understanding and their abilities to recognize and label facial expressions of emotion, understand the external causes of specific emotions, appreciate the role of beliefs and desires in emotion, and distinguish between genuine and dissembled emotions. After controlling for age, their results showed that children's understanding of others' beliefs was positively correlated with their understanding of the causes of others' emotions, but not with emotion labeling and the more complex aspects of emotion understanding assessed. Finally, Ornaghi et al. (2016) showed that there is a positive significant association between 4- and 6-year-old children's ability to infer other people's false beliefs and their understanding of emotion, even when the influence of chronological age is statistically controlled.

Some other studies have examined the relation between young children's understanding of cognitive mental states and emotions in a longitudinal framework (Hughes and Dunn 1998; O'Brien et al. 2011; Seidenfeld et al. 2014). These studies, too, have reported inconsistent findings. O'Brien et al. (2011) used a battery of cognitive and emotional mental state tasks to assess, over a period of 3 and 4 years, the association between children's understanding of cognitive and emotional mental states. Their results showed that children's performance on the tasks assessing emotion labeling, emotion perspective taking and understanding the causes of emotions at age 3, predicted differences in their performance on the tasks assessing false belief understanding and the appearance-reality distinction at age 4. They concluded that children develop basic emotion understanding abilities before they grasp others' cognitive mental states. However, other longitudinal evidence contradicts this conclusion by showing that higher false belief-task performance between 3 and 5 years of age, predicts more elaborate recognition of emotional expressions and understanding of the causes of emotions (Seidenfeld et al. 2014). These results have been interpreted as evidence that cognitive mental state understanding is a necessary foundation in the development of an understanding of emotional mental states.

To summarize, the evidence concerning the association between children's understanding of cognitive mental states and emotions in early childhood is contradictory. Initial research gave support to the view that the two abilities are distinct components of the ToM construct. However, more recent studies have reported findings that are compatible with the view that the two abilities are positively associated and this association cannot be attributed to factors such as age, verbal ability and so forth. Nonetheless, the correlations that have been reported in these studies are weak to moderate in magnitude. Moreover, there is a wide variation in the tasks used to assess each ability, and in some studies only specific subprocesses of the two abilities were found to be positively correlated. From a longitudinal perspective, some studies have shown that children begin to understand emotions before they begin to reason about cognitive mental states. However, other studies have reported the reverse developmental pattern. Taken together, the developmental findings presented in this and the previous section indicate that, although the two abilities follow diverse developmental trajectories, they cannot be treated as completely independent components of the ToM construct. Rather, they should be considered as processes of a complex system which are—at least partially—associated with one another during the early years of life.

10.5 Neuropsychological Evidence

Delineating the development of children's abilities to understand cognitive and emotional mental states requires not only research on their developmental milestones and associations, but also understanding the brain regions involved. Indeed, a number of neuroimaging studies have started investigating the neural substrates that are involved in the cognitive and emotional mental state processing. A recent meta-analysis (Molenberghs et al. 2016) has presented evidence that inferences about cognitive and emotional mental states resulted in consistent activation of the anterior dorsal medial prefrontal cortex and the left and right temporoparietal junction in adults. However, the processing of cognitive mental states resulted also in greater activation in the precuneus, right temporoparietal junction and middle areas of the superior temporal gyrus, whereas the processing of emotional mental states additionally elicited more activation in the left orbito-frontal cortex, bilateral pars opercularis and adjacent ventral premotor cortex.

These results are intriguing in suggesting that inferences about cognitive and emotional mental states activate: (a) an initial brain system that is common to both ToM abilities, and (b) additional neural regions that are specific to the cognitive and emotional ToM respectively. In other words, individuals need to recruit additional distinct neural processes for reasoning about cognitive mental states and emotional mental states beyond those that are common for both classes of mental states (i.e., common to processing e.g., belief, knowledge and emotion). Such an interpretation could possibly explain the developmental findings outlined earlier showing that although the developmental trajectories of children's abilities to understand cognitive and emotional mental states are different, the two ToM abilities share interconnections.

Of course, such a conclusion needs further scrutiny and must be considered in the light of two methodological limitations. First, neuropsychological studies have been carried out with adults and there are no child data available on the brain regions activated when children process emotions, nor are there studies comparing brain activation when children process cognitive states and emotions. As Bowman et al. (2012) phrased it: "it is not possible to determine the developmental process of neural specializations solely from adult research" (p. 619). In other words, even if adult data help us gain an initial understanding of the mature neural substrates of cognitive and emotional ToM, it is possible that children, especially young children, have nothing like them (Wellman 2018). Thus, direct neurocognitive examination of children is needed, especially children aged between 1 and 6 years, when developmental changes in these abilities are pronounced.

Second, the differences in the majority of adult neuroimaging studies comparing brain activation in cognitive mental state and emotion tasks could probably be attributable to differences in the tasks and materials that have been used to assess the two classes of mental states (Molenberghs et al. 2016). As Sabbagh and Bowman (2018) argue, the tasks that have been used to assess brain activity during cognitive mental state-processing (e.g., false belief tasks) are typically theory-based induction tasks—that is, these tasks require inferences about others' mental states on the basis of theoretical knowledge about the nature and the causes of mental states—whereas the tasks that have been used to measure brain activity during emotional mental state processing are immediate-induction tasks (e.g., pictures depicting individuals expressing emotions)—that is, these tasks require inferences about others' mental states on the basis of information that is available on the immediate situation. Therefore, it is unclear whether the differences that have been found are the result of differences in the nature of the tasks or the brain regions involved in cognitive ToM and emotional ToM. Future studies need to compare brain activation when children process matched—in terms of the levels of processing they require—cognitive mental state and emotion understanding tasks.

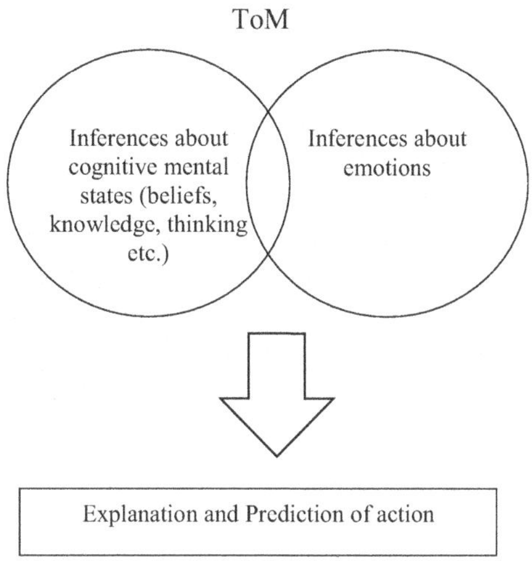

Fig. 10.1 A "nearly decomposable" ToM system: Children's abilities to understand cognitive mental states and emotions are both dissociable and interconnected components of ToM

10.6 Implications for ToM: Is ToM a Nearly Decomposable System?

In the previous sections, work has been reviewed showing that children's abilities to understand cognitive mental states and emotions follow distinct developmental pathways in the early years of life and evidence on their developmental associations. We have also reviewed neuropsychological studies suggesting that common as well as discrete brain regions are involved in cognitive and emotional ToM in adults. What is particularly intriguing about the developmental and the neuropsychological data reported, is that they all converge in suggesting both diversity and unity of the two ToM components. Thus, the whole set of findings reviewed seems to favour the view that the abilities to understand cognitive and emotional mental states are both dissociable and interconnected.

The evidence for both dissociation and interconnection of children's understanding of cognitive mental states and emotions suggests a model such as the one that is outlined in Fig. 10.1. By this model, ToM is a system that is divisible into *at least* two distinct but interdependent components, one for processing cognitive and a second for processing emotional mental states. Simon (1962) has described such systems as being "nearly decomposable", meaning that individual "components perform independent functions but interact in ways that are not negligible" (Bechtel 2012, p. 265). It may be argued that ToM is a nearly decomposable system. Its components—cognitive and emotional ToM—have a "fuzzy" sort of independence: they function independently at the beginning of life (i.e., the existence and function of each component is nearly independent of the existence and function of the other), but in the long run they become coordinated and depend on the exchange of information (i.e., the prediction and explanation of action on the basis of beliefs, knowledge and so forth is being updated in the light of the information about emotions and vice versa). Put simply, the two ToM components dynamically interact with each other, and this probably prevents the system from being broken down into completely separable subsystems.

Clearly, further research is needed to test the hypothesis that ToM is a "nearly decomposable" system. Moreover, further work is required on the complex interplay between the cognitive and emotional ToM components in early childhood. There is also much to learn about the developments that succeed the milestones that occur in the preschool years and the independence and interdependence of these changes in older ages. It is also clear that further distinctions between ToM components need to be considered (see Dennis et al. 2013; Schafsma et al. 2015; Tager-Flusberg and Sullivan 2000) for a more refined and complete model of children's understanding of mind.

10.7 Further Insights: Links of Children's Abilities to Understand Cognitive and Emotional Mental States with Metacognition

A longtime challenge for ToM research is the attempt to forge links between developments in children's ToM and changes in their metacognitive ability. One of the first to advocate a relationship between ToM and metacognition was Wellman (1985), who put forward that "metacognition consists of a large multi-faceted theory of mind" (p. 29). A number of researchers have reported evidence that young children's metacognitive capacities, including metamemory (Lockl and Schneider 2007), metacognitive monitoring (Feurer et al. 2015) and metacognitive vocabulary (Antonietti et al. 2006) are associated with ToM. However, all these studies have treated ToM as a unitary construct. Consequently, their results do not allow one to draw conclusions as to whether the relation between young children's ToM and metacognition is specific either to the cognitive or the emotional ToM component or it can be generalized across both components.

To date, only one study, to our knowledge, has separately examined the relation of cognitive and emotional ToM with children's metacognitive ability in early childhood (Lecce et al. 2015, Experiment 1). This study focused on children's declarative metamemory and showed that at 4 years of age this aspect of metacognition is specifically associated with children's ability to understand cognitive mental states but not with their ability to understand emotions. Moreover, children's cognitive ToM at 4 years of age was found to significantly predict declarative metamemory 6 months later (experiment 2), which led Lecce et al. (2015) to conclude that understanding of cognitive mental states is "a necessary initial step for the development of the other components of metacognition" (p. 68).

Thus, preliminary evidence indicates that the relation between metacognition and ToM in early childhood does not generalize to both ToM components, but holds only for young children's ability to attribute cognitive mental states. This evidence is consistent with the view that the abilities to understand cognitive and emotional mental states are dissociated ToM subsystems. It should be taken in mind however that similarly to ToM, metacognition is a multifaceted ability. The association reported in Lecce et al.'s (2015) study with young children's cognitive ToM, concerned a single aspect of metacognition: declarative metamemory. Thus, it cannot be ruled out that emotional ToM could be related to other aspects of children's metacognitive ability (e.g., metacognitive feelings, Brandl 2012; Efklides 2002).

Further research on the links between young children's abilities to understand cognitive and emotional mental states and metacognition is warranted, to sketch a more accurate description of the interactions between these abilities (Misailidi 2010). Attempts to establish the links between cognitive and emotional ToM with children's metacognitive capacities are expected to provide further insights into the debate regarding the unitary vs. componential structure of ToM. Since both ToM and metacognition are broad, multidimensional constructs, there exists a possibility of different relations among different subprocesses of the two abilities, and also the possibility of change in these relations over developmental time (Misailidi 2010).

10.8 Conclusion

The question that guided the present chapter was this: should young children's abilities to understand cognitive and emotional mental states be considered dissociable or interconnected components of ToM? We approached this question by reviewing findings from recent developmental and neuropsychological studies. The developmental evidence indicates that: (a) the deconstruction of ToM into a cognitive and an emotional component is meaningful; there is evidence suggesting that the two ToM abilities follow distinct developmental trajectories during the early years of life. (b) Nonetheless, this division is not a sharp one; developmental findings also indicate that children's understanding of cognitive and emotional mental states are—at least partially—associated. (c) The neuropsychological data support the developmental findings in showing that common and independent neural substrates are involved in the processing of cognitive and emotional mental states. Overall, the work reviewed in this chapter is consistent with the idea that the abilities to understand cognitive and emotional mental states are both dissociable and interconnected components of a complex system that develops dynamically during the early years of life. This evidence encourages us to think of ToM as a nearly decomposable system.

References

Antonietti, A., Liverta-Sempio, O., Marchetti, A., & Astington, J. (2006). Mental language and understanding of epistemic and emotion mental states. In A. Antonietti, O. Liverta-Sempio, & A. Marchetti (Eds.), *Theory of mind and language in developmental context* (pp. 1–30). New York: Springer.

Apperly, I. A., & Butterfill, S. (2009). Do humans have two systems to track beliefs and belief- like states? *Psychological Review, 116*, 953–970. https://psycnet.apa.org/doi/10.1037/a0016923.

Astington, J. W. (2003). Sometimes necessary, never sufficient: False-belief understanding and social competence. In B. Repacholi & V. Slaughter (Eds.), *Individual differences in theory of mind* (pp. 13–38). New York: Psychology Press.

Astington, J. W., & Hughes, C. (2013). Theory of mind: Self-reflection and social understanding. In P. D. Zelazo (Ed.), *The Oxford handbook of developmental psychology* (pp. 398–424). New York: Oxford University Press.

Bechtel, W. (2012). Referring to localized cognitive operations in parts of dynamically active brains. In A. Raftopoulos & P. Machamer (Eds.), *Perception, realism and the problem of reference* (pp. 262–284). Cambridge: Cambridge University Press.

Bender, P., Pons, F., Harris, P., & de Rosnay, M. (2011). Do young children misunderstand their own emotions? *European Journal of Developmental Psychology, 8*, 331–348. https://doi.org/10.1080/17405629.2010.495615.

Borke, H. (1972). Interpersonal perceptions of young children: Egocentrism or empathy? *Developmental Psychology, 5*, 263–269. https://doi.org/10.1037/h0031267.

Bowman, L. C., Liu, D., Meltzoff, A. N., & Wellman, H. M. (2012). Neural correlates of belief- and desire-reasoning in 7- and 8-year-old children: An event-related potential study. *Developmental Science, 15*, 618–632. https://doi.org/10.1111/j.1467-7687.2012.01158.x.

Boyer, P., & Barrett, H. C. (2005). Domain specificity and intuitive ontology. In D. M. Buss (Ed.), *Handbook of evolutionary psychology* (pp. 96–188). New York: John Wiley & Sons.

Brandl, J. L. (2012). Pretend play in early childhood: The road between mentalism and behaviourism. In M. J. Beran, J. L. Brandl, J. Perner, & J. Proust (Eds.), *Foundations of metacognition* (pp. 146–166). Oxford: Oxford University Press.

Bretherton, I., Fritz, J., Zahn-Waxler, C., & Ridgeway, D. (1986). Learning to talk about emotions: A functionalist perspective. *Child Development, 57*, 529–548. https://doi.org/10.2307/1130334.

Brothers, L., & Ring, B. (1992). A neuroethological framework for the representation of minds. *Journal of Cognitive Neuroscience, 4*, 107–118. https://doi.org/10.1162/jocn.1992.4.2.107.

Carlson, S. M., & Moses, L. J. (2001). Individual differences in inhibitory control and children's theory of mind. *Child Development, 72*, 1032–1053. https://psycnet.apa.org/doi/10.1111/1467-8624.00333.

Cutting, A. L., & Dunn, J. (1999). Theory of mind, emotion understanding, language, and family background: Individual differences and interrelations. *Child Development, 70*, 853–865. https://doi.org/10.1111/1467-8624.00061.

de Rosnay, M., Pons, F., Harris, P. L., & Morrell, J. M. B. (2004). A lag between understanding false belief and emotion attribution in young children: Relationships with linguistic ability and mothers' mental-state language. *British Journal of Developmental Psychology, 22*, 197–218. https://doi.org/10.1348/026151004323044573.

Dennis, M., Simic, N., Bigler, E. D., Abildskov, T., Agostino, A., Taylor, H. G., et al. (2013). Cognitive, affective, and conative theory of mind (ToM) in children with traumatic brain injury. *Developmental Cognitive Neuroscience, 5*, 25–39. https://doi.org/10.1016/j.dcn.2012.11.006.

Dienes, Z., & Perner, J. (1999). A theory of implicit and explicit knowledge. *Behavioral and Brain Sciences, 22*, 735–808. https://doi.org/10.1017/S0140525X99002186.

Dunn, J. (1995). Children as psychologists: The later correlates of individual differences in understanding of emotions and other minds. *Cognition and Emotion, 9*, 187–201. https://doi.org/10.1080/02699939508409008.

Dunn, J., Brown, J., Slomkowski, C., Tesla, C., & Youngblade, L. (1991). Young children's understanding of other people's feelings and beliefs: Individual differences and their antecedents. *Child Development, 62*, 1352–1366. https://doi.org/10.1111/j.1467-8624.1991.tb01610.x.

Dvash, J., & Shamay-Tsoory, S. G. (2014). Theory of mind and empathy as multidimensional constructs: Neurological foundations. *Topics in Language Disorders, 34*, 282–295. https://psycnet.apa.org/doi/10.1097/TLD.0000000000000040.

Efklides, A. (2002). The systemic nature of metacognitive experiences. In P. Chambres, M. Izaute, & P. J. Marescaux (Eds.), *Metacognition: Process, function, and use* (pp. 19–34). Dordrecht: Kluwer Academic Publishers.

Efklides, A., & Misailidi, P. (2019). Emotional self-regulation in the early years: The role of cognition, metacognition and social interaction. In D. Whitebread (Ed.), *The SAGE handbook of developmental psychology and early childhood education* (pp. 502–516). Thousand Oaks: Sage Publications.

Estes, D. (1998). Young children's awareness of their mental activity: The case of mental rotation. *Child Development, 69*, 1345–1360. https://doi.org/10.1111/j.1467-8624.1998.tb06216.x.

Feurer, E., Sassu, R., Cimeli, P., & Roebers, C. (2015). Development of metarepresentations: Procedural metacognition and the relationship to theory of mind. *Journal of Educational and Developmental Psychology, 5*, 6–18. https://doi.org/10.5539/jedp.v5n1p6.

Flavell, J. H., Green, F. L., & Flavell, E. R. (1986). Development of knowledge about the appearance-reality distinction. *Monographs of the Society for Research in Child Development, 51*, 1–68. https://psycnet.apa.org/doi/10.2307/1165866.

Flavell, J. H., Green, F. L., & Flavell, E. R. (1993). Children's understanding of the stream of consciousness. *Child Development, 64*, 387–398. https://doi.org/10.1111/j.1467-8624.1993.tb02916.x.

Flavell, J. H., Green, F. L., & Flavell, E. R. (1995). Young children's knowledge of thinking. *Monographs of the Society for Research in Child Development, 60*, 1–113. https://psycnet.apa.org/doi/10.2307/1166124.

Flavell, J. H., Green, F. L., Flavell, E. R., & Grossman, J. B. (1997). The development of children's knowledge about inner speech. *Child Development, 68*, 39–47. https://doi.org/10.1111/j.1467-8624.1997.tb01923.x.

Flavell, J. H., Green, F. L., & Flavell, E. R. (1998). The mind has a mind of its own: Developing knowledge about mental uncontrollability. *Cognitive Development, 13*, 127–138. https://doi.org/10.1016/S0885-2014(98)90024-7.

Flavell, J. H., Green, F. L., & Flavell, E. R. (2000). Development of children's awareness of their own thoughts. *Journal of Cognition and Development, 1*, 97–112. https://doi.org/10.1207/S15327647JCD0101N_10.

Gopnik, A., & Astington, J. W. (1988). Children's understanding of representational change and its relation to the understanding of false belief and the appearance-reality distinction. *Child Development, 59*, 26–37. https://psycnet.apa.org/doi/10.2307/1130386.

Gopnik, A., & Wellman, H. M. (1994). The theory theory. In L. Hirschfeld & S. Gelman (Eds.), *Domain specificity in cognition and culture* (pp. 257–293). New York: Cambridge University Press.

Gosselin, P., Warren, M., & Diotte, M. (2002). Motivation to hide emotion and children's understanding of the distinction between real and apparent emotions. *The Journal of Genetic Psychology, 163*, 479–495. https://doi.org/10.1080/00221320209598697.

Gross, D., & Harris, P. L. (1988). False beliefs about emotion: Children's understanding of misleading emotional displays. *International Journal of Behavioral Development, 11*, 475–488. https://psycnet.apa.org/doi/10.1177/016502548801100406.

Harris, P. L. (2006). Social cognition. In W. Damon & R. M. Lerner (Eds.), *Handbook of child psychology: Cognition, perception and language* (Vol. 2, 6th ed., pp. 811–858). Hoboken: Wiley.

Harris, P. L. (2008). Children's understanding of emotion. In M. Lewis, J. M. Haviland-Jones, & L. F. Barrett (Eds.), *Handbook of emotions* (3rd ed., pp. 320–331). New York: Guilford Press.

Harris, P. L., Olthof, T., Meerum-Terwogt, M. M., & Hardman, C. E. (1987). Children's knowledge of the situations that provoke emotion. *International Journal of Behavioral Development, 10*, 319–343. https://doi.org/10.1177/2F016502548701000304.

Harris, P. L., Johnson, C. N., Hutton, D., Andrews, G., & Cooke, T. (1989). Young children's theory of mind and emotion. *Cognition and Emotion, 3*, 379–400. https://doi.org/10.1080/02699938908412713.

Harris, P. L., de Rosnay, M., & Ronfard, S. (2014). The mysterious emotional life of little red riding hood. In K. H. Lagattuta (Ed.), *Children and emotion: New insights into developmental affective sciences* (pp. 106–118). Basel: Karger.

Harwood, M. D., & Farrar, M. J. (2006). Conflicting emotions: The connection between affective perspective taking and theory of mind. *British Journal of Developmental Psychology, 24*, 401–418. https://doi.org/10.1348/026151005X50302.

Hughes, C., & Dunn, J. (1998). Understanding mind and emotion: Longitudinal associations with mental-state talk between young friends. *Developmental Psychology, 34*, 1026–1037. https://psycnet.apa.org/doi/10.1037/0012-1649.34.5.1026.

James, W. (1890). *The principles of psychology* (Vol. 1). New York: Henry Holt and Company.

Lane, J. D., Wellman, H. M., Olson, S. L., La Bounty, J., & Kerr, D. C. (2010). Theory of mind and emotion understanding predict moral development in early childhood. *British Journal of Developmental Psychology, 28*, 871–889. https://doi.org/10.1348/026151009X483056.

Lecce, S., Demicheli, P., Zocchi, S., & Palladino, P. (2015). The origins of children's metamemory: The role of theory of mind. *Journal of Experimental Child Psychology, 131*, 56–72. https://psycnet.apa.org/doi/10.1016/j.jecp.2014.11.005.

Liu, D., Wellman, H. M., Tardif, T., & Sabbagh, M. A. (2008). Theory of mind development in Chinese children: A meta-analysis of false-belief understanding across cultures and languages. *Developmental Psychology, 44*, 523–531. https://doi.org/10.1037/0012-1649.44.2.523.

Lockl, K., & Schneider, W. (2007). Knowledge about the mind: Links between theory of mind and later metamemory. *Child Development, 78*, 148–167. https://doi.org/10.1111/j.1467-8624.2007.00990.x.

Luo, Y., & Baillargeon, R. (2007). Do 12.5-month-old infants consider what objects others can see when interpreting their actions? *Cognition, 105*, 489–512. https://psycnet.apa.org/doi/10.1016/j.cognition.2006.10.007.

Misailidi, P. (2006). Young children's display rule knowledge: Understanding the distinction between apparent and real emotions and the motives underlying the use of display rules. *Social Behavior and Personality: An International Journal, 34*, 1285–1296. https://psycnet.apa.org/doi/10.2224/sbp.2006.34.10.1285.

Misailidi, P. (2010). Children's metacognition and theory of mind: Bridging the gap. In A. Efklides & P. Misailidi (Eds.), *Trends and prospects in metacognition research* (pp. 279–291). Boston: Springer.

Mitchell, R. L., & Phillips, L. H. (2015). The overlapping relationship between emotion perception and theory of mind. *Neuropsychologia, 70*, 1–10. https://doi.org/10.1016/j.neuropsychologia.2015.02.018.

Molenberghs, P., Johnson, H., Henry, J. D., & Mattingley, J. B. (2016). Understanding the minds of others: A neuroimaging meta-analysis. *Neuroscience and Biobehavioral Reviews, 65*, 276–291. https://doi.org/10.1016/j.neubiorev.2016.03.020.

Moll, H., & Tomasello, M. (2012). Three-year-olds understand appearance and reality—Just not about the same object at the same time. *Developmental Psychology, 48*, 1124–1132. https://psycnet.apa.org/doi/10.1037/a0025915.

Naito, M. (2004). Is theory of mind a universal and unitary construct? *ISSBD Newsletter, 1*, 9–11.

Naito, M., & Seki, Y. (2009). The relationship between second-order false belief and display rules reasoning: The integration of cognitive and affective social understanding. *Developmental Science, 12*, 150–164. https://doi.org/10.1111/j.1467-7687.2008.00748.x.

O'Brien, M., Miner Weaver, J., Nelson, J. A., Calkins, S. D., Leerkes, E. M., & Marcovitch, S. (2011). Longitudinal associations between children's understanding of emotions and theory of mind. *Cognition and Emotion, 25*, 1074–1086. https://doi.org/10.1080/02699931.2010.518417.

Ong, D. C., Zaki, J., & Goodman, N. D. (2015). Affective cognition: Exploring lay theories of emotion. *Cognition, 143*, 141–162. https://doi.org/10.1016/j.cognition.2015.06.010.

Onishi, K. H., & Baillargeon, R. (2005). Do 15-month-old infants understand false beliefs? *Science, 308*, 255–258. https://psycnet.apa.org/doi/10.1126/science.1107621.

Ornaghi, V., Pepe, A., & Grazzani, I. (2016). False-belief understanding and language ability mediate the relationship between emotion comprehension and prosocial orientation in preschoolers. *Frontiers in Psychology, 7*, 1534. https://doi.org/10.3389/fpsyg.2016.01534.

Perner, J. (1991). *Understanding the representational mind*. Cambridge: MIT Press.

Perner, J., & Ruffman, T. (2005). Infants' insight into the mind: How deep? *Science, 308*, 214–216. https://doi.org/10.1126/science.1111656.

Phillips, A. T., Wellman, H. M., & Spelke, E. S. (2002). Infants' ability to connect gaze and emotional expression to intentional action. *Cognition, 85*, 53–78. https://doi.org/10.1016/S0010-0277(02)00073-2.

Pons, F., Harris, P. L., & de Rosnay, M. (2004). Emotional comprehension between 3 and 11 years: Developmental periods and hierarchical organization. *European Journal of Developmental Psychology, 1*, 127–152. https://doi.org/10.1080/17405620344000022.

Pratt, C., & Bryant, P. (1990). Young children understand that looking leads to knowing (so long as they are looking into a single barrel). *Child Development, 61*, 973–982.

Premack, D., & Woodruff, G. (1978). Does the chimpanzee have a theory of mind? *Behavioral and Brain Sciences, 1*, 515–526. https://doi.org/10.1017/S0140525X00076512.

Repacholi, B. M. (1998). Infants' use of attentional cues to identify the referent of another person's emotional expression. *Developmental Psychology, 34*, 1017–1025. https://doi.org/10.1037/0012-1649.34.5.1017.

Reschke, P. R., Walle, E. A., & Dukes, D. (2017). Interpersonal development in infancy: The interconnectedness of emotion understanding and social cognition. *Child Development Perspectives, 11*, 173–183. https://doi.org/10.1111/cdep.12230.

Ruffman, T. (2014). To belief or not belief: children's theory of mind. *Developmental Review, 34*, 265–293. https://psycnet.apa.org/doi/10.1016/j.dr.2014.04.001.

Sabbagh, M. A. (2004). Understanding orbitofrontal contributions to theory-of-mind reasoning: Implications for autism. *Brain and Cognition, 55*, 209–219. https://psycnet.apa.org/doi/10.1016/j.bandc.2003.04.002.

Sabbagh, M. A., & Bowman, L. C. (2018). Theory of mind. In S. Ghetti (Ed.), *Stevens' handbook of experimental psychology and cognitive neuroscience* (4th ed., pp. 249–288). New York: John Wiley & Sons. https://doi.org/10.1002/9781119170174.epcn408.

Saxe, R., Carey, S., & Kanwisher, N. (2004). Understanding other minds: Linking developmental psychology and functional neuroimaging. *Annual Review of Psychology, 55*, 87–124. https://doi.org/10.1146/annurev.psych.55.090902.142044.

Schaafsma, S. M., Pfaff, D. W., Spunt, R. P., & Adolphs, R. (2015). Deconstructing and reconstructing theory of mind. *Trends in Cognitive Sciences, 19*, 65–72. https://doi.org/10.1016/j.tics.2014.11.007.

Schneider, D., Slaughter, V. P., Becker, S. I., & Dux, P. E. (2014). Implicit false-belief processing in the human brain. *NeuroImage, 101*, 268–275. https://doi.org/10.1016/j.neuroimage.2014.07.014.

Seidenfeld, A. M., Johnson, S. R., Cavadel, E. W., & Izard, C. E. (2014). Theory of mind predicts emotion knowledge development in head start children. *Early Education and Development, 25*, 933–948. https://doi.org/10.1080/10409289.2014.883587.

Shamay-Tsoory, S. G., & Aharon-Peretz, J. (2007). Dissociable prefrontal networks for cognitive and affective theory of mind: A lesion study. *Neuropsychologia, 45*, 3054–3067. https://psycnet.apa.org/doi/10.1016/j.neuropsychologia.2007.05.021.

Simon, H. A. (1962). The architecture of complexity. *Proceedings of the American Philosophical Society, 106*, 467–482.

Skerry, A. E., & Spelke, E. S. (2014). Preverbal infants identify emotional reactions that are incongruent with goal outcomes. *Cognition, 130*, 204–216. https://doi.org/10.1016/j.cognition.2013.11.002.

Smith, N., Hermelin, B., & Tsimpli, I. (2003). Dissociation of social affect and theory of mind in a case of Asperger syndrome. *UCL Working Papers in Linguistics, 15*, 303–322.

Striano, T., & Rochat, P. (2000). Emergence of selective social referencing in infancy. *Infancy, 1*, 253–264. https://psycnet.apa.org/doi/10.1207/S15327078IN0102_7.

Surian, L., Caldi, S., & Sperber, D. (2007). Attribution of beliefs by 13-month-old infants. *Psychological Science, 18*, 580–586.

Tager-Flusberg, H., & Sullivan, K. (2000). A componential view of theory of mind: Evidence from Williams syndrome. *Cognition, 76*, 59–90. https://psycnet.apa.org/doi/10.1016/S0010-0277(00)00069-X.

Tsoi, L. (2016). A unified versus componential view of understanding minds. In J. Sytsma & W. Buckwalter (Eds.), *A companion to experimental philosophy* (pp. 279–291). Malden: Wiley-Blackwell.

Vaillant-Molina, M., Bahrick, L. E., & Flom, R. (2013). Young infants match facial and vocal emotional expressions of other infants. *Infancy, 18*, E97–E111.

Vaish, A., & Striano, T. (2004). Is visual reference necessary? Contributions of facial versus vocal cues in 12-month-olds' social referencing behavior. *Developmental Science, 7*, 261–269. https://doi.org/10.1111/j.1467-7687.2004.00344.x.

Watson, J. K., Gelman, S. A., & Wellman, H. M. (1998). Young children's understanding of the non-physical nature of thoughts and the physical nature of the brain. *British Journal of Developmental Psychology, 16*, 321–335. https://doi.org/10.1111/j.2044-835X.1998.tb00755.x.

Weimer, A. A., Sallquist, J., & Bolnick, R. R. (2012). Young children's emotion comprehension and theory of mind understanding. *Early Education and Development, 23*, 280–301. https://psycnet.apa.org/doi/10.1080/10409289.2010.517694.

Wellman, H. M. (1985). The origins of metacognition. In D. L. Forrest-Pressley, G. E. McKinnon, & T. G. Waller (Eds.), *Metacognition, cognition and human performance* (pp. 1–31). New York: Academic.

Wellman, H. M. (1993). Early understanding of mind: The normal case. In S. Baron-Cohen, H. Tager-Flusberg, & D. J. Cohen (Eds.), *Understanding other minds: Perspectives from autism* (pp. 10–39). New York: Oxford University Press.

Wellman, H. M. (2011). Developing a theory of mind. In U. Goswami (Ed.), *The Blackwell handbook of childhood cognitive development* (2nd ed., pp. 258–284). New York: Blackwell.

Wellman, H. M. (2014). *Making minds: How theory of mind develops*. New York: Oxford University Press.

Wellman, H. M. (2018). Theory of mind: The state of the art. *European Journal of Developmental Psychology, 15*, 728–755. https://doi.org/10.1080/17405629.2018.1435413.

Wellman, H. M., Cross, D., & Watson, J. K. (2001). Meta-analysis of theory-of-mind development: The truth about false-belief. *Child Development, 72*, 655–684. https://psycnet.apa.org/doi/10.1111/1467-8624.00304.

Wilson, D. (2000). Metarepresentation in linguistic communication. In D. Sperber (Ed.), *Metarepresentations: A multidisciplinary perspective* (pp. 411–448). Oxford: Oxford University Press.

Wimmer, H., & Perner, J. (1983). Beliefs about beliefs: Representation and constraining function of wrong beliefs in young children's understanding of deception. *Cognition, 13*, 103–128. https://psycnet.apa.org/doi/10.1016/0010-0277(83)90004-5.

Chapter 11
Influences on the Emergence and Development of Cognitive and Emotional Regulation in Early Childhood

David Whitebread

Abstract It is now well understood that metacognition and self-regulation abilities begin to emerge in children from the first few months of life. It has also been widely reported that these abilities show considerable individual differences by the age at which children enter pre-school or kindergarten, and that these differences continue to grow once the children have entered full-time education. This chapter adopts (Efklides', European Psychologist 13:277–287, 2008) multifaceted and multilevel model of metacognition, including the nonconscious, personal awareness and social processes involved in the early developing stages of cognitive and emotional aspects of self-regulation. In line with this model the final section of the chapter examines the evidence regarding early social experiences, in the home and in school, which are associated with the emergence and development of the individual differences that develop. Research in this area has clear and important implications for early parenting and early childhood education. The chapter concludes with a review of research on interventions designed to support children's early development of cognitive and emotional regulation.

Keywords Nonconscious cognitive regulation · Emotion regulation · Social influences · Early childhood education · Interventions

11.1 Introduction: The Multifaceted and Multilevel Model of Metacognition

As I am sure is true for many, if not all, of the authors in this volume, the empirical and theoretical work of Anastasia Efklides was a major inspiration in my own developing interest and enthusiasm for research in metacognition. In my own case,

D. Whitebread (✉)
Homerton College, University of Cambridge, Cambridge, UK
e-mail: dgw1004@cam.ac.uk

D. Moraitou, P. Metallidou (eds.), *Trends and Prospects in Metacognition Research across the Life Span*, https://doi.org/10.1007/978-3-030-51673-4_11

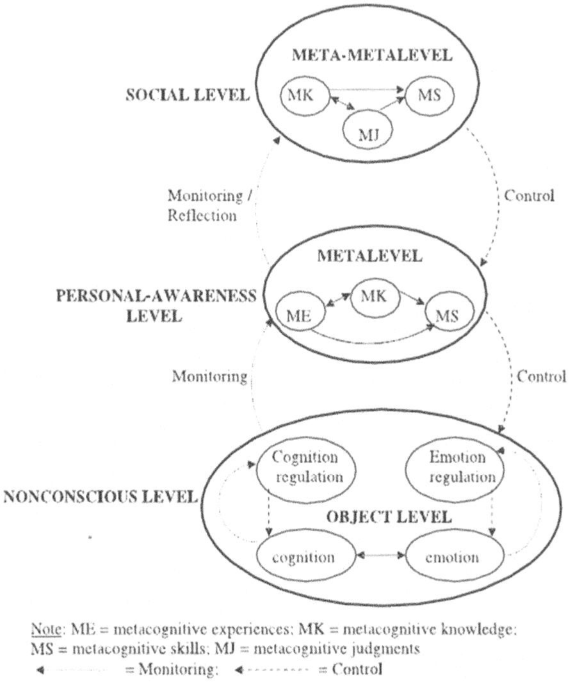

Fig. 11.1 The multifaceted and multilevel model of metacognition. Adapted from Efklides (2008). Metacognition: Defining its facets and levels of functioning in relation to self-regulation and co-regulation. *European Psychologist*, *13*, 277–287

given my early experiences of teaching young children, mostly in the 4–7 age range, it was only natural that I should focus my research on the emergence of metacognitive abilities in its very early stages. This chapter focuses on the research, mainly undertaken over the last two decades, by myself and others, which has established that metacognitive abilities can be detected in very young children. This work has built on Efklides' early recognition that metacognitive experiences have affective as well as purely cognitive components (Efklides 2002, 2006), that they are fundamental to more general, emerging, self-regulatory processes (Efklides 2001), and that their development depends, in its early stages, on nonconscious and social processes (Efklides 2008). Building on the earlier work of Flavell (1979), Brown (1987) and Nelson and Narens (1994), this recognition of the different facets and levels of metacognitive processes led to her proposal of a multifaceted and multilevel model of metacognition (see Fig. 11.1). This model proposes that metacognitive processes, including monitoring and control, and the building of metacognitive knowledge, involve cognitive and emotional elements and occur at nonconscious, personal awareness and social levels. While it is generally true that in the first few years of a child's life there is relatively little personal awareness, it is clear that processes at the social level are active within the first few months (Brinck and Liljenfors 2013) and that conscious awareness begins to emerge for many children between the ages of 3 and 5 years.

This model has guided much of subsequent research, particularly in relation to young children's development of metacognitive and self-regulatory abilities. As such it forms the basis of the structure of this chapter. It begins by examining research which has studied the development of metacognition and self-regulation at the levels of nonconscious and personal awareness, or consciousness, in young children. In the second half of the chapter, addressing research relating to the social level, the influence of young children's social environment on their development of metacognitive and self-regulatory abilities is addressed. The various aspects of young children's social environments and experience result in large individual differences in the development of affective and cognitive regulation within the period of early childhood. They also have significant consequences for their long-term academic achievements and emotional well-being. However, an understanding of the processes which impact on early metacognition and self-regulation also enables the development of practices and interventions which can effectively enhance young children's progress in these vital abilities.

11.2 Nonconscious and Conscious Metacognition in Young Children

The earliest view of metacognition was that it was a set of entirely conscious processes. As Flavell (1979) expressed it:

> Metacognitive experiences are any conscious cognitive or affective experiences that accompany and pertain to any intellectual enterprise. (p. 906)

As Flavell was originally a Piagetian scholar, his view on this might have been influenced by Piagetian theory suggesting that a concept was only properly understood when it was represented in conscious awareness and could be articulated. This position, however, is now recognised to be untenable. Ironically, some of the earliest evidence for nonconscious metacognition came from Piaget's and Flavell's own work. Around the same time as the publication of Flavell's seminal 1979 paper, largely credited with the establishment of metacognition as an area of study, some of Piaget's later work had revealed the existence of nonconscious, unarticulated but accurate procedural knowledge on a range of tasks (Piaget 1977, 1978). On an oddity problem, for example, some children as young as 6 years of age were found to be able to reliably select the object that was the 'odd one out' but were unable to accurately report how they had done it. In Flavell's own earlier studies of children's memory (Flavell et al. 1966) he had found that 25% of 5- and 7-year-old children who could successfully use a rehearsal strategy were unable to report that they had done so.

Other early evidence also cast doubt on the proposition that metacognitive processes were necessarily conscious. Siegler and Shipley (1985), for example, demonstrated that computer simulations, which clearly lack any conscious awareness, could successfully use feedback to choose strategies that solved mathematical calculation problems more efficiently. They also argued that human metacognition necessarily involves mostly nonconscious processes, as the extra work involved in bringing every decision we make into conscious awareness would make the speed at which we decide how to undertake tasks impossible to achieve.

Studies of metacognitive abilities in non-human species, which are also unable to consciously represent and articulate their mental processes, have also demonstrated the possibility of nonconscious metacognition. An early study of metacognition in non-human species, for example, showed that bottlenosed dolphins could indicate when they were uncertain about the correct solution to a problem (Smith et al. 1995), thus indicating some awareness of their own mental states. This study has stimulated a considerable research effort and debate. Section 1 of Beran et al.'s (2012) edited collection on the origins of metacognition, for example, contains six chapters on metacognition in non-human animals. Taken as a whole, the conclusion emerges that, despite extensive critiques and investigations, no study has confirmed an alternative explanation of the uncertainty response in dolphins, monkeys and apes other than that they are capable of nonconscious metacognitive awareness. More recent studies, using sophisticated methodologies more precisely tuned to the capabilities of particular species, have provided evidence of metamemory in rats (Lee et al. 2018) and awareness of knowledge states in pigeons (Iwasaki et al. 2018).

In the research on metacognition in young children, it is now widely accepted that there are nonconscious and conscious processes at play. In an early review of evidence on this issue in adults, Reder and Schunn (1996) presented a wide range of evidence suggesting that the processes of monitoring or metacognitive awareness are overwhelmingly nonconscious, irrespective of age. They also argued that, in line with Siegler and Shipley's (1985) computer simulation studies, within metacognitive control processes in adults, choices between strategies are also nonconscious. In addition to the issue of speed of mental processing raised by Siegler and Shipley, however, they focused on numerous studies showing that when adults are required to verbalise the metacognitive decisions they are making, their performance deteriorates (see Schooler et al. 2014).

However, the processes whereby new strategies are developed, Reder and Schunn (1996) reported, appear to have a conscious element. From a relatively early age, many children and almost all adults are also consciously aware of, and able to articulate, elements of their metacognitive knowledge about their own abilities, about specific mental tasks and about the mental strategies in their developing repertoire (Flavell 1979; Kreutzer et al. 1975; Schneider 2008). This transition, from nonconscious to conscious awareness of their mental strategies is crucial in the long-term development of their metacognitive and self-regulatory abilities. However, there appears to be wide variation in the timing and the extent of this development of conscious awareness, and there are clearly several inter-linked transitional stages involved before the achievement of fully conscious metacognitive processing. Some studies have managed to demonstrate declarative metacognitive knowledge in children as young as 3–5 years of age (Marulis et al. 2016), while numerous studies have shown that it is much later before many children are able to effectively use their metacognitive knowledge to enhance their level of academic achievement (Neuenhaus et al. 2011). A complicating factor in the study of young children's developing metacognitive abilities, as many researchers have reviewed, is the considerable influence of context and social factors on young children's performance on any particular task. For example, more salient, but irrelevant, cues have been shown to influence young children's judgements of their own learning, and young children's metacognitive performance is enhanced when the task is placed in a context that makes sense to them (Schneider and Lockl 2002; Whitebread and Basilio 2012). As is discussed in the final main section of this chapter, the various influences on children's progress in this area are significantly supported at the social level within the Efklides model.

11.2.1 Nonconscious and Conscious Cognitive Regulation

At the nonconscious level in the Efklides model a distinction is made between the regulation of cognition and emotion, and it is now recognised in models of self-regulation that in the first years of life the young child is learning to regulate in both of these areas of development. Bronson (2000) provided a comprehensive review of research addressing the development of cognitive, emotional, motivational and social aspects of self-regulation in young children, as it stood at the turn of the millennium. Fitzsimmon and Bargh (2004) provided a comprehensive review specifically focusing on the nonconscious self-regulation of cognition, emotion and behaviour. Whitebread and Basilio (2012) set out the findings from the considerable new wave of research in the first decade of the new century stimulated by Bronson's review. This included work addressing progress in children up to the age of 6 on executive functioning (EF) and cognitive control, and the socio-emotional development of self-regulation. More recently, Marulis et al. (2019) have set out the most recent research establishing the relationships between EF, metacognition and the cognitive and affective aspects of self-regulation.

The role of EF in the development of early cognitive control was initially established within clinical and neuroscience research (Dajani and Uddin 2015; Kerns et al. 2008; Zelazo and Müller 2002). Within developmental psychological work over the last two decades, the broader role of these fundamental brain processes in the early emergence of metacognitive and self-regulatory processes has been increasingly recognised, following on from the initial insights in this regard developed by Fernandez-Duque et al. (2000). In an integrative review, Garon et al. (2008) concluded that the key EFs were those related to the control of attention (including the ability to focus on relevant rather than more perceptually salient but irrelevant information, and the ability to flexibly switch attention), working memory (holding information in mind while carrying out a task using it), and inhibitory or effortful control (stopping a prepotent or automatic response and replacing it with a different response). They also set out the evidence of the very early emergence of simple forms of each of these key functions, and how they develop through the pre-school period. Initially operating as a single overall function (Wiebe et al. 2011), each of the functions gradually become more distinct and improved in their performance. Thus, during the preschool and primary school years, young children's ability to sustain their attention, hold auditory and visual information in working memory, and inhibit and replace immediate responses each show clear progress. However, as we will outline in the final section of this chapter, this progress is highly dependent upon context and other social influences (Whitebread and Basilio 2012).

There is also evidence that, as the various EF processes become more distinct, their developmental trajectories vary. Working memory has been shown to improve from early childhood and well into adolescence (Gathercole et al. 2004). Whitebread (1999), for example, demonstrated an interaction between working memory and the development of metacognitive strategies on a problem-solving task in 6–10-year-olds. However, the development of inhibitory control appears to be largely complete by 6–7 years of age. Thus, Lyons and Ghetti (2011), in a study of uncertainty monitoring in 3–5-year-olds, indicated an interaction between inhibitory control and metacognitive awareness. Bryce et al. (2015), however, found a highly significant relationship between inhibitory control and metacognitive abilities among 5-year-olds, but no such relationship among 7-year-olds. This suggests, they argued, that once inhibitory control has developed to a certain level, it is necessary but no longer sufficient to explain progress in metacognition. In line with this general finding, other studies have shown the continued impact of EF interventions with children who are weak in this area, but not with the broad population of typically developing children. Thus, Hofmann et al. (2012) reviewed research evidence indicating that the training of EF had significant potential for improving poor self-regulation in children with a range of learning difficulties. However, Jacob and Parkinson (2015), in their review of school-based interventions designed to improve EF in typically developing children, found no evidence of a causal relationship between such improvements and academic achievements. At the same time, a strong relationship has been widely indicated between metacognitive abilities and school success. For example, Hattie (2009), having reported the results of 800 meta-analyses related to a huge range of educational interventions conducted all over the world, concluded that approaches which teach children metacognitive strategies, or which support children's metacognitive awareness, are among the most effective in relation to academic outcomes.

As we shall see in the final section of this chapter, this educational opportunity in regard to metacognition is closely linked to the development of conscious and declarative metacognitive knowledge through a range of social processes. That the processes supporting early cognitive regulation and control are largely nonconscious, as discussed above, is now widely recognised. The processes whereby metacognition enters into the phase of personal awareness, in which metacognitive skills and judgements are fully informed by metacognitive experiences and knowledge, as set out in Efklides' model, appear to be largely dependent on developments in language and in experiences at the social level, as discussed in the final section of this chapter.

In addition to EF, another element of children's early psychological development which has been argued to be a precursor of metacognitive development (Lockl and Schneider 2006) is their developing understanding that other people have minds like theirs, and consequently have different experiences, perceptions and knowledge about the world. This has become to be referred to as children's 'theory of mind' (ToM) and, similarly to metacognition, was initially thought to be fully conscious and declarative. As Hughes and Devine (2019) review, however, this original view, which placed the emergence of ToM at around 4–5 years of age, has more recently been replaced by a recognition that the conscious awareness stage of ToM is preceded by earlier emerging, nonconscious processes. As in the case of early metacognitive processes, this more recent understanding has arisen through methodological developments. Thus, while the original studies of ToM used methods which were dependent upon children's linguistic abilities—for example, the false belief task (Winner and Perner 1983) and the Strange Stories task (Happé 1994)—more recent studies have used non-verbal methods and revealed nonconscious ToM in children from 18 months—for example, an active helping paradigm (Buttelmann et al. 2009) and spontaneous-response tasks (Baillargeon et al. 2010). Once again, as discussed in the final section of this chapter, the achievement of a conscious and articulable level of ToM appears to be largely dependent on developments in language and social experiences.

11.2.2 Nonconscious and Conscious Emotional Regulation

There are also significant early manifestations and development in the socio-emotional aspects of metacognition and self-regulation. This has two elements. First, a distinctive element in Efklides' own research has been the identification of metacognitive feelings as an emotional element which accompanies and supports cognitive regulation (Efklides 2006). This article reviews evidence of the inter-relations between cognitive and affective aspects of metacognitive experiences, particularly focussing on feelings of difficulty (negative affect) and feelings of confidence (positive affect). It also presents evidence that improvements in the accuracy of these elements of metacognitive experience are crucial to the effective self-regulation of learning.

There has been subsequent research investigating the mechanisms which appear to contribute to increases in accuracy of these metacognitive feelings in young children. These include children's developing metacognitive knowledge about tasks, a decrease in children's levels of overconfidence and the development of children's ToM. Thus, Pillow and Pearson (2015), in a study of 1st, 3rd and 5th graders, found a gradual increase with age in the number of distinctions made between common activities (including object recognition, inferential reasoning, counting, and pretending) in relation to their level of controllability, or potential difficulty. In a study of factors leading to increased accuracy in self-evaluations, van Loon et al. (2017) found no developmental increase in what they termed 'the adaptive use of item difficulty' (i.e., children's ability to recognise levels of item difficulty and use this as a guide to more likely errors) between 5/6-year-olds and 7/8-year-olds. However, they did find that the younger children gave inappropriately high rewards to themselves following an incorrect performance, leading them to be more overconfident than the older children. This led to the conclusion that the younger children's more inaccurate self-evaluations arose from self-protective biases, which gradually decrease with age. Danovitch et al. (2019) have more recently differentiated feelings of confidence into two related processes, which they have conceptualised as contributing to intellectual humility (IH). These relate to the decrease in overconfidence about their own abilities or knowledge, as reported by van Loon et al. (2017) and many other researchers, and to children's increasing recognition, through improvements in their ToM capabilities, that others might know more about particular topics than themselves. To test this model, 6–8-year-old children were asked to rate their level of knowledge in relation to biological (e.g., why can fish only live in water?) and technical (how does an elevator work?) questions. Also, in a separate delegation task with the same questions, the same children were placed in a team with two imaginary experts, a doctor and a mechanic, and asked to say who from their team would answer each question. The scores on the two tasks correlated, with lower estimates of own knowledge correlating positively with greater willingness to delegate to the experts, justifying their combination into the measure of IH. The 8-year-olds showed greater IH than the 6-year-olds. Two relations with other measures, however, showed that knowledge self-confidence and recognition that others might be more knowledgeable than oneself were dissociable. First, assessments of the children's IQ correlated with lower self-knowledge ratings, but not with willingness to delegate. Second, the two elements of IH were shown to be related to different neural markers measured during an electroencephalogram (EEG) Go/NoGo task, measuring error monitoring.

The second element in emotional regulation relates to the self-regulation of emotions themselves. Whitebread and Basilio (2012) have set out the significant research in this area related to development in infancy and toddlerhood. As they note, socio-emotional regulation at these stages is also influenced by the development of EF, and particularly inhibitory control. Developments in early emotional self-regulation, as they indicate, involve:

> the ability to control and modulate emotional expressions (positive or negative) and interacting with others in increasingly more complex ways in accordance with social rules. It also refers to the ability to adapt to emotionally challenging situations, to inhibit behaviours perceived as inappropriate in a given context and to privilege behaviours that are perceived as the socially expected, even when they do not correspond to the individual's first response or may not be pleasant to undertake. (Whitebread and Basilio 2012, p. 20)

While these authors note that there are genetic factors which influence the early development of these capabilities, these biological mechanisms have been shown to significantly interact with social aspects of young children's experience, particularly related to the quality of early mother-child interactions (Kochanska et al. 2009), to which we return in the final section of this chapter.

In a more recent review of the research on emotional self-regulation in young children, Efklides and Misailidi (2019) also recognise the role of early social interactions but point to other influential developments including improvements in young children's EF and ToM. They go on to argue that, as in the area of cognitive self-regulation, improvements in EF through the first few years of life appear to predict emotional self-regulation. In particular, they review research showing that the regulation of emotion by the age of 4 years recruits midfrontal and anterior cingulate brain regions known to be involved in the full range of EF and metacognitive activity (Rothbart et al. 2011). In a similar, more recent study, with even younger children, Perry et al. (2016) found that early neurophysiological processes measured during an attention task during infancy, at 10 months, predicted the children's ability to regulate emotion when they were 3 years old.

As regards ToM, while the early developing ability of young children to understand that others might have knowledge they do not have has been very widely researched, there has been relatively little research addressing their understanding of others' emotions. However, as Efklides and Misailidi (2019) review, this has also been shown to begin to develop in very young children. Thus, by the end of their first year, infants have been shown to recognise their parents' facial or vocal emotional expressions, and to use these to guide how they respond to ambiguous situations. By the age of 3 years children can label facial expressions of basic emotions, and by 6 years of age they can recognise that the outward expression of emotion may not match a person's internal feelings. While it seems theoretically likely that children's developing ToM and understanding of others' emotions would contribute to their emotional self-regulation, this has not been demonstrated empirically with any certainty. In an extensive investigation of relationships between ToM, EF and cognitive, behavioural and emotional aspects of self-regulation, Jahromi and Stifter (2008), for example, found no direct relation between measures of ToM and emotion regulation. However, it seems likely that a strong relation exists, but mediated, as discussed earlier, through children's language abilities. Cole et al. (2010) provided an extensive review of four distinct lines of evidence which suggest that expressive language is related to emotional self-regulation. First, they cite numerous studies showing associations between language delays and emotional regulation difficulties. Second, they argue that both expressive language and emotion regulation are dependent on limited cognitive resources, and this leads to a developing relationship between them. Thus, if a young child is highly emotionally expressive, regulating their emotions will consume excessive proportions of their available resources, which will then limit the resources available to support their expressive language development, and vice versa in the case of expressive language difficulties. Evidence that verbal processing in very young children requires widespread neural processing (Redcay et al. 2008) is cited in support of this view. Third, a number of studies have shown a relationship between children's internal state language, including emotion terms, and their socio-emotional competence (e.g., Denham et al. 2003). This clearly relates to evidence, to which we return in the final section of this chapter, that parent-child conversations relating to emotions appears to scaffold young children's emotional self-awareness and hence their ability to self-regulate their emotions (Shields et al. 2001). Finally, the extensive evidence of the self-regulatory function of young children's self-directed, or private, talk (e.g., Winsler et al. 2009), has led to its effective use in therapeutic work fostering socio-emotional competence.

11.3 The Social Level: Supporting the Emergence of Self-Regulation

As noted at the outset of this chapter, research on the early emergence of metacognition and self-regulation has found profound and significant individual differences. While there are differences related to early EF and self-regulation at the level of genetics (Kochanska et al. 2009), and temperament (Frick et al. 2018), these differences have been shown to be largely moderated by early social influences. Evidence of the impacts of family income levels (Evans and Rosenbaum 2008), social class (Lawson et al. 2018) and maternal education level (Montroy et al. 2016) attest to the effect of the young child's early social environment on their early self-regulation development. However, the considerable body of research investigating the early antecedents and social influences on self-regulation development have not painted a depressing picture of children's fate being fixed and pre-determined. Rather, the study of early parenting and educational practices has revealed a range of features of early social environments that can beneficially be manipulated to support children's early metacognitive and self-regulatory development. The most encouraging evidence even suggests that some interventions in this area can particularly benefit children who are most at risk of developing weak self-regulation abilities. In this final section of the chapter research is reviewed which has investigated the impact of factors in the home and in early schooling on children's self-regulation development. Interventions designed to address these various influential aspects of the young child's social environment are also reviewed. The success of these various interventions, particularly with children who are disadvantaged in some way, and who would otherwise be weak in their developing self-regulatory abilities, indicates the importance of the social level in Efklides' model of metacognition, particularly as it relates to the emergence of affective and cognitive regulation.

11.3.1 Social Influences in the Home

Given the evidence that EF, metacognition and self-regulation abilities begin to emerge from very early in life, and that they have a profound influence on an individual's short- and long-term outcomes, there has been a considerable research effort to investigate the social features within children's early home life that effect their early abilities in these areas. These studies have predominantly focused on the quality of parent-child interactions. In one of the earliest longitudinal studies of the role of early parent–child relationships in the development of child EF, for example, Bernier et al. (2010) investigated the impact of three aspects of mother-child relationships which had emerged from the literature relating to early frontal brain development, and its relationship to early EF development (Zelazo et al. 2008). These comprised maternal sensitivity, mind-mindedness (the extent to which the mother includes reference to mental states in her discourse with her children) and autonomy support, which were assessed based on 70–90 min observations of mothers with their young children on four occasions. The children's EF was assessed at 18 and 26 months, using assessments identified by Carlson (2005) as developmentally sensitive at those ages. Their results indicated that all three aspects of early mother-child interactions at 12–15 months predicted EF when the children were 18 and 26 months.

In a wider systematic review of studies examining the impact of parenting on children's emerging self-regulation, Pino-Pasternak and Whitebread (2010) identified 22 scientifically rigorous studies, carried out between 1980 and 2009, involving pre-school and primary school-aged children. Their analysis identified three parenting dimensions (challenge, autonomy and contingency) and six parenting cognitive and socio-emotional behaviours (metacognitive talk; active participation; understanding of control; shifts in responsibility; emotional responsiveness, and contingent instructional scaffolds) related to various aspects of cognitive and motivational self-regulation. More recently, Barker et al. (2014), in a study focusing on the level of autonomy support afforded to 6-year-olds within the family, examined the impact of the amount of time spent in 'less-structured' activities during out-of-school times in children's daily, annual and typical schedules. Children who experienced more less-structured time showed enhanced performance on teacher reported and direct measures of cognitive self-regulation (or 'self-directed EF', as Barker et al. 2014 described it), while children with higher proportions of their out-of-school time engaged in structured activities showed weaker levels of cognitive self-regulation. These relationships held up even when controlling for age, verbal ability, and household income. A more in-depth analysis of specific subgroups of children, depending on the nature of their less-structured activities at home, further revealed that time spent in unguided practice, enrichment outings (to the zoo, beach, museum etc.) and some forms of play was the strongest predictor of self-regulation performance in the classroom.

Other studies have focused more on the general home environment, in an attempt to uncover the psychological processes whereby general sociological factors such as poverty or SES impact upon children's early self-regulation and school performance. The key factor emerging from this work concerns levels of personal stress. Blair (2010), for example, provided an extensive review of research examining the neurobiological mechanisms whereby extended high stress levels in the context of poverty impact upon the psychological health and mental functioning of children and their parents. As Evans and Kim (2013) review, disadvantaged children are more likely than those in wealthier households to experience an array of physical and psychological stressors, including substandard housing, a chaotic home environment, family turmoil and separation from adult caregivers, all of which contribute to deleterious effects on their school adjustment, performance and self-regulation.

In a more recent longitudinal study, Pino-Pasternak et al. (2019) have examined the impact of home environment and parenting factors combined on the development of young children's self-regulation development during their first 2 years of schooling (i.e., between the ages of 5 and 7 years). This study of 98 children combined observed and reported data assessing the quality of the home and school environments and examined the relationships of these aspects of the children's experience with their developing EF, self-regulation and academic progress. The study is ongoing and only the initial data is currently reported. In line with the previous literature, however, their preliminary analysis of data collected at the beginning of the study confirmed that higher levels of cognitive stimulation and lower levels of chaos in the home were associated with more autonomy supporting parenting, and this, in turn, was associated with higher levels of social and cognitive self-regulation. At the same time, lower levels of self-regulation overall were associated with observed parent-child conflict. Higher levels of social self-regulation, measured through the teachers' observations of children's abilities to work co-operatively and negotiate with themselves and other children, were associated with lower levels of chaos in the home and higher incidence of shared parent-child activities.

11.3.2 Interventions with Parents

What clearly emerges from the whole range of studies examining social influences on young children's metacognitive and self-regulatory abilities is that these crucial aspects of early development are highly sensitive to the quality of the home environment. Blair and Raver (2015) have concluded from the accumulated evidence in this area that individual differences in early self-regulation are the '*primary mechanism through which poverty affects school readiness*' (p. 722). As a consequence of this recognition of the fundamental importance of the quality of the home and parenting practices, a considerable body of research has been undertaken examining the efficacy of parenting programs to improve child programs. Sanders and Mazzucchelli (2013) have provided a comprehensive review of work in this area, addressing the known benefits of children developing strong self-regulatory abilities in early childhood, the characteristics of effective parental interventions, reviews of particular parenting programs and effective techniques used within them. The key approach, which is richly evidenced within this paper, is to support the development of self-regulation abilities in the parents which, in turn, supports their abilities to support these same competencies in their children. As an example of this approach, the paper reviews studies using the Triple P-Positive Parenting Program, including several independent meta-analyses finding positive parental and child outcomes (Nowak and Heinrichs 2008).

Intervention studies of this kind have identified some of the psychological roots of self-regulation weaknesses in parents living in poverty or experiencing other stressors within the family context. Patterson and Chamberlain (1994), for example, described parents who have low self-efficacy and self-management skills, are reluctant to set goals for their children or themselves, attribute their child's and their own behaviour to factors outside their control and tend to look to others to solve their problems. Among the elements of programs successfully helping such parents to develop improved self-regulation abilities are practices which convey respect in an emotionally supportive context, which convey positive expectations that change is possible, use a guided participation approach, challenge beliefs about needing to be rescued and self-defeating behaviour, and establish expectancies that promote self-regulation by setting achievable goals for the parent.

Pears et al. (2015) reported a study that employed a randomised control study examining the effectiveness of a school readiness intervention (the Kids in Transition to School or KITS Program) focusing on parenting and children's self-regulatory abilities at the point of transition into kindergarten, when the children were just 5 years of age. The sample of 209 participating families each had a child with significant developmental or behavioural problems. One hundred and seven families and children were randomly assigned to the KITS program and 102 to the services-as-usual (SAU) group. The KITS program ran for 2 months before and 2 months after kindergarten entry, and comprised sessions related to early literacy skills, prosocial skills and self-regulatory abilities. The latter involved three elements directed to the three aspects of early EF abilities—handling frustration and disappointment (inhibitory control), following multistep directions (working memory) and making appropriate transitions (control of attention). The parenting program for the KITS group focused on parenting skills of the type outlined above, preparing their child for school (early literacy and routines around school activities) and becoming involved in the school. The results indicated an interesting chain of effects, with a significant positive effect of the intervention on parenting skills by the end of the intervention, which then had a significant positive effect on the children's self-regulation by the end of kindergarten.

11.3.3 Social Influences and Interventions in Early Childhood Education

Many of the insights gained from studies of the home environment and mother-child interactions are also, unsurprisingly, echoed in the considerable body of research in this area carried out in the context of early childhood education. Pre-eminent in this field is the work of Perry (1998, 2013) who carried out a series of detailed observational studies in 2nd and 3rd grade classrooms. From the extensive data collected, she identified characteristics of classrooms that supported self-regulation. These included giving children opportunities for decision making, setting their own challenges, assessing their own work, encouraging positive feelings towards challenging tasks, and emphasising personal progress rather than social comparisons. By contrast, classrooms that did not support the development of children's self-regulation were characterised by limited choices of activities, teacher-controlled assessment procedures, with an emphasis on performance and comparisons between children. It is clear that the emotional and motivational climate in these classrooms and the level of support for the children's autonomy was very different.

Numerous other studies have identified the emotional climate of the classroom and support for children's autonomy as key predictors of gains in young children's self-regulatory abilities. Fuhs et al. (2013), for example, in a study with over 800 preschool children, found that higher levels of children's cognitive self-regulation developed in classrooms where the teachers more frequently expressed approval of children's behaviour and established a positive emotional climate. Cadima et al. (2016) similarly found in a study of just over 200 preschool children that, over the course of the school year, teacher-child closeness predicted improvements in observed self-regulation abilities. They also found that children with low initial self-regulation abilities benefitted the most from higher classroom quality in this regard. While early studies of attempts to directly teach metacognitive and self-regulatory abilities to young children showed this to be generally effective (Dignath et al. 2008), the growing evidence of the impact of the emotional aspects of early childhood classroom environments have led to a move away from direct teaching in this area and towards a clearer emphasis on providing an emotionally positive and supportive experience for young children in early childhood education (Boekaerts and Corno 2005).

In addition to this provision of an emotionally supportive classroom environment, which is vital in children's early development generally, I have previously argued that the three key elements in high quality early childhood pedagogy comprise a style of teacher-child interaction which supports the development of early self-regulation, support for children's oral language development, and the provision of a full range of opportunities to play, (Whitebread 2018; Whitebread et al. 2015a, b). Of relevance to the purpose of the current chapter, however, is that, in addition to their unique contribution to quality in early childhood education, language development and play have an important role in supporting the early development of self-regulation.

There is extensive evidence of the impact of oral language development on children's self-regulatory abilities. For example, Vallotton and Ayoub (2011) showed a strong relationship between vocabulary size and a range of observed self-regulatory behaviours in children at ages 14, 24 and 36 months. In a very recent study with pre-school children, Cadima et al. (2019) found that self-regulation abilities were predicted by autonomy support, while the relation between teacher-child closeness and the children's self-regulation development was moderated by their receptive vocabulary. In addition, they found a bi-directional relationship between vocabulary and self-regulation.

A possible explanation of the close relation between early language development and metacognitive and self-regulatory development emerges from studies showing a disjunction in the trajectories between metacognitive experience or monitoring and the use of the accrued metacognitive knowledge to inform the choice of cognitive strategies. A range of studies have shown that, while monitoring skills appear to develop more or less chronologically, children's developing abilities to make effective choices of cognitive strategies in relation to tasks shows considerable individual differences (Bryce and Whitebread 2012). For example, various studies have shown that high-achieving children's monitoring abilities are average for their age but their ability to make effective strategy choices in relation to different tasks are considerably advanced (Eme et al. 2006; Puustinen 1998). A study exemplifying the role of language in this individual difference in effective strategy choice was carried out by Fabricius and Hagen (1984). In a study paralleling the early work of Flavell et al. (1966) they administered a memory task to 6- and 7-year-olds before and after teaching them a grouping strategy, and found that the children could use the strategy and it improved their performance on the task. In this case, however, before they were asked to undertake the task on a third occasion, the children were asked to articulate how they had improved their performance. Of those who were able to do so, 99% then used the grouping strategy again on the new task and maintained their improved level of performance. For the children who were not able to articulate the strategy correctly, 69% failed to use the strategy again and did not maintain an improved performance.

This kind of evidence of the link between being able to articulate one's own mental processes and the effective use of accrued metacognitive knowledge provides important insights into the processes whereby metacognition transitions from the nonconscious level in Efklides' model to the level of personal awareness, or consciousness. It has also led to a range of interventions, within early childhood educational contexts, which have required children to articulate their thinking by various means, and thus supported the development of their metacognitive and self-regulatory skills. These have included requiring children to give self-explanations of their thinking in relation to solving mathematical problems (Siegler and Lin 2010), holding discussions with children about what might be useful memory strategies in relation to particular tasks (Ornstein et al. 2010), and engaging children in collaborative group problem-solving, so that they need to explain their ideas and reasoning, and thus 'co-regulate' one another and jointly involve themselves in 'socially-shared regulation' of the group (Grau and Whitebread 2012; Volet and Vauras 2013). In my own research group, a one-year longitudinal study in which 5- and 6-year-old children were taught to follow 'rules for talk' (Mercer and Littleton 2007) to effectively collaborate on problem-solving tasks showed this approach to very significantly enhance the children's ability to articulate their own thinking and their metacognitive skills (Pino-Pasternak et al. 2014).

As I have argued in previous publications, young children's play also has an important role as a contributor of metacognitive experiences which enhance their metacognitive and self-regulatory abilities (Whitebread 2010). Within my own research group we have demonstrated this in relation to a number of play types, including social pretend play (Whitebread and O'Sullivan 2012), musical play (Zachariou and Whitebread 2017), and constructional play (Spektor-Levy et al. 2017). In each of these play areas and in others, the mechanisms involved appear to include an increase in engagement, and the opportunity to explore different approaches, or strategies, in a 'safe' context in which mistakes are purely a source of learning without any serious consequences. The seminal study by Sylva et al. (1976), illustrated these two mechanisms clearly. The experimental group of 3–5-year old children were given the opportunity to play with some objects which had to be joined together in a particular way to solve a problem-solving task. The control group were instructed by an adult how to join these objects together so they could solve the problem. When they were then presented with the problem, an equal number of children in the two groups succeeded initially. However, when all of the control group had given up, children in the play group continued to be engaged by the task and continued trying out different ways to put the objects together to solve the problem, and many more eventually succeeded.

Numerous studies have demonstrated the enhanced motivation effect of placing tasks in play contexts. In a recent study reported by White, Prager et al. (2017), children showed greatly enhanced ability to regulate their attention on a vigilance task when they were pretending to be Batman than when they were simply doing it as themselves. In a much earlier study, Istomina (1975) demonstrated that young children could remember a greater number of food items when these were presented in the context of a shopping game than when they were presented as part of a memory task. In her report, furthermore, she included transcripts of the children's attempts to remember the items when they were pretending to go shopping. These transcripts illustrated the children monitoring their memory while they were walking over to the pretend shop and, in some cases, when they realised they had forgotten some items, returning to the experimenter and asking for the list again. Most significantly, the transcripts reveal the ineffectual strategies these children used initially (e.g., listening carefully and nodding their head as they were told each food item), and the more successful ones they used when they were told the list again (e.g., whispering the names of the food items to themselves). The transition from nonconscious to conscious metacognition, and the role of language, is once again clearly illustrated in the transcripts, as the children are recorded speaking to themselves as they struggled to remember all the food items. This use of 'private speech' has been frequently observed and reported when young children are engaged in engaging play scenarios, and has been widely recognised as a transitional phase of language use supporting children's early efforts to regulate their own emotions and cognitions (Winsler et al. 2009).

11.4 Conclusion

The work of Efklides has clearly stimulated a huge quantity of research in metacognition and its related conceptual areas and has introduced an array of important theoretical insights which have had a considerable influence on the shape of the research and on its rapid development. As I have attempted to illustrate in this chapter, in relation to the emergence of metacognitive abilities in young children, this is abundantly the case in regard to her multifaceted and multilevel model of metacognition. This has provided a framework through which the development of metacognitive processes can be conceptualised, from the early nonconscious processes exhibited by infants and toddlers to the emerging personal awareness achieved by young children. It has also provided a model of how social processes can support this development through childhood. So, it is both a developmental model and also a model of the fully realised metacognitive and self-regulatory processes achieved by adults who are both emotionally and cognitively in full control, as far as is humanly possible, of their mental activity. We owe a huge debt to Efklides for the outstanding leadership she has provided for this important area of research within developmental psychology, and I hope that this chapter has illustrated, in some small way, the range and significance of the research which has been been inspired over recent decades by her work,

References

Baillargeon, R., Scott, R. M., & He, Z. (2010). False-belief understanding in infants. *Trends in Cognitive Sciences, 14*, 110–118.

Barker, J. E., Semenov, A. D., Michaelson, L., Provan, L. S., Snyder, H. R., & Munakata, Y. (2014). Less-structured time in children's daily lives predicts self-directed executive functioning. *Frontiers in Psychology, 5*, 593.

Beran, M. J., Brandl, J. L., Perner, J., & Proust, J. (Eds.). (2012). *Foundations of metacognition*. Oxford: Oxford University Press.

Bernier, A., Carlson, S. M., & Whipple, N. (2010). From external regulation to self-regulation: Early parenting precursors of young children's executive functioning. *Child Development, 81*, 326–339.

Blair, C. (2010). Stress and the development of self-regulation in context. *Child Development Perspectives, 4*, 181–188.

Blair, C., & Raver, C. C. (2015). School readiness and self-regulation: A developmental psychobiological approach. *Annual Review of Psychology, 66*, 711–731.

Boekaerts, M., & Corno, L. (2005). Self-regulation in the classroom: A perspective on assessment and intervention. *Applied Psychology: An International Review, 54*, 199–231.

Brinck, I., & Liljenfors, R. (2013). The developmental origin of metacognition. *Infant and Child Development, 22*, 85–101.

Bronson, M. B. (2000). *Self-regulation in early childhood*. New York: The Guilford Press.

Brown, A. L. (1987). Metacognition, executive control, self-regulation and other more mysterious mechanisms. In F. E. Weinert & R. H. Kluwe (Eds.), *Metacognition, motivation and understanding* (pp. 65–116). London: Erlbaum.

Bryce, D., & Whitebread, D. (2012). The development of metacognitive skills: Evidence from observational analysis of young children's behaviour during problem-solving. *Metacognition and Learning, 7*, 197–217.

Bryce, D., Whitebread, D., & Szucs, D. (2015). The relationships among executive functions, metacognitive skills and educational achievement in 5- and 7-year-old children. *Metacognition and Learning, 10*, 181–198.

Buttelmann, D., Carpenter, M., & Tomasello, M. (2009). Eighteen-month-old infants show false belief understanding in an active helping paradigm. *Cognition, 112*, 337–342.

Cadima, J., Barros, S., Ferreira, T., Serra-Lemos, M., Leal, T., & Verschueren, K. (2019). Bidirectional associations between vocabulary and self-regulation in preschool and their interplay with teacher–child closeness and autonomy support. *Early Childhood Research Quarterly, 46*, 75–86.

Cadima, J., Verschueren, K., Leal, T., & Guedes, C. (2016). Classroom interactions, dyadic teacher-child relationships, and self-regulation in socially disadvantaged young children. *Journal of Abnormal Child Psychology, 44*, 7–17.

Carlson, S. M. (2005). Developmentally sensitive measures of executive function in preschool children. *Developmental Neuropsychology, 28*, 585–615.

Cole, P. M., Armstrong, L. M., & Pemberton, C. K. (2010). The role of language in the development of emotion regulation. In S. D. Calkins & M. A. Bell (Eds.), *Child development at the intersection of emotion and cognition* (pp. 59–77). Washington: American Psychological Association.

Dajani, D. R., & Uddin, L. Q. (2015). Demystifying cognitive flexibility: Implications for clinical and developmental neuroscience. *Trends in Neurosciences, 38*, 571–578.

Danovitch, J. H., Fisher, M., Schroder, H., Hambrick, D. Z., & Moser, J. (2019). Intelligence and neurophysiological markers of error monitoring relate to children's intellectual humility. *Child Development, 90*, 924–939.

Denham, S. A., Blair, K. A., DeMulder, E., Levitas, J., Sawyer, K., Auerbach-Major, S., & Queenan, P. (2003). Preschool emotional competence: Pathway to social competence? *Child Development, 74*, 238–256.

Dignath, C., Buettner, G., & Langfeldt, H. P. (2008). How can primary school students learn self-regulated learning strategies most effectively? A meta-analysis on self-regulation training programs. *Educational Research Review, 3*, 101–129.

Efklides, A. (2001). Metacognitive experiences in problem solving: Metacognition, motivation, and self-regulation. In A. Efklides, J. Kuhl, & R. M. Sorrentino (Eds.), *Trends and prospects in motivation research* (pp. 297–323). Dordrecht: Springer.

Efklides, A. (2002). The systemic nature of metacognitive experiences: Feelings, judgements and their interrelations. In M. Izaute, P. Chalbres, & P. J. Marescaux (Eds.), *Metacognition: Process, function and use* (pp. 19–34). Boston: Springer.

Efklides, A. (2006). Metacognition and affect: What can metacognitive experiences tell us about the learning process? *Educational Research Review, 1*, 3–14.

Efklides, A. (2008). Metacognition: Defining its facets and levels of functioning in relation to self-regulation and co-regulation. *European Psychologist, 13*, 277–287.

Efklides, A., & Misailidi, P. (2019). Emotional self-regulation in the early years: The role of cognition, metacognition and social interaction. In D. Whitebread, V. Grau, K. Kumpulainen, M. McClelland, N. Perry, & D. Pino-Pasternak (Eds.), *The Sage handbook of developmental psychology and early childhood education* (pp. 502–516). London: Sage Publications Limited.

Eme, E., Puustinen, M., & Coutelet, B. (2006). Individual and developmental differences in reading monitoring: When and how do children evaluate their comprehension? *European Journal of Psychology of Education, 21*, 91–115.

Evans, G. W., & Kim, P. (2013). Childhood poverty, chronic stress, self-regulation, and coping. *Child Development Perspectives, 7*, 43–48.

Evans, G. W., & Rosenbaum, J. (2008). Self-regulation and the income-achievement gap. *Early Childhood Research Quarterly, 23*, 504–514.

Fabricius, W. V., & Hagen, J. W. (1984). Use of causal attributions about recall performance to assess metamemory and predict strategic memory behaviour in young children. *Developmental Psychology, 20*, 975–987.

Fernandez-Duque, D., Baird, J. A., & Posner, M. I. (2000). Executive attention and metacognitive regulation. *Consciousness and Cognition, 9*, 288–307.

Fitzsimmons, G. M., & Bargh, J. A. (2004). Automatic self-regulation. In R. F. Baumeister & K. D. Vohs (Eds.), *Handbook of self-regulation: Research, theory and applications* (pp. 151–170). New York: The Guilford Press.

Flavell, J. H. (1979). Metacognition and cognitive monitoring: A new area of cognitive developmental inquiry. *American Psychologist, 34*, 906–911.

Flavell, J. H., Beach, D. R., & Chinsky, J. M. (1966). Spontaneous verbal rehearsal in a memory task as a function of age. *Child Development, 37*, 283–299.

Frick, M. A., Forslund, T., Fransson, M., Johansson, M., Bohlin, G., & Brocki, K. C. (2018). The role of sustained attention, maternal sensitivity, and infant temperament in the development of early self-regulation. *British Journal of Psychology, 109*, 277–298.

Fuhs, M. W., Farran, D. C., & Nesbitt, K. T. (2013). Preschool classroom processes as predictors of children's cognitive self-regulation skills development. *School Psychology Quarterly, 28*, 347–359.

Garon, N., Bryson, S. E., & Smith, I. M. (2008). Executive function in preschoolers: A review using an integrative framework. *Psychological Bulletin, 134*, 31–60.

Gathercole, S. E., Pickering, S. J., Ambridge, B., & Wearing, H. (2004). The structure of working memory from 4 to 15 years of age. *Developmental Psychology, 40*, 177–190.

Grau, V., & Whitebread, D. (2012). Self and social regulation of learning during collaborative activities in the classroom: The interplay of individual and group cognition. *Learning and Instruction, 22*, 401–412.

Happé, F. G. (1994). An advanced test of theory of mind: Understanding of story characters' thoughts and feelings by able autistic, mentally handicapped, and normal children and adults. *Journal of Autism and Developmental Disorders, 24*, 129–154.

Hattie, J. (2009). *Visible learning: A synthesis of 800 meta-analyses relating to achievement*. London: Routledge.

Hofmann, W., Schmeichel, B. J., & Baddeley, A. D. (2012). Executive functions and self-regulation. *Trends in Cognitive Sciences, 16*, 174–180.

Hughes, C., & Devine, R. T. (2019). Learning to read minds: A synthesis of social and cognitive perspectives. In D. Whitebread, V. Grau, K. Kumpulainen, M. McClelland, N. Perry, & D. Pino-Pasternak (Eds.), *The Sage handbook of developmental psychology and early childhood education*. London: Sage Publications Limited.

Istomina, Z. M. (1975). The development of voluntary memory in preschool-age children. *Soviet Psychology, 13*, 5–64.

Iwasaki, S., Watanabe, S., & Fujita, K. (2018). Pigeons (*Columba livia*) know when they will need hints: Prospective metacognition for reference memory? *Animal Cognition, 21*, 207–217.

Jacob, R., & Parkinson, J. (2015). The potential for school-based interventions that target executive function to improve academic achievement: A review. *Review of Educational Research, 85*, 512–552.

Jahromi, L. B., & Stifter, C. A. (2008). Individual differences in pre-schoolers' self-regulation and theory of mind. *Merrill-Palmer Quarterly, 54*, 125–150.

Kerns, J. G., Nuechterlein, K. H., Braver, T. S., & Barch, D. M. (2008). Executive functioning component mechanisms and schizophrenia. *Biological Psychiatry, 64*, 26–33.

Kochanska, G., Philibert, R. A., & Barry, R. A. (2009). Interplay of genes and early mother-childrelationship in the development of self-regulation from toddler to preschool age. *Journal of Child Psychology and Psychiatry, 50*, 1331–1338.

Kreutzer, M. A., Leonard, S. C., & Flavell, J. H. (1975). An interview study of children's knowledge about memory. *Monographs of the Society for Research in Child Development, 40*, 1–60.

Lawson, G. M., Hook, C. J., & Farah, M. J. (2018). A meta-analysis of the relationship between socioeconomic status and executive function performance among children. *Developmental Science, 21*, e12529.

Lee, K. A., Preston, A. J., Wise, T. B., & Templer, V. L. (2018). Testing for metacognitive responding using an odor-based delayed match-to-sample test in rats. *Journal of Visualized Experiments, 136*, e57489.

Lockl, K., & Schneider, W. (2006). Precursors of metamemory in young children: The role of theory of mind and metacognitive vocabulary. *Metacognition and Learning, 1*, 15–31.

Lyons, K. E., & Ghetti, S. (2011). The development of uncertainty monitoring in early childhood. *Child Development, 82*, 1778–1787.

Marulis, L., Baker, S., & Whitebread, D. (2019). Integrating metacognition and executive function to enhance young children's perception of and agency in their learning. *Early Childhood Research Quarterly, 50*, 46–54. https://doi.org/10.1016/j.ecresq.2018.12.017.

Marulis, L. M., Palincsar, A. S., Berhenke, A. L., & Whitebread, D. (2016). Assessing metacognitive knowledge in 3–5-year olds: The development of a metacognitive knowledge interview (McKI). *Metacognition and Learning, 11*, 339–368.

Mercer, N., & Littleton, K. (2007). *Dialogue and the development of children's thinking: A sociocultural approach*. London: Routledge.

Montroy, J. J., Bowles, R. P., Skibbe, L. E., McClelland, M. M., & Morrison, F. J. (2016). The development of self-regulation across early childhood. *Developmental Psychology, 52*, 1744–1762.

Nelson, T. O., & Narens, L. (1994). Why investigate metacognition? In J. Metcalfe & A. P. Shimamura (Eds.), *Metacognition: Knowing about knowing* (pp. 1–25). Cambridge: The MIT Press.

Neuenhaus, N., Artelt, C., Lingel, K., & Schneider, W. (2011). Fifth graders' metacognitive knowledge: General or domain-specific? *European Journal of Psychology of Education, 26*, 163–178.

Nowak, C., & Heinrichs, N. (2008). A comprehensive meta-analysis of triple P-positive parenting program using hierarchical linear modeling: Effectiveness and moderating variables. *Clinical Child and Family Psychology Review, 11*, 114–144.

Ornstein, P. A., Grammer, J. K., & Coffman, J. L. (2010). Teachers' "mnemonic style" and the development of skilled memory. In H. S. Waters & W. Schneider (Eds.), *Metacognition, strategy use and instruction* (pp. 23–53). New York: The Guilford Press.

Patterson, G. R., & Chamberlain, P. (1994). A functional analysis of resistance during parent training therapy. *Clinical Psychology: Science and Practice, 1*, 53–70.

Pears, K. C., Kim, H. K., Healey, C. V., Yoerger, K., & Fisher, P. A. (2015). Improving child self-regulation and parenting in families of pre-kindergarten children with developmental disabilities and behavioral difficulties. *Prevention Science, 16*, 222–232.

Perry, N. E. (1998). Young children's self-regulated learning and contexts that support it. *Journal of Educational Psychology, 90*, 715–729.

Perry, N. E. (2013). Understanding classroom processes that support children's self-regulation of learning. In D. Whitebread, N. Mercer, C. Howe, & A. Tolmie (Eds.), *Self-regulation and dialogue in primary classrooms. British journal of educational psychology monograph series II: Psychological aspects of education – Current trends, no. 10* (pp. 45–67). British Psychological Society: Leicester.

Perry, N. B., Swingler, M. M., Calkins, S. D., & Bell, M. A. (2016). Neurophysiological correlates of attention behaviour in early infancy: Implications for emotion regulation during early childhood. *Journal of Experimental Child Psychology, 142*, 245–261.

Piaget, J. (1977). *The grasp of consciousness*. London: Routledge and Kegan Paul.

Piaget, J. (1978). *Success and understanding*. London: Routledge and Kegan Paul.

Pillow, B. H., & Pearson, R. H. (2015). Children's and adults' judgments of the controllability of cognitive activities. *Metacognition and Learning, 10*, 231–244.

Pino-Pasternak, D., Basilio, M., & Whitebread, D. (2014). Interventions and classroom contexts that promote self-regulated learning: Two intervention studies in United Kingdom primary classrooms. *Psykhe, 23*, 1–13.

Pino-Pasternak, D., Valcan, D., & Malpique, A. (2019). Associations between the home environment, parenting and self-regulation in early childhood. In D. Whitebread, V. Grau, K. Kumpulainen, M. McClelland, N. Perry, & D. Pino-Pasternak (Eds.), *The Sage handbook of developmental psychology and early childhood education* (pp. 487–501). London: Sage Publications Limited.

Pino-Pasternak, D., & Whitebread, D. (2010). The role of parenting in children's self-regulated learning. *Educational Research Review, 5*, 220–242.

Puustinen, M. (1998). Help-seeking behaviour in a problem-solving situation: Development of self-regulation. *European Journal of Psychology of Education, 23*, 271–282.

Redcay, E., Haist, F., & Courchesne, E. (2008). Functional neuroimaging of speech perception during a pivotal period in language acquisition. *Developmental Science, 11*, 237–252.

Reder, L. M., & Schunn, C. D. (1996). Metacognition does not imply awareness: Strategy choice is governed by implicit learning and memory. In L. M. Reder (Ed.), *Implicit memory and metacognition* (pp. 45–77). Mahwah: Erlbaum.

Rothbart, M. K., Sheese, B. E., Rueda, M. R., & Posner, M. I. (2011). Developing mechanisms of self-regulation in early life. *Emotion Review, 3*, 207–213.

Sanders, M. R., & Mazzucchelli, T. G. (2013). The promotion of self-regulation through parenting interventions. *Clinical Child and Family Psychology Review, 16*, 1–17.

Schneider, W. (2008). The development of metacognitive knowledge in children and adolescents: Major trends and implications for education. *Mind, Brain, and Education, 2*, 114–121.

Schneider, W., & Lockl, K. (2002). The development of metacognitive knowledge in children and adolescents. In T. J. Perfect & B. L. Schwartz (Eds.), *Applied metacognition* (pp. 224–257). Cambridge: Cambridge University Press.

Schooler, J. W., Ryan, R. S., & Reder, L. (2014). The costs and benefits of verbally rehearsing memory for faces. In D. J. Herrmann, C. McEvoy, C. Hertzog, P. Hertel, & M. K. Johnson (Eds.), *Basic and applied memory research: Volume 2: Practical applications* (pp. 51–66). London: Routledge.

Shields, A., Dickstein, S., Seifer, R., Giusti, L., Magee, K. D., & Spritz, B. (2001). Emotional competence and early school adjustment: A study of pre-schoolers at risk. *Early Education and Development, 2*, 73–96.

Siegler, R. S., & Lin, X. (2010). Self-explanations promote children's learning. In H. S. Waters & W. Schneider (Eds.), *Metacognition, strategy use and instruction* (pp. 85–112). New York: The Guilford Press.

Siegler, R. S., & Shipley, C. (1985). Variation, selection, and cognitive change. In T. Simon & G. Halford (Eds.), *Developing cognitive competence: New approaches to process modelling* (pp. 31–76). Hillsdale: Erlbaum.

Smith, J. D., Schull, J., Strote, J., McGee, K., Egnor, R., & Erb, L. (1995). The uncertain response in the bottlenosed dolphin (*Tursiops truncates*). *Journal of Experimental Psychology: General, 124*, 391–408.

Spektor-Levy, O., Basilio, M., Zachariou, A., & Whitebread, D. (2017). Young children's spontaneous manifestation of self-regulation and metacognition during constructional play tasks. *Teachers College Record, 119*, n13.

Sylva, K., Bruner, J. S., & Genova, P. (1976). The role of play in the problem-solving of children 3–5 years old. In J. S. Bruner, A. Jolly, & K. Sylva (Eds.), *Play: Its role in development and evolution* (pp. 55–67). Harmondsworth: Penguin.

Vallotton, C., & Ayoub, C. (2011). Use your words: The role of language in the development of toddlers' self-regulation. *Early Childhood Research Quarterly, 26*, 169–181.

van Loon, M., Destan, N., Spiess, M. A., de Bruin, A., & Roebers, C. M. (2017). Developmental progression in performance evaluations: Effects of children's cue-utilization and self-protection. *Learning and Instruction, 51*, 47–60.

Volet, S., & Vauras, M. (Eds.). (2013). *Interpersonal regulation of learning and motivation: Methodological advances*. London: Routledge.

White, R. E., Prager, E. O., Schaefer, C., Kross, E., Duckworth, A. L., & Carlson, S. M. (2017). The "batman effect": Improving perseverance in young children. *Child Development, 88*, 1563–1571.

Whitebread, D. (1999). Interactions between children's metacognitive processes, working memory, choice of strategies and performance during problem solving. *European Journal of Psychology of Education, 14*, 489–507.

Whitebread, D. (2010). Play, metacognition and self-regulation. In P. Broadhead, J. Howard, & E. Wood (Eds.), *Play and learning in the early years* (pp. 161–176). London: Sage Publications.

Whitebread, D. (2018). Quality in early childhood education: The contribution of developmental psychology. In M. Fleer & B. van Oers (Eds.), *International handbook of early childhood education* (Vol. I, pp. 319–334). Dordrecht: Springer.

Whitebread, D., & Basilio, M. (2012). The emergence and early development of self-regulation in young children. *Profesorado: Journal of Curriculum and Teacher Education, Monograph issue: Learn to learn. Teaching and Evaluation of Self-Regulated Learning, 16*, 15–34.
Whitebread, D., Kuvalja, M., & O'Connor, A. (2015a). *Quality in early childhood education: An international review and guide for policy makers. Report for the world innovation summit for education*. Dohar: WISE.
Whitebread, D., & O'Sullivan, L. (2012). Preschool children's social pretend play: Supporting the development of metacommunication, metacognition and self-regulation. *International Journal of Play, 1*, 197–213.
Whitebread, D., Pino-Pasternak, D., & Coltman, P. (2015b). Making learning visible: The role of language in the development of metacognition and self-regulation in young children. In S. Robson & S. Quinn (Eds.), *The Routledge international handbook of young children's thinking and understanding* (pp. 199–214). London: Routledge.
Wiebe, S. A., Sheffield, T., Nelson, J. M., Clark, C. A. C., Chevalier, N., & Espy, K. A. (2011). The structure of executive function in 3-year-olds. *Journal of Experimental Child Psychology, 108*, 436–452.
Wimmer, H., & Perner, J. (1983). Beliefs about beliefs: Representation and constraining function of wrong beliefs in young children's understanding of deception. *Cognition, 13*, 103–128.
Winsler, A. E., Fernyhough, C. E., & Montero, I. E. (2009). *Private speech, executive functioning, and the development of verbal self-regulation*. Cambridge: Cambridge University Press.
Zachariou, A., & Whitebread, D. (2017). A new context affording for regulation: The case of musical play. *International Journal of Educational Psychology, 6*, 212–249.
Zelazo, P. D., Carlson, S. M., & Kesek, A. (2008). The development of executive function in childhood. In C. Nelson & M. Luciana (Eds.), *Handbook of developmental cognitive neuroscience* (2nd ed., pp. 553–574). Cambridge: MIT Press.
Zelazo, P. D., & Müller, U. (2002). Executive function in typical and atypical development. In U. Goswami (Ed.), *Blackwell handbook of childhood cognitive development* (pp. 445–469). Oxford: Blackwell.

Chapter 12
Strategic, Emotional, and Motivational Influences on Metacognition in Older Adulthood

Shannon McGillivray

Abstract While older adulthood is often associated with a decline in cognitive functions, there are numerous studies that suggest that metacognitive functioning remains relatively intact. This disparity between, for example, explicit memory functioning and ones' insight and control over memory among older adults raises some interesting questions. Can older adults use metacognitive strategies to help compensate for declining memory functions? What role do interest, emotions, and knowledge have on metacognitive judgments? The current chapter discusses both intrinsic and extrinsic motivational influences, and the role of strategy, in older adults' metacognitive processes.

Keywords Metacognition · Older adults · Emotion · Strategic control · Motivation

12.1 Introduction

Explicit memory abilities have been shown to decline during normal aging (Craik and Salthouse 2008; Kausler 1994), but a growing body of evidence suggests that metamemory process may remain largely intact (for reviews, see Castel et al. 2016; Hertzog 2016; Hertzog and Dunlosky 2011). Metacognition, or metamemory, simply refers to one's awareness and insight about one's own memory and how it works. Metamemory includes, but is not limited to, beliefs about one's memory skills and task demands, strategies one uses to remember information, insight into memory changes, feelings and emotions about one's memory, and knowledge of memory functioning (Dunlosky and Metcalfe 2009).

Specific metamemory measures typically assess either memory monitoring or control (Nelson and Narens 1990). Metacognitive monitoring involves the assessment of ongoing memory encoding and retrieval processes. Monitoring can be

S. McGillivray (✉)
Department of Psychological Science, Weber State University, Ogden, UT, USA
e-mail: smcgillivray@weber.edu

D. Moraitou, P. Metallidou (eds.), *Trends and Prospects in Metacognition Research across the Life Span*, https://doi.org/10.1007/978-3-030-51673-4_12

assessed by asking participants to explicitly report on their beliefs regarding what information is more memorable, or feelings of confidence that what one remembered was accurate. Metacognitive control, which can be influenced by monitoring (Hertzog and Dunlosky 2011), includes behaviors and actions implemented to achieve desired memory-related goals such as restudying information one feels is less well learned, or utilizing mnemonic strategies to enhance later recall. Beliefs that older and younger adults have about their memory abilities (e.g., belief that one will be able to remember important, interesting information) can influence expectations for memory performance (e.g., this information will be remembered), effort exerted during a memory task (e.g., engagement of more elaborative processing or strategy usage), and thus can influence one's actual performance.

This disparity between impaired explicit memory functioning and relatively intact insight and control over memory among older adults raises some interesting questions. Can older adults use metacognitive strategies to help compensate for declining memory functions? The selective optimization with compensation theory suggests that successful aging is related to the ability to strategically focus limited cognitive resources into areas that yield optimal returns (Baltes and Baltes 1990). Furthermore, it has been suggested that older adults may often be more selective compared with younger adults in how they choose to engage their cognitive resources (Hess 2006). Thus, it could be the case that older adults could use metacognitive insight to selectively control cognitive operations based on their goals, motivation, and the meaningfulness of information. Thus, older adults may be able to compensate for impairments by optimizing performance in specific, goal-related domains (Riediger et al. 2006). The current chapter will examine the role that interest, emotions, motivation, and prior knowledge (which have been shown to reduce or eliminate age-related memory deficits; see Castel 2008; Hess and Emery 2012; McGillivray and Castel 2017; McGillivray et al. 2015) have on metacognitive judgments. The current chapter also discusses both intrinsic and extrinsic motivational influences, and the role of strategy and importance, in older adults' memory and metacognitive processes.

12.2 Strategic Metacognitive Monitoring

The ability to recall information that is more important or valuable is essential to healthy memory functioning, and functioning in everyday life. For example, if older adults are not able to recall as much information as younger adults, but are able to recall the most important information, then perhaps quality of memory functioning remains intact despite deficits in memory quantity. Previous studies have investigated older and younger adults' ability to recall objectively more important information and have no age-related deficits in memory for more valuable information (e.g., Castel et al. 2002), truthful versus false information (Rahhal et al. 2002) or medically important information (May et al. 2005; Middlebrooks et al. 2016).

Taking a closer look at value, Castel and colleagues (Castel et al. 2002) have examined both older and younger adults' ability to remember words paired with varying point values. In this "value-directed remembering" paradigm, participants studied 6 lists of different word-value pairs (e.g., book—12, chair—3) and were told the goal was to maximize their score, which was the sum of the point values associated with remembered words. Thus, there was an external incentive to recall the words paired with higher point values, and some information was more "important" to remember. Although younger adults recalled more words than older adults, recall for the words associated with the highest point values showed no age-related differences. These results suggest that older adults are able to remember high-value information to the same extent as younger adults, although it may be at the expense of lower-value information. Older adults seem to be able to shift attention and strategically recall the high-value information at the expense of lower value information, maximizing memory efficiency (Castel 2008; Castel et al. 2002; Friedman and Castel 2013; Hennesse et al. 2019), although this pattern typically only emerges with task experience. These findings also suggest that metacognition may play an important role in older adults' adoption of effective strategies that lead them to attend to and recall higher value information.

Strategy usage is often a product of goal-directed behavior, an element that is typically examined in metacognitive control studies, but not captured in traditional metacognitive monitoring paradigms. One common measure of metacognitive monitoring is a judgment of learning (JOL). During JOL tasks participants are asked to assign some piece of information a numerical value (e.g., 0–100), and this value indicates how likely they think it is that they will later remember that information. These judgments can then be compared to actual memory performance in order to assess absolute and/or relative accuracy. Absolute accuracy of JOLs is typically measured by calculating the average JOL rating (e.g., 70% if the scale was from 0 to 100%), and comparing it with the average percentage of information recalled (e.g., 40%). Absolute accuracy allows for insight into whether individuals display a general pattern of over-or-under confidence in memory abilities (e.g., if the average JOL was 70, but a person only recalled 40% of the material this would indicate overconfidence). Relative accuracy examines whether the JOLs assigned by an individual can distinguish between what information is later remembered versus forgotten, and higher relative accuracy occurs when higher JOLs are given to information later recalled, and lower JOLs are given to information forgotten at test.

In most JOL tasks, there are no actual consequences or outcomes tied to these predictions. However, in the real world there are often consequences associated with whether or not our monitoring judgments are accurate. For example, if you believe you will remember important health information told to you by your doctor, you may decide you do not need to write it down. However, if you are incorrect in your initial assessment of your ability to remember this information, it could have negative repercussions. In order to examine a more strategic form of metacognitive monitoring, some studies have introduced consequences tied to metacognitive predictions (McGillivray and Castel 2011, 2017).

McGillivray and Castel (2011) used a modified value-directed remembering paradigm in which older and younger adults were asked to "bet" on the likelihood they would recall an item, and there were consequences associated with the accuracy of those bets. Participants were given six different lists of words paired with varying point values and were told the point value indicated how much the word was worth. As participants were shown each word, they had to "bet" (yes or no) which items they thought they would be able to remember. If participants bet on an item, then they received whatever points were associated with that item if they later recalled it, but lost those points if they failed to recall it. Participants were told the goal was to maximize their score, and score was the sum of all of the words bet on and recalled, minus the sum of the words bet on and not recalled. Thus, there were rewards associated with accurately monitoring and predicting which items would be recalled, and penalties if one failed to do so.

McGillivray and Castel (2011) found that both younger and older adults' betting and recall performance were significantly driven by the objective point value associated with the words and strategically bet on and recalled more of the high value relative to the low value items (see Fig. 12.1). In regard to metacognitive accuracy, both younger and older adults were highly overconfident on initial lists (i.e., they bet on more items than they were actually able to recall), but this was reduced with task experience. Overall point scores on each list improved with task experience, and in fact older and younger adults' scores were comparable on later lists, despite the fact that older adults recalled less information overall.

The ability of older adults to achieve scores compared to those of younger adults suggests that older adults were implementing strategies that actually led to the marginally better metacognitive accuracy on the later lists, in order to achieve goal-relevant outcomes.

The findings from McGillivray and Castel (2011) indicate that the introduction of negative consequences may have served to enhance motivation to accurately monitor and update performance expectations with task experience, perhaps even to a larger extent for older adults relative to younger adults. While McGillivray and Castel (2011) explicitly indicated which items were more valuable to recall, more recent studies have utilized a similar "betting" paradigm to examine strategic monitoring when participants were allowed to decide what information was more or less "valuable" (McGillivray and Castel 2017). In doing so, it allowed for an examination of potential age-related differences in internally driven strategic metacognitive monitoring.

McGillivray and Castel (2017) presented older and younger adults with either six lists of unrelated words (Experiment 1), mixed lists of related and unrelated word pairs (Experiment 2), or lists of items related to a particular scenario (Experiment 3; e.g., items one might want to take on a camping trip). As participants saw each item, they assigned it a point value from 0 to 10, and if they later recalled the item, they received whatever points were assigned to it, but lost those points if they failed to recall it. Requiring participants to assign a value is more similar to standard JOL paradigms, and allowed for more direct comparisons with prior metacognitive monitoring and aging research. The "bet" (i.e., point value) assigned in McGillivray

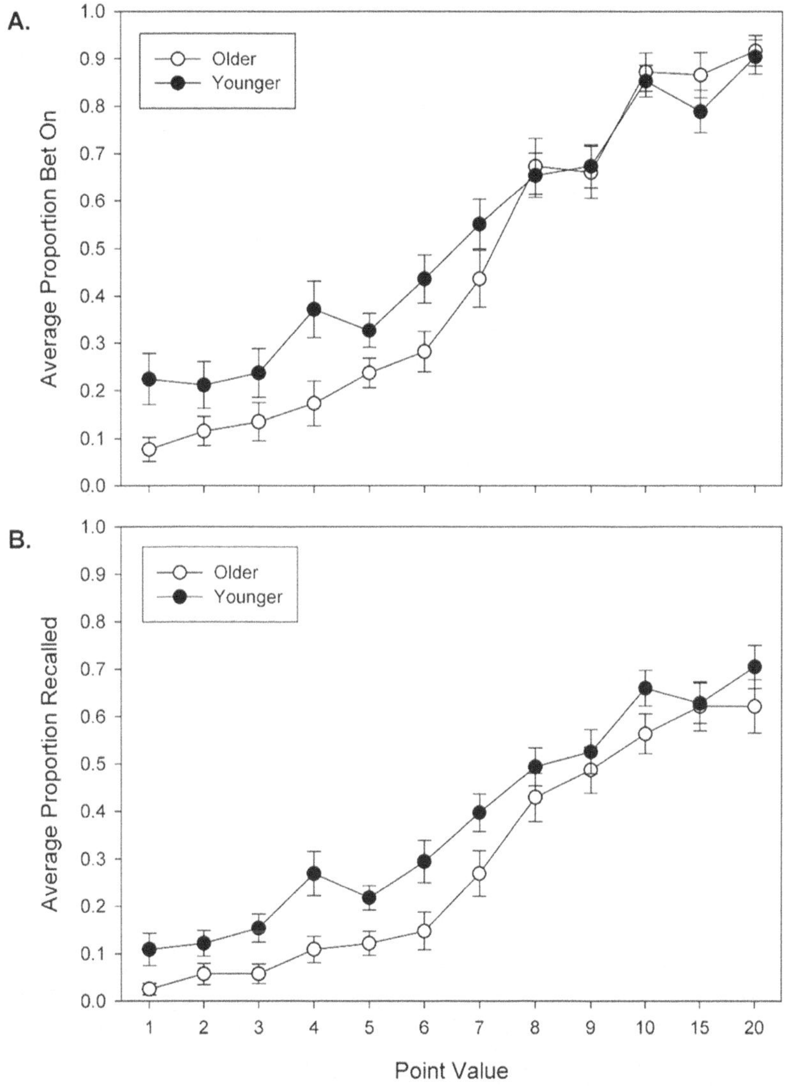

Fig. 12.1 Shows the average proportion of items bet on (top panel A) and recalled (bottom panel B) as a function of point value by older and younger adults. Error bars represent standard error of the mean. Copyright © 2011 by the American Psychological Association. Reproduced with permission. (McGillivray and Castel 2011)

and Castel's (2017) studies is similar to a judgment of how likely a participant believes an item will be recalled. That is, if one thinks an item will be recalled later, a higher value should be given. However, the use of "bets" required one to be strategic, and thus the use of metacognitive control processes during encoding.

McGillivray and Castel (2017) found that when the materials were unrelated single words (Experiment 1) both younger and older adults were able to successfully recall words they had assigned higher subjective values, and were able to improve metacognitive accuracy and reduce initial overconfidence with task experience. When the to-be-learned material were unrelated and related word pairs (Experiment 2), it was found that older adults bet on fewer items, recalled fewer items, and achieved lower point scores compared with younger adults. However, age-related memory differences were eliminated for the related word pairs.

The finding that age-related differences were prominent for the unrelated word pairs is consistent with older adults' deficits in associative learning (Naveh-Benjamin 2000; Naveh-Benjamin et al. 2003; Old and Naveh-Benjamin 2008). However, age-related associative deficits for the related word pairs were not present. It is likely that the related words pairs allowed older individuals to strategically rely on verbal or semantic knowledge, which is less susceptible to age-related declines (McCabe et al. 2010; Naveh-Benjamin et al. 2003). Older adults also displayed better overall metacognitive accuracy than younger adults. This finding of better monitoring abilities in this experiment is somewhat consistent with the finding from Hertzog and colleagues (Hertzog et al. 2002) who have reported that older individuals were more likely to utilize semantic relatedness as a cue when making JOLs. This suggests that older adults may be able to utilize their prior verbal knowledge in an advantageous way when it comes to metacognitive monitoring and optimizing memory-related outcomes.

Experiment 3 (McGillivray and Castel 2017) utilized lists of items that pertained to particular scenarios, such as going on a camping trip. It was found that younger and older adults performed comparable on all of the measures, including overall metacognitive accuracy and recall, although task experience had no impact on performance. In this task, items on each list varied in terms of how central they were to the scenario. For example, on the "camping" list there were, objectively, more important items such as tent and sleeping bag, and also some less important items such as whistle and playing cards. The data suggested that both younger and older adults were able to capitalize on this prior knowledge to effectively assign monitoring judgments, and then later recall the more central information. These findings are consistent with evidence that schemas and prior knowledge (e.g., knowledge of items one might usually take camping) can serve to mitigate typically observed age-related memory deficits (Castel 2005). The results also suggest that when the materials are more realistic, and thus enable one to use prior knowledge, older and younger adults can implement effective strategic learning and monitoring behaviors from the onset.

In regards to strategic metacognitive monitoring abilities of older adults, studies that have implemented consequences associated with monitoring judgments may make individuals feel more accountable for their judgments, which could increase motivation for accuracy and strategy usage. At present, there is growing evidence that the ability to utilize one's metacognitive monitoring (and control) abilities is intact during older adulthood, and that proper motivation and accountability of one's memory predictions can lead one to accurately and strategically monitoring one's memory processes. This suggests that older adults could effectively utilize metacognitive strategies and awareness to help compensate for age-related changes in memory abilities that in turn can enable older individuals to function successfully in everyday life.

12.3 Strategic Metacognitive Control

Metacognitive control includes behaviors and actions implemented to achieve desired memory-related goals, such as restudying information one feels is less well learned, or utilizing mnemonic strategies to enhance later recall. Metacognitive monitoring and control are thought to have a reciprocal relationship (e.g., Nelson and Narens 1990). Specifically, if one is able to effectively monitor what information is more or less likely to be recalled, then that knowledge can be used to engage strategies to enhance memory for information deemed less well learned. Beliefs that older and younger adults have about their memory abilities (e.g., belief that one will be able to remember important information) can influence expectations for memory performance (e.g., this information will be remembered), effort exerted during a memory task (e.g., engagement of more elaborative processing or strategy usage), and thus can influence one's actual performance. The evidence that older adults can successfully monitor memory operations also suggests that as one ages, intact monitoring abilities could allow one to implement effect control strategies in order to successfully achieve goal-related memory outcomes (Hertzog and Dunlosky 2011).

In regard to age-related changes in metacognitive control, Dunlosky and Connor (1997) observed that when older and younger adults were allowed to restudy words at their own pace, all participants spent more time studying items that they had assigned lower JOLs (i.e., words they judged as more difficult to recall) compared with those words that had been given higher JOLs. However, younger adults exhibited this effect to a greater extent, indicating that some age-related differences were present in the degree to which monitoring was used to effectively allocate study time. Furthermore, Tullis and Benjamin (2012) found that while older adults' study selection choices are similar to younger adults', they may not always lead to optimal memory-related outcomes. That being said, Dunlosky and Hertzog (1997) found that younger and older adults used a "functionally identical algorithm" in their selection of items for restudy, and both younger and older individuals strategically selected items to restudy that they believed were not as well learned (Dunlosky and Hertzog 1997; Hines et al. 2009). While some researchers have observed some age-related deficits in metacognitive control, there are many studies that have found age-related sparing of these processes (for a more comprehensive review of aging a metacognitive control, see Hertzog 2016).

Further evidence of age-related sparing of more *strategic* metacognitive control operations was found by Castel and colleagues (Castel et al. 2013) in a task in which the objective value of the to-be-learned information was varied. The purpose of using value in this context was to assess the extent to which a salient external cue (i.e., point value) could effectively be used by older and younger adults to guide study choices. In this study, participants were given 2 min to study a list of 30 words, and each word was associated with a different point value (values ranged from 1 to 30). Participants were allowed to study as few or as many of the items as they wanted, they were allowed to study items multiple times, and could control how long they studied each item. Importantly, in this task participants were told the goal was not necessarily to recall as many items as one could, but to obtain a high point score. Scores were the sum of the point values associated with words recalled, and thus some items were more valuable and important to remember. As is shown in Fig. 12.2, both older and younger adults were strategic in terms of studying higher point value words more often, and for longer periods of time, suggesting value or objective importance can be used as a cue to guide strategic and selective metacognitive control behaviors during the learning process.

Examining strategy use further, an important question is how or what do younger and older individuals prioritize during the learning process? Under limited time conditions (as is often the case in experimental studies and in real life), there are a number of different factors that may influence what one chooses to study, such as difficulty level of the material, or importance of the material.

Studies that have manipulated the difficulty of the material have generally found that both younger and older adults tend to study easier items first (Price and Murray 2012), a strategy consistent with the region of proximal learning framework (Kornell and Metcalfe 2006; Metcalfe 2002). The region of proximal learning framework suggests that individuals strategically choose to devote study time to information that one has the greatest likelihood of later remembering. For example, if one had limited time to study, and could either study something very difficult (that might take a while to learn), or something easier (that one had a greater likelihood of mastering), it might be more advantageous to study the somewhat easier information.

While there is evidence that older and younger adults may prioritize easier items first during study processes, how might the importance of the material impact this pattern? If some information is objectively more valuable, but difficult, will individuals selectively focus on this information? Price and colleagues (Price et al. 2010, Experiment 2) presented both younger and older adults with Spanish-English vocabulary word pairs. The vocabulary terms were clearly labeled for participants as being "easy", "medium", or "difficult" to learn, and the point value associated with each term was also manipulated such that for some participants either the easier or harder items were worth more points (there was also a neutral condition in which points were equivalent for all items). In addition, participants were either given a goal of either achieving a higher or lower overall point score. It was found that both younger and older adults still studied easier items first overall, but both age groups were sensitive to point value in their study choices. However, older adults were somewhat less likely than younger adults to study high value, difficult items, and this pattern was related to older adults' memory self-efficacy. These findings indicate that, at times, internal beliefs and knowledge of one's capabilities may influence study choices to a greater extent than do external, goal-relevant cues. Thus, if one believes

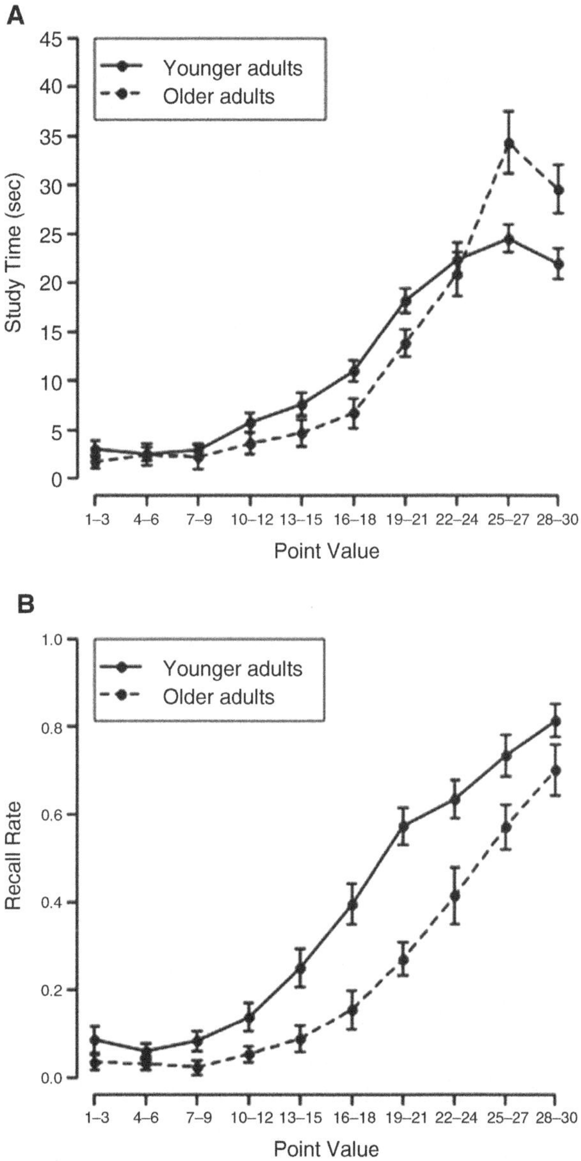

Fig. 12.2 Shows in A (top panel) the mean study time (in seconds), averaged across lists, as a function of binned point values for younger and older adults. B (bottom panel) shows the mean proportion recalled, averaged across lists, as a function of binned point values for younger and older adult. Copyright © 2013 by the American Psychological Association. Reproduced with permission. (Castel et al. 2013)

they might not be able to remember challenging, but important, information, then one either may not attempt to try to remember that information, or might instead turn to a more external strategy, such as writing it down (McDougall 1995).

The finding from Price et al. (2010) that older adults were somewhat less sensitive to value of information in their metacognitive control behaviors suggests that aging may detrimentally impact self-regulated learning strategies, at least under some conditions. Additional age-related deficits in study time allocation have been observed by Tullis and Benjamin (2012). In their study, younger and older adults studied word pairs, and then were allowed to select half of the items for restudy. During restudy, participants either restudied the word pairs they had selected (honor condition) or those they had not selected (dishonor condition). It was found that younger individuals recalled more in the honor compared to dishonor condition, suggesting that they were fairly accurate in their assessment of which items warranted additional study. Older adults, however, recalled more word pairs in the dishonor condition, suggesting older adults may exhibit some age-related deficits in implementing effective study choices, even if their memory monitoring abilities remain intact.

Contrary to what was found by Tullis and Benjamin (2012), Li and colleagues (Li et al. 2018), utilizing a similar honor and dishonor procedure, found that both younger and older adults were more likely to recall information in honor condition (i.e., when they were allowed to restudy their selected choices). Importantly, Li et al. (2018) also examined the effect of point value on item restudy choice. In this study word pairs were associated with either 1 or 5 points. It was found that older adults were more likely to choose to restudy the 5-point value items, regardless of whether they felt these were well-learned items (i.e., had given higher or lower JOLs), whereas younger adults were more likely to restudy the 1-point items they felt were less well learned. This is further evidence suggesting that importance of material can have an impact on what older adults may choose to focus on, and that older adults may choose to selectively focus on higher value information, at the expense of less valuable information.

While there is some research on how value and importance impact metacognitive control operations, there are some inconsistencies in regards to what effect, if any, aging has on these processes. In general, the patterns of results suggest that older adults do strategically select and choose to focus on valuable or important information that leads to goal-relevant outcomes, and, at times, may demonstrate slightly more selectivity in their metacognitive control behaviors than do younger adults. In the real world, this would suggest that older adults may be more likely to attend to information they deem more important, but this could be at the expense of less important information.

12.4 Metacognition and Subjective Interest and Importance

While there is evidence suggesting that older adults are able to recall more objectively high value information, and metacognitive monitoring and control processes are also sensitive to objective value, it is often one's own interest or goals that determine the overall worth or "value" of information. Older adults, in particular, might place an even greater emphasis on remembering information they think is more important or valuable compared with information they are told is important. For example, it was found that older adults were better able to recall side effects of medications that they subjectively rated as more severe compared to those they deemed milder, whereas younger adults recalled mild and severe side effects equally (Friedman et al. 2015).

Other studies have examined the influence of this more subjective measure of importance on memory in older and younger adults by manipulating personal relevance of the to-be-remembered information. For example, Hess et al. (2001) found that older adults were more accurate in their recollection of information related to a narrative describing an older target person (increased relevance) compared with one describing a younger target person; younger adults showed the opposite effect. Furthermore, older adults benefitted to a greater extent from increasing relevance than did younger adults. Germain and Hess (2007) found this pattern of better memory for more personally relevant information held true and also demonstrated that increased relevance was strongly associated not only with memory performance, but with more efficient processing (i.e., the ability to ignore irrelevant information). This suggests that interest or relevance of information can have an even larger positive effect on memory processes for older adults compared with younger adults, and that metacognitive monitoring and control processes might also be sensitive to degree of personal interest or importance.

The effect of subjective interest on memory has previously been examined in younger adults (Kang et al. 2009). Within this study, interest was defined as curiosity to learn unknown information. Curiosity is thought to be driven by an awareness of a gap between desired knowledge, and one's current level of understanding (Loewenstein 1994). Thus, in a sense, curiosity may be modulated by a combination of metacognitive appraisals of our level of knowledge and of our level of certainty in our ability to obtain that knowledge. Kang et al. (2009) presented younger adult participants with trivia question, and had participants rate how curious they were to learn the answer, after which participants were shown the answer. When given a later recall test, participants recalled more answers to the trivia questions that initially elicited higher levels of curiosity.

While previous studies have examined the impact of curiosity on memory for younger adults, there has been an increasing body of research examining the effects of curiosity on older adult's memory and metacognitive processes. One might suspect that if older adults are more selective about what information they attend to, then curiosity or interest could potentially be a larger predictor of memory performance, and may also have a greater influence on metacognitive monitoring judgments. Specifically, if one thought something was very important or interesting, then it is probable that one might also believe that information will be remembered, or perhaps even engage in additional strategies to try to effectively learn it.

McGillivray et al. (2015) examined the effect of initial curiosity to learn, and subjective interest on memory and metacognition in younger and older adults. In their study participants were presented with a large number of obscure trivia questions, and after being shown each question participants indicated their curiosity to learn the answer before they were shown the correct answer. After learning the answer, participants were asked to indicate how interesting they thought the answer was (post-answer interest) and also provided a judgment of learning (JOL) to indicate how well they thought they would be able to later remember that answer.

It was found that intrinsic post-answer interest was the largest predictor of later memory for the information for both younger and older adults. In addition, decreasing effects of interest from a short-delay to long-delay memory tests for younger adults were observed, but there were increasing predictive effects of interest on memory for older adults, suggesting interest may have increasing effects on memory for older adults with time.

McGillivray et al. (2015) also observed that both initial curiosity to learn answers, and to a larger extent, post-answer interest, predicted judgments of learning for both younger and older adults. This suggests that curiosity and interest are a cue that both younger and older adults may use when deciding what one is more or less likely to remember. New analysis of the data reported in this study examined JOL accuracy (using gamma correlations) for both high and low interest-eliciting questions for younger and older adults in order to determine if accuracy of metacognitive monitoring judgments is influenced by the subjective interest in the material. For each participant, the mean interest rating was calculated and the data were divided into high and low interest questions, and accuracy of the JOLs for these two categories of questions were examined. Among older adults, JOL accuracy was comparable for low-interest evoking questions ($G = 0.38$) and high interest evoking questions ($G = 0.34$). However, for younger adults JOL accuracy was better for low-interest evoking questions ($G = 0.58$) compared to high interest evoking questions ($G = 0.33$). While this could suggest that younger adults are better at monitoring their memory compared with older adults when they are less interested, these should be interpreted with some caution. It should be noted that the mean-split analysis resulted in a restricted range of scores, which could be obscuring the observed relationship between interest and accuracy of one's monitoring judgments. That being said, the ability to accurately monitor performance related to what one finds interesting seems to be relatively unaffected during later adulthood (Hargis et al. 2017; McGillivray et al. 2015).

In addition to the observed effects curiosity has on memory, it has been proposed that curiosity can serve many adaptive functions, particularly as individuals age (Sakaki et al. 2018). Specifically, prior studies have found that curiosity engages the dopaminergic system (Kang et al. 2009) and increases activity in the striatum, substantia nigra and ventral tegmental area (Gruber et al. 2014). In addition, factors such as novelty and uncertainty (which are likely associated with curiosity) may also activate noradrenergic systems (Devauges and Sara 1990; Gompf et al. 2010; Lavin et al. 2014). Sakaki et al. (2018) put forth evidence that suggest that curiosity's activation of the dopaminergic noradrenergic systems may have both direct and indirect effects on hippocampal, prefrontal cortex, and working memory function, as well as general feelings of well-being and health (see Fig. 12.3). The researchers also suggest that chronic activation of curiosity (i.e., trait curiosity) could lead one to engage in stimulating behaviors and activities that may protect against cognitive decline, as well as activate neurological circuits that could further expand upon the benefits that might be associated more momentary feelings of curiosity outlined in Fig. 12.3. Further, evidence of the benefits of curiosity, beyond just for the information that one might be curious about, were found by Galli and colleagues (Galli

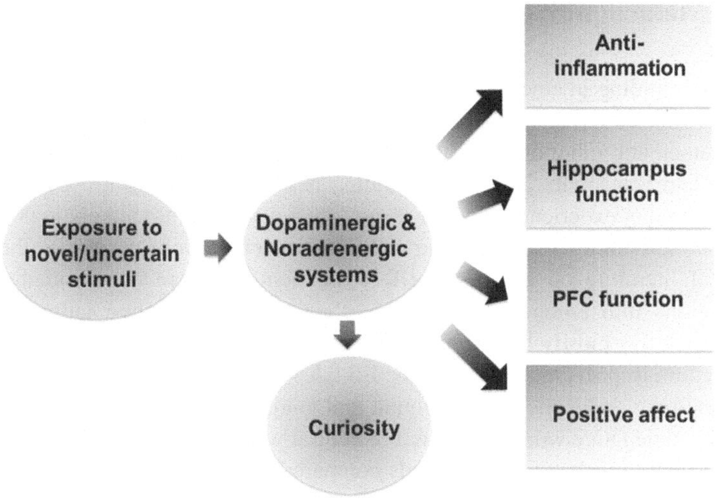

Fig. 12.3 Shows the proposed effects of feeling curiosity when exposed to something novel and/or uncertain. Reprinted from Neuroscience and Behavioral Reviews, Vol. 88, Sakaki, Yagi, and Murayama, Curiosity in old age: A possible key to achieving adaptive aging, p. 109, © 2018, with permission from Elsevier. (Sakaki et al. 2018)

et al. 2018). In this study, older and younger adult participants were shown trivia questions and indicated their level of curiosity to find out the answer.

In addition, task-irrelevant faces were shown after participants saw each question, but before they were shown the answer to the question. It was found that both younger and older adults were more likely to recall answers to trivia questions they were more curious about, and were also more likely to correctly recognize faces presented with the questions that had elicited higher levels of curiosity. These finding offer additional support for the potentially expansive benefits that feelings of curiosity may elicit, at least in memory-related domains.

In summary, as individuals age, factors such as subjective interest or curiosity could have an even larger effect on memory. In addition to interests' impact on memory, subjective feelings of interest may also impact metacognitive monitoring judgments, although it is unclear how they may impact metamemory control behaviors. It is likely that interest might serve to rally and direct attentional resources or lead one to engage in more elaborative encoding, which in turn benefits long-term memory and could also benefit strategic metacognitive control operations. Importantly, a person's interests can be linked with satisfaction in life, and thus a better understanding of how, precisely interest impacts cognitive operations is warranted.

12.5 Metacognitive Monitoring and Emotional Material

A common finding in emotion and memory literature is that individuals, of all ages, are somewhat more likely to (although not always, see Dougal and Rotello 2007) better remember emotional information compared to neutral information (e.g., Murphy and Isaacowitz 2008). This finding is consistent with most people's subjective everyday experiences, in that seems like we are just more likely to notice and remember something if it elicits an emotional reaction from us. While there is a wealth of literature on emotions' effect on memory, there are decidedly fewer examinations into emotional materials' effect on metacognitive judgments, and this research has mostly been conducted with only younger adults (for a review of how emotion impacts metamemory see Efklides 2016).

Zimmerman and Kelley (2010) found that younger adults' JOLs were higher for positive and negative words compared to neutral words, and participants were more likely to freely recall emotional words compared to neutral words. However, on a cued recall test, only the positive words were remembered better, despite high JOLs for both negative and positive information. Other studies with younger adults utilizing positive and neutral pictures (Hourihan and Bursey 2017) and neutral and negative faces (Witherby and Tauber 2018 Experiment 1) have found that participants' JOLs, but not memory, for emotional materials were higher. This suggests that emotional content may be a strong cue that individuals rely on when forming their metacognitive judgements, but this cue may be, at times, misleading when it comes to accuracy of these judgments.

Before discussing the few research studies on metacognition, emotion, and aging, it is important to note some of the age-related differences in standard memory tasks for emotional materials. For example, there have been a number of studies that have found a positivity bias in older adults' memories (but see Fernandes et al. 2008). The positivity bias refers to the finding that older adults seem to be more likely to remember positive compared to negative information (Carstensen and Mikels 2005; Charles et al. 2003; Mather and Carstensen 2005; Schlagman et al. 2006). Interestingly, it has been suggested that this positivity bias may be the result of older adults' chronically-activated goal to maintain a positive emotional state (Mather and Knight 2005). That is, older adults to some extent may choose to attend to positive information, and perhaps even work to down-regulate negative information. An important question, as it relates to metacognition, is whether this goal to attend to and remember more positive information is more implicit or explicit in nature. If a positivity effect exists in older adults' memories, will conscious, explicit metacognitive judgements of emotional materials reflect this?

Across two experiments Tauber and Dunlosky (2012) investigated both younger and older adults' metacognitive accuracy for emotional words. Using a similar paradigm as Zimmerman and Kelley (2010), participants were shown positive (e.g., bunny, diamond), negative (e.g., assault, bomb), and neutral (e.g., fabric, cork) words. Immediately after each word participants were asked to provide a JOL from 0% (certain the words would not be recalled) to 100% (certain the word

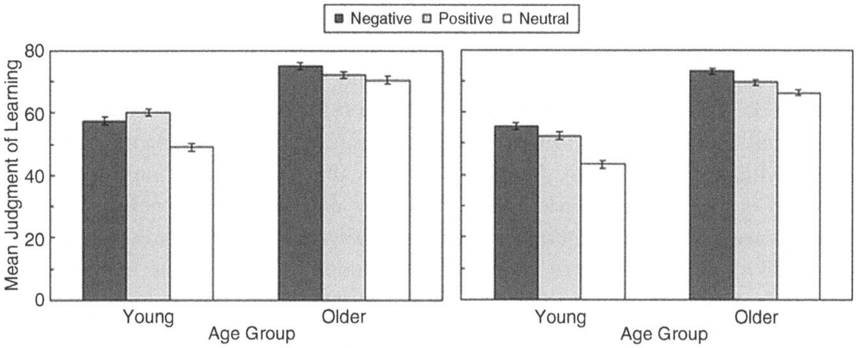

Fig. 12.4 Shows the average judgment of learning (JOL) for positive, negative, and neutral word type from Experiment 1 (left panel) and Experiment 2 (right panel). Error bars are standard errors of the mean. Copyright © 2012 by the American Psychological Association. Reproduced with permission. Tauber and Dunlosky (2012)

would be recalled). After this the participants were asked to freely recall as many words as they could. As is shown in Fig. 12.4, Tauber and Dunlosky (2012) found that younger adults' JOLs were higher for both positive and negative words compared to neutral words, but older adults only gave higher JOLs to negative, but not positive, words compared to neutral words. Furthermore, both age groups recalled more positive and negative words compared to neutral words, but did not recall more negative compared to positive words. In regards to the accuracy of metacognitive judgments, the researchers examined whether higher JOLs were given to information later recalled, and lower JOLs to information not recalled (i.e., relative accuracy using gamma correlations). The results across the two experiments were somewhat mixed, but indicated that both younger and older adults' judgments were relatively accurate in predicting recall of negative information, but that older adults were in fact less accurate in their predictions of their ability to recall positive information. Although overall accuracy of judgments did not differ significantly for emotional compared to neutral information. This suggests that the ability to accurate judge what one is likely to recall may not be affected by the emotional content of the information.

The results of this study are somewhat puzzling as they run counter to the literature that has found a positivity bias in older adults' memories. If anything, Tauber and Dunlosky (2012) found that older adults displayed more of a negativity bias in both their JOLs and recall. While older and younger adults' metacognitive monitoring judgments were somewhat sensitive to the effects of emotion, older adults' judgments were in fact less sensitive to the effects of positive emotions. Mather and Knight (2005) suggested that the positivity bias may, in part, be due to a chronically activated goal to maintain a positive emotional state.

While older adults did recall more positive (and negative) compared to neutral information, this pattern did not seem to be captured in their JOLs. This could indicate that if a positivity goal exists, it may at times operate on a more implicit level that does not affect older adults' explicit judgments. It could also be the case that the need to provide a JOL became a more salient than the goal to maintain a positive emotional state. Mather and Knight (2005) found that older adults under divided attention do not exhibit a positivity bias in memory, and it has also been suggested that asking individuals to provide judgments may actually alter memory performance (Mitchum et al. 2016). Another possibility that Tauber and Dunlosky (2012) proposed is that the materials (i.e., words) may not be as emotionally salient as materials used in other emotional memory paradigms (e.g., pictures). Thus, if an individual experienced less of an emotional reaction to some of the material, and perhaps in particular the positive material, there may be no reason to suspect that judgments or memory performance would be impacted.

In order to examine older adults' metamemory monitoring for more emotionally arousing information, Tauber and colleagues (Tauber et al. 2017) presented younger and older adults with positive and neutral images. It has been suggested that pictures may be more likely to elicit emotional responses than single words (Kensinger and Schacter 2006). Importantly, the emotional intensity of the images varied and were either classified as positive and high arousal (e.g., skydiving), positive and low arousal (e.g., fishing), neutral and high arousal (e.g., lava) or neutral and low arousal (e.g., a rock formation; Tauber et al. 2017). As participants studied each picture, they provided a JOL from 0 to 100. After a short delay, participants took part in a free recall test in which they had to describe the images they remembered. It was found that both younger and older adults' JOLs were higher for both high and low arousal positive images compared to high and low arousal neutral images, but JOLs did not seem to differentiate between high and low arousal positive images. A similar pattern was observed with older and younger adults' recall performance, with both younger and older adults remembering more positive images, regardless of arousal level, compared to neutral images. Lastly, the accuracy of metacognitive judgments appeared to be unaffected by image type, arousal level, or age.

The findings from Tauber and colleagues (2012, 2017) suggest that older adults are, in fact, effectively able to monitor their encoding of positive emotional information, provided the material contains richer emotional cues. Put simply, age does not seem to negatively impact one's ability to realize that positive information is more likely to be remembered than neutral information. Furthermore, it suggests that emotion can, at times, be a salient cue that both younger and older adults use to form memory judgements, although these cues might be misleading at times, particularly when it comes to correctly recognizing emotional material (see Comblain et al. 2004; Kapucu et al. 2008). However, Tauber and colleagues (2012, 2017) found that the ability to accurately monitor positive information does not appear to be any better than the ability to monitor neutral information (i.e., measures of resolution were similar for emotional and neutral information). What this indicates is that emotional content neither enhances nor diminishes one's ability to judge what is more or less likely to be recalled. What is still unclear though is whether metamemory judgments would be impacted when both positive and negative emotion-inducing material is present. As was previously mentioned, most of the studies that have found a positivity bias in older adults' memories have used positive and negative images.

To date no studies have utilized similar materials to study older adult metacognitive monitoring judgments, and this is an important area for future research.

12.6 Summary and Future Directions

Declines in cognitive functioning have been well documented in aging literature. While, of course, it is vital to understand the limitations older individuals may face, and potential causes of deficits, it is equally as important to fully explore and understand the constellation of factors that mitigate deficits and speak to older individuals' ability to maintain a high quality of life and healthy functioning. The findings of intact metacognitive functioning in many studies suggest that insight into, and understanding of one's memory capabilities is not negatively impacted during the aging process, or at least is impacted to a lesser extent than other cognitive functions.

A central and perhaps quite critical memory-related goal in many individual's lives, and perhaps particularly older adults, is to be able to remember information that is important (either subjectively or objectively) information one is interested in, or more emotional-relevant information. Evidence suggests that that the mechanisms that lead one to be able to recall more important or interesting information are intact during the aging process, and interest, prior knowledge, and the emotional content of the material may mitigate some of typically observed age-related decrements in memory processes.

While there is a growing body of evidence that suggests factors such as emotion, motivation, interest, and prior knowledge impact memory, there is still relatively little research on how these impact metacognitive monitoring and control during older adulthood. Some of the studies discussed in this chapter suggest that older adults are able to strategically monitor and control memory processes, and that metamemory judgments are sensitive to subjective interest and emotional content, but many questions remain unanswered. For example, do older and younger adults differ in regards to metacognitive control processes (e.g., item selection or strategy usage) when learning emotional or "interesting" material? Are older adults more likely to implement strategic control behaviors or mnemonic strategies when motivated to learn either valuable or interesting information? Additional research into the impact that interest, emotions, motivation, and prior knowledge have on metamemory monitoring and control is warranted and could further inform and improve theories of cognitive aging, and well as theories of learning and memory more generally.

In addition, this relative sparing of metacognitive abilities, in light of some deficits in explicit memory abilities, suggests that older adults may be able to use metacognitive strategies or awareness to help overcome or compensate for age-related declines in memory performance. In fact, it has been suggested that training metamemory monitoring and control could serve to better inform or perhaps be even more beneficial than general memory training strategies for older adults

(Hertzog and Dunlosky 2011; see also Bampa et al., Chap. 13 this volume). For example, Troyer (2001) found that educating older individuals how memory works as well as memory strategies increased older adults' knowledge of and satisfaction with their memory, as well their memory functioning on everyday task. This line of research has implications not only for memory training programs, but also speaks to older adults' ability to maintain healthy cognitive functioning in everyday life.

In conclusion, there are numerous factors, including but not limited to value, emotion, and importance, that have the capacity to moderate one's memory and metacognitive judgments. It is crucial to fully explore and understand the relationships between these various memory-moderating factors as well as the degree to which they affect metamemory, particularly for older adults. Older adulthood is often accompanied by a number of major life-decisions in areas such as health care, retirement, and financial planning. Making effective decisions often requires learning new information, being aware of one's knowledge level, and ultimately prioritizing and organizing that information. Once the factors and mechanisms supporting the facilitation of memory, as well as metamemory monitoring and control are better understood and fully explored, they could serve to assist fields such as information dissemination in a way that assists learning, prioritization and enhances quality of everyday functioning for older adults.

Acknowledgments I would like to thank my mentor and colleague Dr. Alan D. Castel for his unwavering support of, and contribution to, the research reviewed in this chapter.

References

Baltes, P. B., & Baltes, M. M. (1990). Psychological perspectives on successful aging: The model of selective optimization with compensation. In P. B. Baltes & M. M. Baltes (Eds.), *Successful aging: Perspectives from the behavioral sciences* (pp. 1–34). New York, NY: Cambridge University Press.

Carstensen, L. L., & Mikels, J. A. (2005). At the intersection of emotion and cognition: Aging and the positivity effect. *Current Directions in Psychological Science, 14*, 117–121. https://doi.org/10.1111/j.0963-7214.2005.00348.x.

Castel, A. D. (2005). Memory for grocery prices in younger and older adults: The role of schematic support. *Psychology and Aging, 20*, 718–721. https://doi.org/10.1037/0882-7974.20.4.718.

Castel, A. D. (2008). The adaptive and strategic use of memory by older adults: Evaluative processing and value-directed remembering. In A. S. Benjamin & B. H. Ross (Eds.), *The psychology of learning and motivation* (pp. 225–270). London: Academic.

Castel, A. D., Benjamin, A. S., Craik, F. I. M., & Watkins, M. J. (2002). The effects of aging on selectivity and control in short-term recall. *Memory & Cognition, 30*, 1078–1085. https://doi.org/10.3758/BF03194325.

Castel, A. D., Murayama, K., Friedman, M. C., McGillivray, S., & Link, I. (2013). Selecting valuable information to remember: Age-related differences and similarities in self-regulated learning. *Psychology and Aging, 28*, 232–242. https://doi.org/10.1037/a0030678.

Castel, A. D., Middlebrooks, C. D., & McGillivray, S. (2016). Monitoring memory in old age: Impaired, spared, and aware. In J. Dunlosky & S. K. Tauber (Eds.), *Oxford handbook of metacognition* (pp. 519–535). New York: Oxford University Press.

Charles, S. T., Mather, M., & Carstensen, L. L. (2003). Aging and emotional memory: The forgettable nature of negative images for older adults. *Journal of Experimental Psychology: General, 132*, 310–324. https://doi.org/10.1037/0096-3445.132.2.310.

Comblain, C., D'Argembeau, A., Van der Linden, M., & Aldenhoff, L. (2004). The effect of ageing on the recollection of emotional and neutral pictures. *Memory, 12*, 673–684. https://doi.org/10.1080/09658210344000477.

Craik, F. I. M., & Salthouse, T. A. (2008). *Handbook of aging and cognition* (3rd ed.). Mahwah: Lawrence Eribaum.

Devauges, V., & Sara, S. J. (1990). Activation of the noradrenergic system facilitates an attentionalshift in the rat. *Behavioral Brain Research, 39*, 19–28. https://doi.org/10.1016/0166-4328(90)90118-x.

Dougal, S., & Rotello, C. M. (2007). "Remembering" emotional words isbased on response bias, not recollection. *Psychonomic Bulletin & Review, 14*, 423–429. https://doi.org/10.3758/BF03194083.

Dunlosky, J., & Connor, L. T. (1997). Age differences in the allocation of study time account for age differences in memory performance. *Memory & Cognition, 25*, 691–700. https://doi.org/10.3758/BF03211311.

Dunlosky, J., & Hertzog, C. (1997). Older and younger adults use a functionally identical algorithm to select items for restudy during multitrial learning. *Journal of Gerontology: Psychological Sciences, 52*, 178–186. https://doi.org/10.1093/geronb/52B.4.P178.

Dunlosky, J., & Metcalfe, J. (2009). *Metacognition*. Thousand Oaks: Sage Publications.

Efklides, A. (2016). Metamemory and affect. In J. Dunlosky & S. K. Tauber (Eds.), *Oxford handbook of metacognition* (pp. 245–267). New York: Oxford University Press.

Fernandes, M., Ross, M., Wiegand, M., & Schryer, E. (2008). Are the memories of older adults positively biased? *Psychology and Aging, 23*, 297–306. https://doi.org/10.1037/0882-7974.23.2.297.

Friedman, M. C., & Castel, A. D. (2013). Memory, priority encoding, and overcoming high-value proactive interference in younger and older adults. *Aging, Neuropsychology, and Cognition, 20*, 660–683. https://doi.org/10.1080/13825585.2012.762083.

Friedman, M. C., McGillivray, S., Murayama, K., & Castel, A. D. (2015). Memory for medication side effects in younger and older adults: The role of subjective and objective importance. *Memory & Cognition, 43*, 206–215. https://doi.org/10.3758/s13421-014-0476-0.

Galli, G., Sirota, M., Gruber, M. J., Ivanof, B. E., Ganesh, J., Materassi, M., et al. (2018). Learning facts during aging: The benefits of curiosity. *Experimental Aging Research, 44*, 311–328. https://doi.org/10.1080/0361073X.2018.1477355.

Germain, C. M., & Hess, T. M. (2007). Motivational influences on controlled processing: Moderating distractibility in older adults. *Aging Neuropsychology and Cognition, 14*, 462–486. https://doi.org/10.1080/13825580600611302.

Gompf, H. S., Mathai, C., Fuller, P. M., Wood, D. A., Pedersen, N. P., Saper, C. B., & Lu, J. (2010). Locus coeruleus and anterior cingulate cortex sustain wakefulness in a novel environment. *The Journal of Neuroscience, 30*, 14543–14551. https://doi.org/10.1523/jneurosci.3037-10.2010.

Gruber, M. J., Gelman, B. D., & Ranganath, C. (2014). States of curiosity modulate hippocampus-dependent learning via the dopaminergic circuit. *Neuron, 84*, 486–496. https://doi.org/10.1016/j.neuron.2014.08.060.

Hargis, M. B., Yue, C. L., Kerr, T., Ikeda, K., Murayama, K., & Castel, A. D. (2017). Metacognition and proofreading: The roles of aging, motivation, and interest. *Aging, Neuropsychology, and Cognition, 24*, 216–226. https://doi.org/10.1080/13825585.2016.1182114.

Hennessee, J. P., Patterson, T. K., Castel, A. D., & Knowlton, B. J. (2019). Forget me not: Encoding processes in value-directed remembering. *Journal of Memory and Language, 106*, 29–39. https://doi.org/10.1016/j.jml.2019.02.001.

Hertzog, C. (2016). Aging and metacognitive control. In J. Dunlosky & S. K. Tauber (Eds.), *Oxford handbook of metacognition* (pp. 537–558). New York: Oxford University Press.

Hertzog, C., & Dunlosky, J. (2011). Metacognition in later adulthood: Spared monitoring can benefit older adults' self-regulation. *Current Directions in Psychological Science, 120*, 67–173. https://doi.org/10.1177/0963721411409026.

Hertzog, C., Dunlosky, J., Powell-Moman, A., & Kidder, D. P. (2002). Aging and monitoring associative learning: Is monitoring accuracy spared or impaired? *Psychology and Aging, 17*, 209–225. https://doi.org/10.1037/0882-7974.17.2.209.

Hess, T. M. (2006). Adaptive aspects of social cognitive functioning in adulthood: Age-related goal and knowledge influences. *Social Cognition, 24*, 279–309. https://doi.org/10.1521/soco.2006.24.3.279.

Hess, T., & Emery, L. (2012). Memory in context: The impact of age-related goals on performance. In M. Naveh-Benjamin & N. Ohta (Eds.), *Memory and aging: Current issues and future directions* (pp. 183–214). New York: Psychology Press.

Hess, T. M., Rosenberg, D. C., & Waters, S. J. (2001). Motivation and representational processes in adulthood: The effects of social accountability and information relevance. *Psychology and Aging, 16*, 629–642. https://doi.org/10.1037/0882-7974.16.4.629.

Hines, J. C., Touron, D. R., & Hertzog, C. (2009). Metacognitive influences on study time allocation in an associative recognition task: An analysis of adult age differences. *Psychology and Aging, 24*, 462–475. https://doi.org/10.1037/a0014417.

Hourihan, K. L., & Bursey, E. (2017). A misleading feeling of happiness: Metamemory for positive emotional and neutral pictures. *Memory, 25*, 35–43. https://doi.org/10.1080/09658211.2015.1122809.

Kang, M. J., Hsu, M., Krajbich, I. M., Loewenstein, G., McClure, S. M., Wang, J. T., et al. (2009). The wick in the candle of learning: Epistemic curiosity activates reward circuitry and enhances memory. *Psychological Science, 20*, 963–973. https://doi.org/10.1111/j.1467-9280.2009.02402.x.

Kapucu, A., Rotello, C. M., Ready, R. E., & Seidl, K. N. (2008). Response bias in "remembering" emotional stimuli: A new perspective on age differences. *Journal of Experimental Psychology: Learning, Memory, and Cognition, 34*, 703–711. https://doi.org/10.1037/0278-7393.34.3.703.

Kausler, D. H. (1994). *Learning and memory in normal aging*. San Diego: Academic.

Kensinger, E. A., & Schacter, D. L. (2006). Processing emotional pictures and words: Effects of valence and arousal. *Cognitive, Affective, & Behavioral Neuroscience, 6*, 110–126. https://doi.org/10.3758/CABN.6.2.110.

Kornell, N., & Metcalfe, J. (2006). Study efficacy and the region of proximal learning framework. *Journal of Experimental Psychology: Learning, Memory, and Cognition, 32*, 609–622. https://doi.org/10.1037/0278-7393.32.3.609.

Lavin, C., San Martín, R., & Rosales-Jubal, E. (2014). Pupil dilation signals uncertainty and surprise in a learning gambling task. *Frontiers in Behavioral Neuroscience, 7*, 218. https://doi.org/10.3389/fnbeh.2013.00218.

Li, P., Zhang, Y., Li, W., & Li, X. (2018). Age-related differences in effectiveness of item restudy choices: The role of value. *Aging, Neuropsychology, and Cognition, 25*, 122–131. https://doi.org/10.1080/13825585.2016.1267326.

Loewenstein, G. (1994). The psychology of curiosity: A review and reinterpretation. *Psychological Bulletin, 116*, 75–98. https://doi.org/10.1037/0033-2909.116.1.75.

Mather, M., & Carstensen, L. L. (2005). Aging and motivated cognition: The positivity effect in attention and memory. *Trends in Cognitive Sciences, 9*, 496–502. https://doi.org/10.1016/j.tics.2005.08.005.

Mather, M., & Knight, M. (2005). Goal-directed memory: The role of cognitive control in older adults' emotional memory. *Psychology and Aging, 20*, 554–570. https://doi.org/10.1037/0882-7974.20.4.554.

May, C. P., Rahhal, T., Berry, E. M., & Leighton, E. A. (2005). Aging, source memory, and emotion. *Psychology and Aging, 20*, 571–578. https://doi.org/10.1037/0882-7974.20.4.571.

McCabe, D. P., Roediger, H. L., McDaniel, M. A., Balota, D. A., & Hambrick, D. Z. (2010). The relationship between working memory capacity and executive functioning: Evidence for a

common executive attention construct. *Neuropsychology, 24*, 222–243. https://doi.org/10.1037/a0017619.
McDougall, G. J. (1995). Memory self-efficacy and strategy use in successful elders. *Educational Gerontology, 21*, 357–373. https://doi.org/10.1080/0360127950210406.
McGillivray, S., & Castel, A. D. (2011). Betting on memory leads to metacognitive improvement in younger and older adults. *Psychology and Aging, 26*, 137–142. https://doi.org/10.1037/a0022681.
McGillivray, S., & Castel, A. D. (2017). Older and younger adults' strategic control of metacognitive monitoring: The role of consequences, task experience, and prior knowledge. *Experimental Aging Research, 43*, 233–256. https://doi.org/10.1080/0361073X.2017.1298956.
McGillivray, S., Murayama, K., & Castel, A. D. (2015). Thirst for knowledge: The effects of curiosity and interest on memory in younger and older adults. *Psychology and Aging, 30*, 835–841. https://doi.org/10.1037/a0039801.
Metcalfe, J. (2002). Is study time allocated selectively to a region of proximal learning? *Journal of Experimental Psychology: General, 131*, 349–363. https://doi.org/10.1037/0096-3445.131.3.349.
Middlebrooks, C. D., McGillivray, S., Murayama, K., & Castel, A. D. (2016). Memory for allergies and health foods: How younger and older adults strategically remember critical health information. *Journal of Gerontology: Psychological Sciences, 71*, 389–399. https://doi.org/10.1093/geronb/gbv032.
Mitchum, A. L., Kelley, C. M., & Fox, M. C. (2016). When asking the question changes the ultimate answer: Metamemory judgments change memory. *Journal of Experimental Psychology: General, 145*, 200–219. https://doi.org/10.1037/a0039923.
Murphy, N. A., & Isaacowitz, D. M. (2008). Preferences for emotional information in older and younger adults: A meta-analysis of memory and attention tasks. *Psychology and Aging, 23*, 263–286. https://doi.org/10.1037/0882-7974.23.2.263.
Naveh-Benjamin, M. (2000). Adult age differences in memory performance: Tests of an associative deficit hypothesis. *Journal of Experimental Psychology: Learning, Memory, and Cognition, 26*, 1170–1187. https://doi.org/10.1037/0278-7393.26.5.1170.
Naveh-Benjamin, M., Hussain, Z., Guez, J., & Bar-On, M. (2003). Adult age differences in episodic memory: Further support for an associative-deficit hypothesis. *Journal of Experimental Psychology: Learning, Memory, and Cognition, 29*, 826–837. https://doi.org/10.1037/0278-7393.29.5.826.
Nelson, T. O., & Narens, L. (1990). Metamemory: A theoretical framework and some new findings. In G. H. Bower (Ed.), *The psychology of learning and motivation* (pp. 125–173). New York: Academic.
Old, S. R., & Naveh-Benjamin, M. (2008). Differential effects of age on item and associative measures of memory: A meta-analysis. *Psychology and Aging, 23*, 104–118. https://doi.org/10.1037/0882-7974.23.1.104.
Price, J., & Murray, R. G. (2012). The region of proximal learning heuristic and adult age differences in self-regulated learning. *Psychology & Aging, 27*, 1120–1129. https://doi.org/10.1037/a0029860.
Price, J., Hertzog, C., & Dunlosky, J. (2010). Self-regulated learning in younger and older adults: Does aging affect metacognitive control? *Aging, Neuropsychology, and Cognition, 17*, 329–359. https://doi.org/10.1080/13825580903287941.
Rahhal, T. A., May, C. P., & Hasher, L. (2002). Truth and character: Sources that older adults can remember. *Psychological Science, 13*, 101–105. https://doi.org/10.1111/1467-9280.00419.
Riediger, M., Li, S. C., & Lindenberger, U. (2006). Selection, optimization, and compensation as developmental mechanisms of adaptive resource allocation: Review and preview. In J. E. Birren & K. W. Schaie (Eds.), *Handbook of the psychology and aging* (6th ed., pp. 289–313). Amsterdam: Elsevier.

Sakaki, M., Yagi, A., & Murayama, K. (2018). Curiosity in old age: A possible key to achieving adaptive aging. *Neuroscience and Behavioral Reviews, 88*, 106–116. https://doi.org/10.1016/j.neubiorev.2018.03.007.

Schlagman, S., Schulz, J., & Kvavilashvili, L. (2006). A content analysis of involuntary autobiographical memories: Examining the positivity effect in old age. *Memory, 14*, 161–175. https://doi.org/10.1080/09658210544000024.

Tauber, S. K., & Dunlosky, J. (2012). Can older adults accurately judge their learning of emotional information? *Psychology and Aging, 27*, 924–933. https://doi.org/10.1037/a0028447.

Tauber, S. K., Dunlosky, J., Urry, H. L., & Opitz, P. C. (2017). The effect of emotion of younger and older adults' monitoring of learning. *Aging, Neuropsychology, and Cognition, 24*, 555–574. https://doi.org/10.1080/13825585.2016.1227423.

Troyer, A. K. (2001). Improving memory knowledge, satisfaction, and functioning via an education and intervention program for older adults. *Aging, Neuropsychology, and Cognition, 8*, 256–268. https://doi.org/10.1076/anec.8.4.256.5642.

Tullis, J. G., & Benjamin, A. S. (2012). Consequences of restudy choices in younger and older learners. *Psychonomic Bulletin & Review, 19*, 743–749. https://doi.org/10.3758/s13423-012-0266-2.

Witherby, A. E., & Tauber, S. K. (2018). Monitoring of learning for emotional faces: How do fine-grained categories of emotion influence participants' judgments of learning and beliefs about memory? *Cognition and Emotion, 32*, 860–866. https://doi.org/10.1080/02699931.2017.1360252.

Zimmerman, C. A., & Kelley, C. M. (2010). "I'll remember this!" Effects of emotionality on memory predictions versus memory performance. *Journal of Memory and Language, 62*, 240–253. https://doi.org/10.1016/j.jml.2009.11.004.

Chapter 13
Metacognition in Cognitive Rehabilitation in Adults: A Systematic Review

Grigoria Bampa, Despina Moraitou, and Panayiota Metallidou

Abstract Numerous studies have provided evidence for the positive effects of cognitive training rehabilitation programs targeting multiple aspects of cognition. However, their limitations, such as lack of transfer effects or limited maintenance over time of the training-related gains, have driven the scientific community to search for other conceptual frameworks that could inform rehabilitation efforts. Metacognition was such an alternative theoretical approach. Metacognition refers to higher-level cognitive processes responsible for the monitoring and control of cognitive behavior. Even though research about the impact of metacognition in cognitive rehabilitation is still in its infancy, the available studies have provided some promising results. In order to gain a better overview of these findings, we conducted a literature review based on recent studies that investigated the efficacy of metacognitive training programs in older and younger adults with cognitive deficits. The results of these studies as well as the structure of the applied training programs are discussed.

Keywords Cognitive deficits · Metacognitive training · Older adults · Randomized control trials · Young adults

---

G. Bampa (✉) · D. Moraitou
Laboratory of Psychology, Section of Cognitive and Experimental Psychology, School of Psychology, Aristotle University of Thessaloniki, Thessaloniki, Greece

Laboratory of Neurodegenerative Diseases, Center of Interdisciplinary Research and Innovation (CIRI-AUTH), Thessaloniki, Greece
e-mail: grigoria@psy.auth.gr

P. Metallidou
Laboratory of Psychology, Section of Cognitive and Experimental Psychology, School of Psychology, Aristotle University of Thessaloniki, Thessaloniki, Greece

D. Moraitou, P. Metallidou (eds.), *Trends and Prospects in Metacognition Research across the Life Span*, https://doi.org/10.1007/978-3-030-51673-4_13

13.1 Introduction

Over the last decades, plenty of research has been conducted to investigate the efficacy of cognitive training programs (CTPs) in clinical and non-clinical populations such as patients who suffered stroke or patients with an acquired brain injury (Cicerone et al. 2011). CTPs have also been applied in older adults with or without dementia (Acevedo and Loewenstein 2007; Kelly et al. 2014).This line of research suggests that CTPs can be an effective means for the improvement of various aspects of cognition. However, recent meta-analytic studies revealed significant limitations of CTPs in cognitively healthy older adults (Kelly et al. 2014) and in older adults with or without cognitive impairment (Reijnders et al. 2013). Specifically, one of the main limitations is that training-related gains are limited to the trained domains and do not generalize to other cognitive domains or to everyday life situations (Kelly et al. 2014). Another limitation is that training-related gains are not sufficiently maintained over time. Considering that the core objective of CTPs is to train patients with cognitive deficits to cope with their difficulties and improve their daily life, the abovementioned limitations are significant obstacles in the attainment of this goal.

To deal with these limitations, several studies investigated the potential contribution of metacognition in cognitive rehabilitation. Metacognition refers to higher-order cognitive processes that monitor and control cognition. It was introduced by John Flavell (1976) and further elaborated by Nelson (1996). Metacognition comprises both knowledge a person has about cognition and its functions (metacognitive knowledge), and strategies to monitor and control cognitive processing and behavior (metacognitive regulation) (Flavell 1976; Schraw and Moshman 1995). Specifically, metacognitive knowledge (MK) refers to a person's declarative knowledge and beliefs about cognition, cognitive strategies and cognitive tasks, as well as to a person's awareness of their cognitive capabilities. Metacognitive regulation (MR) comprises online monitoring of cognitive processing as well as self-reflective cognitive processes including appraisal of cognitive processing and its outcome and regulation of cognitive behavior when automatic cognitive processing fails.

Recent research evidence within the tradition of age differences in metamemory monitoring and control suggests that at least some aspects of metacognitive monitoring and control remain intact in older adults, despite certain impairments in their actual memory functioning. When, though, are observed age-related differences in self-regulation in adults, we are far from explaining these differences (for reviews see Castel et al. 2016; Hertzog 2016). The evidence suggests that age-related changes in cognitive mechanisms, such as working memory declines due to neurobiological aging, could not explain the older adults' intact metacognitive monitoring in various memory tasks and would not suffice for explaining their constraints in self-regulatory behavior. Older adults consistently show a well-preserved self-regulatory flexibility (e.g., they invest effort to select and study highly-valued to be remembered information in experimental tasks), even though sometimes this does not compensate for their lower actual performance. This definitely calls for locating the factors that may affect the use of their metacognitive control resources and leaves ample space for implementing interventions that make use of such compensatory mechanisms. In line with the growing promising evidence for older adults' insights in their cognitive functioning the last 15 years many interventions have been designed and implemented which employ metacognition as a means to enhance adults' cognitive functioning and well-being.

Specifically, recent studies suggest that incorporating metacognitive components in CTPs can facilitate transfer of training and maintenance of effects over time (Bottiroli et al. 2017; Carretti et al. 2011; Cavallini et al. 2010). In their study Bottiroli et al. (2017) found that providing older adults with instructions on how to approach a cognitive task and on how to use memory strategies can help them improve their daily functioning. Similarly, in their study Cavallini et al. (2010) found that providing older adults with instructions on how to apply trained memory strategies on new tasks, can promote transfer effects. A different approach was used in the case of patients with traumatic brain injury (TBI). TBI patients often have significantly impaired self-awareness making them incapable to function independently in their daily life (Ciurli et al. 2010). Teaching them metacognitive strategies that support monitoring of cognitive performance helped them become aware of their difficulties and anticipate such difficulties. Specifically, use of external aids (e.g., calendars, notes, electrical devices etc.) improved TBI patients' daily functioning (Ownsworth 2010; Ownsworth et al. 2010).

Another approach proved helpful in the self-regulation of cognitive performance in patients suffering from stroke was intervention to improve metacognitive knowledge about one's abilities and self-efficacy beliefs (Bandura 1986). A person's subjective beliefs regarding their cognitive capacities interferes with actual performance (Beaudoin 2018) as well as with psychological variables of well-being (Aben et al. 2008; Kit et al. 2007). In their study Aben et al. (2008) found that the reduced memory self-efficacy that patients who suffered from stroke tend to report was related to psychiatric symptoms like depression and neuroticism.

To sum up, incorporation of metacognitive components in CTPs appears to be a promising approach; however, the contribution of metacognition in CTPs is not yet clear. The aim of this review is to provide an overview of studies that investigated the efficiency of metacognitive training programs (metaCTPs) in adults with cognitive deficits. More specifically, with this overview we intend to provide a better understanding regarding: first, the specific characteristics of metaCTPs (such as the content of these trainings and the targeted aspects of metacognition and/or cognition) and second, the results of these training programs concerning transfer effects and gains maintenance over time.

It should be noted that goal management training (GMT) is another approach in cognitive rehabilitation that also targets metacognitive skills such as self-monitoring and self-evaluation processes. More specifically, during GMT sessions patients learn how to set realistic goals and how to monitor and regularly appraise their cognitive behavior in order to achieve the predefined goal. Goal management training was developed by Robertson (1996) and originated from the theory of goal-directed behavior (Duncan 1986). However, for the purpose of the present review we decided to focus only on studies that were based on the theoretical framework of metacognition. The review is divided in two main sections. The first section focuses on the effects of metaCTPs in older adults with cognitive difficulties due to aging, while the second part focuses on adults with cognitive deficits as a result of a neurological condition. The results of these studies as well as the structure of the applied training programs will be discussed.

13.2 Method

To conduct the present literature review, the databases PubMed, PsychInfo, and Scopus were searched in February 2018. The following keywords were used: metacognitive intervention OR metacognitive training OR metacognitive skills training OR metamemory training OR metacognitive strategy training. Only randomized controlled trials (RCTs) published from 2008 onward in English language were included. Based on these criteria a total of 1151 results were retrieved. A detailed description of the screening process is illustrated in Fig. 13.1.

After an extensive screening procedure, a total of nine (five for older adult people and four for adult neurological patients) studies were selected for further analysis (see Table 13.1).

13.2.1 Older Adults

Cognitive decline is often associated with aging, even in healthy older adults. This has implications for everyday life functioning and, oftentimes, gives rise to anxiety and depression resulting to significantly impaired quality of life. Five out of nine studies that were included in this review tested the results of metaCTPs in older adults.

The first study was conducted by Bailey et al. (2010). They examined whether older adults could benefit from an at-home metamemory training. The rationale of their study originates from a previous study that was conducted by Dunlosky et al. (2013). Dunlosky et al. (2013) tested whether training older adults in self-testing promotes associative learning. To do so, they recruited 95 older adults and randomly assigned them to three groups (waiting list control group, strategy control group, and regulation group). The waiting list control group did not receive any training, while the rest two groups learned how to use two cognitive strategies (mental imagery and sentence generation) to learn word pairs. In addition to the cognitive strategies, the regulation group was trained in self-testing. They were instructed to monitor their learning process and to decide which items were sufficiently learned and which were not. Then, participants were instructed to restudy the non-learned items. In order to efficiently use self-testing, one can control study time. If study time is limited it is expected that it would compensate one's monitoring skills. Therefore, researchers

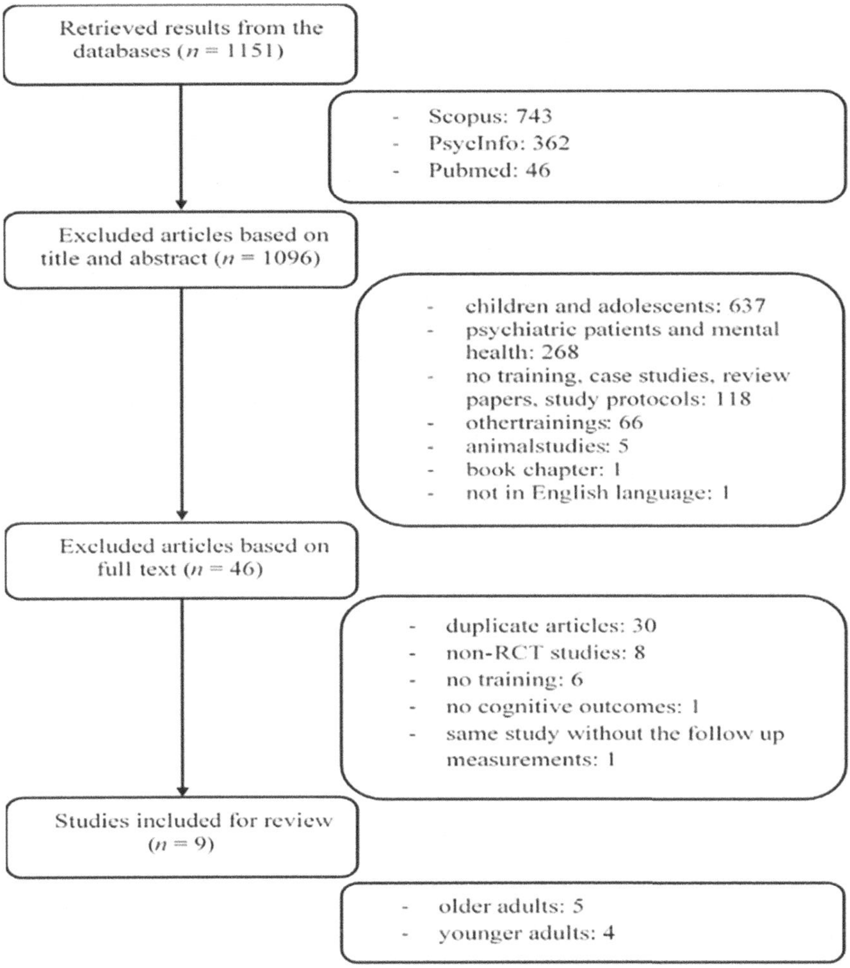

Fig. 13.1 Diagram of the process of studies' selection

provided all participants with two versions (experimenter-paced versus self-paced version) of an associative learning task (list of associative paired-words) and a list learning task (list of single words). The tasks were administered before and after the training period which consisted of two sessions (2-h duration each) and three homework assignments. In the experimenter-paced version the items to learn were presented on a computer screen at a fix rate, while in the self-paced version participants were given 20 min for each task to study the lists. The results showed that the regulation group performed better at post training compared to the strategy group and the waiting list control group. In addition, the gains of the training were greater in the self-paced version of the tasks. It is important to mention that the total amount of time participants invested in the self-paced version did not differ

Table 13.1 The included studies in this review

Study	Metacognitive Training	Population
1. Bailey et al. (2010)	At-home Metamemory Training	Cognitively healthy older adults
2. McDougall et al. (2010)	Cognitive Behavioral Model of Every-day Memory training	Cognitively healthy older adults
3. Youn et al. (2011)	Multi-strategic Memory Training	Subjective Cognitive Impairment
4. Vranic et al. (2013)	Multifactorial Memory Training	Cognitively healthy older adults
5. Wiegand et al. (2013)	Multidimensional Memory Training	Community-dwelling, Cognitively healthy older adults
6. Zucchella et al. (2013)	Cognitive training program with metacognitive components	Inpatients with Primary Brain Tumor in early phase after surgery
7. Aben et al. (2014)	Memory Self-Efficacy Training program	Stroke patients
8. Hanssen et al. (2016)	Metacognitive Intervention based on Goal Attainment Scaling method	Multiple Sclerosis patients
9. McDonald et al. (2017)	Memory and Attention Adaptation Training	Traumatic Brain Injury patients

significantly among the three groups. This means that the performance of the regulation group was improved in the self-paced version not because participants invested more time, but because they sufficiently allocated study time. These findings indicate that training older adults in self-testing enhance their learning skills and it is more efficient than training them only in cognitive strategies. Bailey et al. (2010) applied the same procedure only instead of training participants in the laboratory they provided them with a manual to train themselves at home. The manual included instructions for two cognitive strategies (mental imagery and sentence creation) and four assignments with paired-word lists. It also included instructions on how to monitor learning process via self-testing and study time allocation. To test the results of the training 56 cognitively healthy older adults were randomly assigned to a training group ($n = 29$, *mean age* = 70) or to a waiting list control group ($n = 27$, *mean age* = 73). The results were in line with Dunlosky et al. (2013). Specifically, older adults who received the metamemory training significantly improved their performance in the self-paced version of the paired-word list task. Interestingly, even those participants who were classified as self-testers (as self-testers were classified those participants who reported that self-testing is a strategy they already use in their everyday life) benefitted from the metamemory training. A possible explanation is that participants learned to apply self-testing in a more conscious and goal-oriented way rather than automatically. In summary, older adults can benefit from self-regulated learning and the gains are greater when they have the opportunity to regulate study time. Unfortunately, no follow up measures were obtained to test whether training related gains lasted over time. Furthermore, it would be of a great interest to investigate whether training older adults in monitoring skills would improve their performance in cognitive tasks other than associative learning. The next study, tested the results of a Multistrategic Memory Training (MMT) in more than one cognitive domain using a variety of neuropsychological tasks.

The efficacy of a MMT in 32 older adults with subjective memory complaints (SMC) was tested by Youn et al. (2011). All participants underwent a neuropsychiatric and a neuropsychological assessment in order to exclude dementia and history of neurological or psychiatric disorders. Then, participants were randomly assigned to an experimental ($n = 16$, *mean age* = 69) or a control group ($n = 16$, *mean age* = 69). The experimental group received ten training sessions (once per week for 1½ h), while the control group received a non-cognitive specific intervention of the same duration. During the MMT training sessions participants received information regarding memory and its subsystems, perception and attention, aging, and stress, and they learned cognitive strategies. In order to experience and become aware that different strategies might lead to different outcomes, the participants were instructed to practice the learned strategies and to test their results. At the end of each session, there was discussion about the learned strategies and on how to use them properly in daily life situations. Neuropsychological measures were obtained before and after the training in order to test for training-related differences. The results showed that memory was improved after the training, and so did attention and verbal fluency. In comparison to the metacognitive training that was tested by Bailey et al. (2010), the MMT targeted not only monitoring skills but also skills of cognitive control (decide which cognitive strategy to use based on the experience that different strategies lead to different results) and MK about memory function and cognitive strategies. The findings of the MMT showed positive effects on more than one cognitive domain indicating transfer effects. However, no follow up measures were obtained to estimate for their maintenance over time.

The next study was conducted by Vranic et al. (2013), in order to test the efficacy of a multifactorial memory training in cognitively healthy older adults living in residential care centers. Fifty-one older adults were recruited and randomly assigned to an experimental group ($n = 31$, *mean age* = 72) or a control group ($n = 20$, *mean age* = 75). The experimental group received the multifactorial memory training while the control group participated in group sessions discussing various topics of interest to older adults. The training period included nine group sessions of 90 min duration each, taking place once per week. Each session included discussion of the previous topic and homework, and introduction to the new topic via interactive discussion and relevant activities. The first six sessions were about providing participants with educational material about memory related topics (i.e., memory and its subsystems, aging, memory self-efficacy), while the last three sessions focused on strategy training (external aids and internal cognitive strategies such as mental imagery, story generation and reiteration). Homework assignments were related to each session's topic (for example, the homework assignment for the session about short-term and long-term memory session was for the participants to remember phone numbers or word lists) and were given between the training sessions. To test the efficacy of the training a practiced task (immediate recall list), unpracticed tasks for short-term memory, long-term memory, and working memory as well as two self-report scales (Need for Cognition scale and Subjective Memory Complaints Questionnaire) were given before and after the training period, and at 7 months follow-up. Training-related gains were found for the experimental group for the practiced as well as for the unpracticed tasks and these gains were maintained after 7 months. Furthermore, the experimental group showed statistically significant higher scores on the Need for Cognition scale (at both post-test and follow up) and on the Subjective Memory Complaints Questionnaire (only at post-test). No significant differences were found for the control group on any of the outcome measures (cognitive tasks or the self-report scales).

The next two studies are based on the theoretical framework of self-efficacy (henceforth, self-efficacy oriented training programs), meaning that the primary focus of their training programs is about subjective memory beliefs and quality of life. Specifically, McDougall et al. (2010) tested the efficacy of a Cognitive Behavioral Model of Everyday Memory (CBMEM) training. The aim of the CBMEM-based memory training was to promote quality of life by enhancing memory self-efficacy. The training included 8 weekly group training sessions and four booster sessions. During the CBMEM training sessions, participants received information regarding factors that affect memory functioning, external and internal strategies (use of external aids such as calendars or alarms and internal cognitive strategies such as mental imagery, association etc.), and information regarding stereotypes about aging via discussion and exercises. Homework was given in-between the training sessions. One month after completion of the training sessions, four booster sessions followed (one every 2 weeks). The aim of the booster sessions was to provide participants with additional practice and assistance on how to transfer memory strategies to everyday life situations. To test the efficacy of the CBMEM training a total sample size of 265 cognitively healthy older adults were recruited and randomly assigned to the CBMEM training ($n = 135$, *mean age* = 75) or to health promotion training ($n = 130$, *mean age* = 75). Both training programs had the same duration. Participants of the health promotion training engaged in interactive discussion regarding a variety of age-related topics without targeting memory. They did not receive any practical exercises or homework. Measures of memory performance and daily functioning as well as self-reported scores on memory self-efficacy, subjective beliefs about one's memory function (Metamemory in Adulthood questionnaire, MIA) and symptoms of depression and anxiety were obtained at baseline (pre-training) at 2 months (post-training session), at 6 months (after the booster sessions), at 12 and at 26 (end of the study) months follow up. The results showed that for both groups daily functioning was significantly improved from baseline to post-training sessions. Furthermore, both the experimental and the control group maintained their performance on all the cognitive, metacognitive and functional outcome measures (Direct Assessment of Functional Status) over time (24 months follow up). Significant differences between the two groups (experimental versus the active control group) were found from baseline to end of study for the overall cognition (Mini Mental State Examination, MMSE) and memory complaints (Metamemory in Adulthood questionnaire, MIA, complaint subscale) in favor of the experimental group.

Wiegand et al. (2013) assessed the efficacy of a Multidimensional Memory Training. The aim of the training was to promote healthy lifestyle behaviors in order to improve cognitive functioning. Forty-two community-dwelling older adults with no cognitive impairments were recruited and randomly assigned to either an experimental ($n = 21$, *mean age* = 70) or a waiting list control group ($n = 20$, *mean age* = 72). The multidimensional memory training included five group sessions of 2 h duration each on a weekly basis. The first half of the training included interactive group discussion, educational material and exercises regarding the relationship between aging, lifestyle behaviors (physical activities, cognitive engagement, social interaction, stress coping, and nutrition) and memory functioning. The aim was the participants to learn, practice and eventually apply healthier lifestyle habits that promote memory functioning. The last half of the training focused on teaching memory strategies and how to apply them to everyday life situations. All participants underwent three testing sessions (before, right after and 1 month after training). Reported changes in lifestyle behaviors and in intention to seek medical care were used as primary outcome measures, while metamemory self-reports (metamemory knowledge, use of strategies, perceived memory ability, contentment and controllability) and memory performance (name-learning task and face-learning task) were used as secondary outcome measures. The results showed that compared to the control group, the experimental group reported changes in lifestyle habits and reduced intention to seek medical care. Moreover, the experimental group showed improved metamemory self-reports (metamemory knowledge and memory contentment), and these gains were maintained after 1 month. No significant differences were found for the two groups in objective memory performance. According to the researchers of this study, subjective rather than objective memory changes were of their primary focus. In addition, they highlight the need for the development of neuropsychological tools that can detect and assess changes regarding one's cognitive performance in everyday life situations and not only in the laboratory.

To summarize, a total of five studies that tested the efficacy of a metacognitive training in older adults have been analyzed. The recruited sample size of these studies varies from 32 (Youn et al. 2011) to 265 participants (McDougall et al. 2010) and the age range was from 60 to 89 years. Four out of five studies, applied the metacognitive training in older adults with an average for their age cognitive status or with non-objectively measured cognitive deficits (Bailey et al. 2010; McDougall et al. 2010; Vranic, et al. 2013; Wiegand, et al. 2013), and Youn et al. (2011) recruited older adults with subjective cognitive impairment (SCI). An overview of the characteristics of the above analyzed studies is presented in Table 13.2. Regarding the structure and the content of the applied training programs, the training programs were mainly provided in group sessions (except the at-home metacognitive training of Bailey et al. 2010) and each session included the following components: educational material, practical exercises and paradigms, interactive discussion and homework. However, there is an important difference in the primary focus and the specific targeted domains of these studies. To be more specific, the aim of the training programs tested by Bailey et al. (2010), Youn et al. (2011), and Vranic et al. (2013) was to enhance participants' metacognitive knowledge as regards to

Table 13.2 Characteristics of studies in older adults

Study	Sample size (EG/CG)	Mean Age (EG/CG)	Population	Outcome measures	EG vs. CG at post-raining	EG vs. CG at follow up
Bailey et al. (2010)	29/27	70/73	Cognitively healthy	Self-paced paired-word list task	+	No follow up
				Experimenter-paced paired-word list task	n. s.	
McDougall et al. (2010)	135/130	75/75	Cognitively healthy	Mini Mental State Examination	+	n. s.
				Hopkins Verbal Learning Test—Revised	n. s.	n. s.
				Direct Assessment of Functional Status	n. s.	n. s.
				Brief Visuospatial Memory Test	n. s.	n. s.
				Rivermead Behavioral Memory Test	n. s.	n. s.
				Memory Self-Efficacy Questionnaire	n. s.	n. s.
				Metamemory in Adulthood	+	+
				Spielberger State–Trait Anxiety Inventory	n. s.	n. s.
				Centers for Epidemiologic Studies Scale	n. s.	n. s.
Youn et al. (2011)	16/16	69/69	Subjective Cognitive Impairment	Elderly Verbal Learning Test:		No follow up
				Short-term delayed free recall/ cued recall/ long-term delayed free recall/ cued recall/recognition	+/+ +/+ n. s.	
				Simple Rey Figure Test:		
				Copy/immediate/delayed/recognition	n. s./n. s./ n. s./+	
				Digit Span Test: forward/backward	n. s./n. s.	
				Verbal Span Test: forward/backward	+/n. s.	
				Phonemic Fluency Test	n. s.	
				Categorical Fluency Test	+	
				SMCQ	n. s.	
				Geriatric Depression Scale—Short form	n. s.	

Vranic et al. (2013)	31/20	72/75	Cognitively Healthy	Immediate recall list	+	+
				Digit Span Test: forward/backward	+/+	+/+
				Listening Span Test	+	+
				Delayed Story recall	+	+
				Delayed Story recognition	+	+
				Need for cognition	n. s.	+
				SMCQ	n. s.	n. s.
Wiegand et al. (2013)	21/20	70/72	Community-dwelling, Cognitively Healthy	Lifestyle changes	+	+
				Intention to seek medical care	n. s.	+
				Memory knowledge	+	+
				Strategy Toolbox	+	+
				Name Learning Task	n. s.	n. s.
				Face Learning Task	n. s.	n. s.
				MMQ: Contentment/Ability/Strategy	+/n. s./n. s.	+/n. s./n. s.
				Memory Controllability	n. s.	n. s.

Notes: EG, experimental group; CG, control group; +, statistically significant improved score in favor of the EG; n. s., nonsignificant difference between the two groups; SMCQ, Subjective Memory Complaints Questionnaire; MMQ, Multifactorial Memory Questionnaire memory function and cognitive strategies, as well as to improve metacognitive regulation by encouraging participants to monitor and evaluate the efficacy of the trained cognitive strategies and finally to apply them in different cognitive tasks. As a result of these training programs, participants' cognitive performance was improved, but no changes in subjective beliefs about memory or psychological aspects of well-being were reported. The opposite results were found in the studies of McDougall et al. (2010) and Wiegand et al. (2013), meaning that the training programs that they applied promoted significant changes in participants' subjective beliefs (memory contentment, strategy use) and psychological well-being (depression, lifestyle habits), while only minor or no changes were found for objectively measured cognitive performance. The primary aim of these training programs was to improve older adults' memory self-efficacy and to encourage them to apply habits that promote well-being, such as relaxation techniques, social and cognitive engagement, exercising etc. Even though, these training programs also included discussion and exercises about cognitive strategies, they did not achieve to promote changes in cognitive performance. One possible explanation could be that unlike the self-efficacy oriented training programs, the first three studies applied strategy training in a more systematic way and provided participants with practical exercises and feedback in every session. This approach seems to be more beneficial for objective cognitive performance. However, it is important to highlight that gains in objective cognitive performance as measured by neuropsychological tests do not automatically lead to transfer effects in everyday life. Another possible explanation for these findings could be that the training period was too short to affect both aspects (subjective and objective) of older adults' cognitive behavior and to promote lifestyle changes. Considering that subjective beliefs of one's cognitive capacities as well as objective cognitive performance are substantial for one's well-being and everyday functioning, a suggestion for future research and for clinicians would be to incorporate both components in training programs.

According to an experimental study that conducted by Hertzog et al. (2012), older adults even though are able to monitor the efficacy of different cognitive strategies, it is less likely for them to adopt a new and more efficient strategy (in that case mental imagery versus repetition) than younger adults. One possible explanation authors offered is that older adults may avoid adopting a new strategy due to low self-efficacy and they tend to stick with the one they already know and it is less cognitively demanding. Therefore, it might be more meaningful and efficient for a training program to start with self-efficacy enhancement and then target control and regulatory skills. Otherwise, negative beliefs of one's cognitive capacities might compromise one's cognitive engagement and motivation to learn and adopt new cognitive strategies.

13.2.2 Adult Patients with a Neurological Condition

Younger adults can also experience cognitive difficulties. This is a common and severe consequence of a neurological condition. In this section, four studies that have examined the effects of metaCTPs in younger adults with a neurological condition (brain tumor, stroke, multiple sclerosis and brain injury) are presented and analyzed.

In their study Zucchella et al. (2013) tested the results of a cognitive training program with metacognitive components in inpatients with primary tumor during the early phase after surgery. For the purpose of their study, 53 inpatients were recruited and they were randomly assigned to a training group ($n = 25$, *mean age* = 59) or a control group, ($n = 28$, *mean age* = 53). Patients with disabilities such as aphasia, severe behavioral or psychiatric symptoms, and severe visual deficits were excluded. The aim of the training was to test whether an early cognitive intervention could promote cognitive functions in neuro-oncological inpatients. The training included 16 individual sessions of 1-h duration each (four sessions per week). The sessions were guided by two experienced psychologists. The intervention combined computer exercises with a metacognitive training. Specifically, the training sessions included forty-five minutes of computer-based cognitive exercises targeting a variety of cognitive functions such as memory, executive functions, orientation in time and space, and visual attention. To promote self-monitoring and self-regulation, the psychologist guided and encouraged participants to use metacognitive strategies such as thinking about how to proceed with a task or checking whether they understood the task demands etc. During the last 15 min the patient and the psychologist engaged in a discussion regarding any difficulties or questions the participant might have. Furthermore, the psychologist provided the patient with guidance on how to transfer the learned strategies to everyday life situations. In order to test the efficacy of the training, all participants underwent neuropsychological assessment before and after the training. The results showed training-related gains in the cognitive domains of verbal memory, speed of processing and attention.

Aben et al. (2014) tested the efficiency of a Memory Self-Efficacy (MSE) training program in patients who suffered from stroke. The goal of the training was to provide participants with stroke-related information and with guidance on how to cope with the subsequent memory deficits. A total number of 153 stroke patients were recruited from two rehabilitation centers in the Netherlands. They were randomly assigned to a training ($n = 77$) or an active control group ($n = 76$) and the mean age of the total population was 58 years. The experimental group received the MSE training which consisted of three main parts: (1) information about stroke and memory, (2) instructions about cognitive strategies (external and internal) in order to adjust for deficits in memory function, and (3) information regarding affective and cognitive factors (mood and constant worries about one's memory performance) that can compromise memory function. Participants also received a written manual with educational material and homework assignments to practice between sessions. The control group participated in group meetings where they talked about stroke, its causes and its consequences. The duration was the same for both groups, i.e., nine group sessions of 1-h duration each, spread over a month. To assess training-related gains and their maintenance over time, all participants underwent an assessment before the training, right after the training, after 6 months and after 12 months. The assessment consisted of two memory tasks (delayed recall condition from the Auditory Verbal Learning Test, AVLT, and the delayed recall condition from the Rivermead Behavioral Memory Test, RBMT) and self-report scales measuring metamemory (memory self-efficacy and strategy use), quality of life, and depression. The memory self-efficacy score was significantly higher in the experimental group at the end of the program compared to the control group, and the difference was maintained over time (at the 6- and 12-months follow up). Furthermore, even though the quality of life score had increased in the experimental group after training, the difference reached statistical significance only in the younger-adults' subgroup of the experimental group (< 65 years old). No significant difference was found neither for memory performance nor for depression score between the two groups after the training or at the follow up assessments. As regard to memory performance, it is possible that cognitive functioning got better over time even without training. Finally, as regard to depression score, it is likely that social interaction and sharing stroke-related experiences during the group meetings of the control group resulted to a decline in depressive symptoms.

The next study was conducted by Hanssen et al. (2016). The aim of the study was to test whether a metacognitive intervention could improve cognitive coping and quality of life in patients with multiple sclerosis (MS).To do so, 120 MS patients with reported cognitive difficulties were recruited and randomly assigned to either an experimental ($n = 60$, *mean age* $= 54$) or a control group ($n = 60$, *mean age* $= 53$). All participants received a 4-week rehabilitation program according to the therapeutic protocol of the rehabilitation center. In addition to the standard rehabilitation program, the experimental group received a metacognitive intervention, which included three group sessions and five individual sessions. During the individual sessions, each participant received personal feedback on their cognitive status and guidance on how to posit and achieve realistic goals in everyday life situations. To do so, participants were taught the method of Goal Attainment Scaling (GAS) (Kiresuk and Sherman 1968), which is based on the metacognitive strategies of self-monitoring and self-evaluation. During the group sessions, participants received educational material via lectures, discussion and exercises. The content of the educational material included information about cognitive functions and the importance of goal management, about executive functions such as planning and monitoring, and about difficulties in communication and related coping strategies. After the 4 weeks of the training sessions, participants received six phone calls over a period of 3 months (one phone call every 2 weeks). The aim was to encourage participants and offer additional guidance on how to use the GAS method in their daily life. In order to test for training-related differences between the groups and the maintenance of training effects over time, both groups underwent a neuropsychological assessment (Behavior Rating Inventory of Executive Functions—Adult version, General Executive Composite, Metacognition Index, Hopkins Symptoms

Checklist, and Multiple Sclerosis Impact Scale) before and after the rehabilitation period, at 4 and at 7 months after the start of the rehabilitation program. According to the results of the study, all participants showed improved performance on general executive functioning from baseline to 4 and 7 months after the start of the rehabilitation. However, only the experimental group showed improvements in psychological aspects such as quality of life (Hopkins Symptoms Checklist) and psychological well-being (Multiple Sclerosis Impact Scale). No outcome measures regarding specific cognitive domains were obtained.

The last study included in this review was conducted by McDonald et al. (2017). The aim was to test the efficacy of two CTPs combined or not with pharmacotherapy (methylphenidate, MPH) in patients with traumatic brain injury (TBI). The tested CTPs were the Memory and Attention Adaptation Training (MAAT) (developed by Ferguson and Mittenberg 1996) and the Attention Builders Training (ABT) (developed by Berg et al. 1991). The total duration of the training period was approximately 6 months, including four individual sessions of 50 min duration each and three brief phone calls. The MAAT is a metacognitive training that targets self-awareness and self-regulation. Specifically, during the training sessions participants received information regarding TBI and subsequent cognitive deficits as well as guidance on how to compensate for these deficits using cognitive strategies. In addition, the patients were guided to think of situations in which they were more likely to face cognitive difficulties and learned relaxation techniques to cope with stress symptoms. Finally, they received a manual with educational material and written instructions about cognitive strategies and how to use them properly. Participants of the ABT program practiced cognitive tasks and received general information regarding TBI and its cognitive consequences. However, they did not receive any information regarding compensatory strategies or how to cope with cognitive difficulties in everyday life situations. All participants received biweekly phone calls. During these phone calls only participants of the MAAT program received further guidance regarding the use of compensatory strategies. The participants of the ABT program received a simple evaluation of their homework assignments. For the purpose of the study, a total number of 71 participants were randomly assigned to four different groups (MAAT–MPH, $n = 17$, *mean age* = 43, MAAT placebo, $n = 17$, *mean age* = 37, ABT–MPH, $n = 19$, *mean age* = 43, ABT–placebo, $n = 18$, *mean age* = 37). All participants underwent a neuropsychological assessment before and after the training. The assessment included neuropsychological evaluation of multiple cognitive domains (attention, memory and executive functions) and filling in a self-report scale regarding cognitive abilities (Multiple Abilities Self-Report Questionnaire). The findings showed that the metacognitive training was more effective compared to the ABT training. Specifically, participants of the MAAT–placebo group performed better on verbal learning compared to the ABT–placebo group and participants of the MAAT–MPH performed better than the participants of the other three groups on divided attention and memory tasks.

To sum up, a total of four studies that investigated the efficacy of metaCTPs in adults with cognitive deficits have been analyzed. The sample size of these studies varied from 53 (Zucchella et al. 2013) to 153 patients (Aben et al. 2014) and the age of participants from 37 (McDonald et al. 2017) to 59 years (Zucchella et al. 2013). The findings suggest that metaCTPs can lead to beneficial effects on several domains of cognition such as memory and attention (McDonald et al. 2017; Zucchella et al. 2013), executive functioning (Hanssen et al. 2016; McDonald et al. 2017; Zucchella et al. 2013), on metacognitive domains (Aben et al. 2014; Hanssen et al. 2016) as well as on psychological well-being (Aben et al. 2014; Hanssen et al. 2016). Furthermore, based on the fact that the neurological conditions of the participants in the studies differed, it can be argued that metacognitive training can be effective in persons confronting various neurological conditions such as patients with brain tumor (Zucchella et al. 2013), patients who had suffered stroke (Aben et al. 2014), patients with MS (Hanssen et al. 2016) and patients with TBI (McDonald et al. 2017). An overview of the characteristics of the above studies is presented in Table 13.3.

Regarding the structure of the applied training programs, all four studies used a similar structure based on three main components: (1) educational material regarding the special needs and the consequences of each clinical condition, (2) exercises to practice cognitive strategies, (3) discussion and guidance for transferring the learned skills to everyday life. According to the findings of these four studies, the gains of a metaCTP were more prominent in the studies of Zucchella et al. (2013) and McDonald et al. (2017), while for the studies of Aben et al. (2014) and Hanssen et al. (2016) no significant differences were reported between the experimental and the control group. A common characteristic among the recruited neurological populations of these four studies is their reduced ability in self-awareness regarding their cognitive deficits (anosognosia). Hanssen et al. (2016) recruited MS patients with reported cognitive difficulties. Thus, these participants were already aware of their cognitive deficits—that probably indicates individuals with developed metacognitive skills—and they had most likely found their own ways to compensate for these deficits. If that is true, it is reasonable why no significant changes were detected. In the study of Aben et al. (2014) the lack of significant differences between the two groups in memory performance could be partly explained by the fact that cognitive functioning in patients who suffered stroke improves to some extend over time even without specific training.

13.3 General Discussion

The aim of the current review was to present an overview of the available scientific evidence on the efficacy of metaCTPs in older adults and in younger adults with a neurological condition. We analyzed nine studies and their findings provide some promising evidence regarding the beneficial effects of metaCTPs in multiple domains such as cognition, metacognition and psychological well-being. The current review is based on studies that were conducted during the last decade. A similar search for studies before 2008 using the same keywords did not reveal any randomized controlled trial studies to match the criteria for this review.

Table 13.3 Characteristics of studies in adult patients with a neurological condition

Study	Sample size (EG/CG)	Mean age (EG/CG)	Population	Outcome measures	EG vs. CG at post-training	EG vs. CG at follow-up
Zucchella et al. (2013)	25/28	59/53	Inpatients with Primary Brain Tumor in early phase after surgery	Mini Mental State Examination	n. s.	No follow up
				Digit Span Test	n. s.	
				Corsi's Test	n. s.	
				RAVLT: Immediate recall/ Delayed Recall	n. s./+[a]	
				LMT: Immediate recall/ Delayed Recall	+/+	
				Frontal Assessment Battery	n. s.	
				Raven's Coloured Progressive Matrices—47	n. s.	
				Trail Making Test: Part A/ Part B	+/+	
				Attentive Matrices	+	
				Phonological Fluency	n. s.	
				Semantic fluency	n. s.	
				Rey–Osterrieth Figure, copy	n. s.	
Aben et al. (2014)	77/76	58 (total population mean age)	Stroke patients	Metamemory in Adulthood Questionnaire:		
				Memory Self-Efficacy/ Strategy use	+/n. s.	+/n. s.
				Depression	n. s.	n. s.
				Quality of Life:		
				Visual Analogue score/ Psycho-logical/ Social	n. s./n. s./n. s.	n. s./n. s./n. s.
				Social Support List (Social participation)	n. s.	n. s.

(continued)

Table 13.3 (continued)

Study	Sample size (EG/CG)	Mean age (EG/CG)	Population	Outcome measures	EG vs. CG at post-training	EG vs. CG at follow-up
				Impact on Participation and Autonomy:		
				Problem experience	n. s.	n. s.
				Delayed Recall AVLT	n. s.	n. s.
				Delayed Recall RBMT	n. s.	n. s.
Hanssen et al. (2016)	60/60	54/53	Multiple Sclerosis	BRIEF—A	n. s.	n. s.
				General Executive Composite	n. s.	n. s.
				Metacognition Index	n.s.	n. s.
				HSCL—25	n. s.	+
				MSIS—29: Psychological subscale	n.s.	+
McDonald et al. (2017)	MAAT–MPH = 17 MAAT–placebo = 17 ABT–MPH=19 ABT–placebo = 18	MAAT–MPH = 43 MAAT–placebo = 37 ABT–MPH=43 ABT–placebo = 37	Traumatic Brain Injury	CVLT (Trials 1–5)	+[b]	No follow up
				PASAT	+[c]	
				Digit Symbol Coding Test	n. s.	
				Trail Making Test A	n. s.	
				MASQ	n. s.	
				Craft Stories, Immediate recall	n. s.	
				Brown Location Test	+[c]	
				D–KEFS, Sorting Test	n. s.	

Notes: EG, experimental group; CG, control group; n. s., non-significant difference between the two groups; RAVLT, Rey Auditory Verbal Learning Test; [a]+, statistically significant improved score in favor of the EG; LMT, Logical Memory Test; AVLT, Auditory Verbal Learning Test; RBMT, Rivermead Behavioral Memory Test; BRIEF—A, Behavior Rating Inventory of Executive Functions—Adult Version; HSCL, Hopkins Symptoms Checklist—25; MSIS, Multiple Sclerosis Impact Scale; MAAT, Memory and Attention Adaptation Training; MPH, methylphenidate; CVLT, California Verbal Learning Test; [b]+, statistically significant improved score in favor of the MAAT–placebo versus ABT–placebo group; PASAT, Paced Auditory Serial Addition Test; [c]+, statistically significant improved score in favor of the MAAT–MPH versus the rest three groups; ABT, Attention Builders Training; MASQ, Multiple Abilities Self-Report Questionnaire; D–KEFS, Delis–Kaplan Executive Function System

All nine studies applied training programs that targeted both aspects of metacognition, that is, metacognitive knowledge and metacognitive regulation. Specifically, theoretical information was provided to help participants to gain awareness regarding their condition and its consequences on several domains (cognition, mood, and daily functioning). In addition, declarative knowledge about coping strategies (how, when and why use them) was enhanced in order to facilitate the transfer of these strategies in participants' everyday life. Furthermore, metacognitive regulation was promoted through feedback and discussion upon the exercises and the homework assignments. This process encouraged participants to evaluate their performance and to experience that different strategies may lead to different outcomes. It is also important to note that the efficacy of these training programs was tested with several populations such as healthy older adults, patients with brain tumor or brain injury, patients with multiple sclerosis and patients who suffered from stroke, suggesting that a metacognitive approach in cognitive rehabilitation is suitable for a variety of conditions.

However, the aforementioned results should be interpreted with caution. The available number of analyzed studies is very limited and the applied interventions varied widely among these studies. Only four out of nine studies used a set of neuropsychological tasks to test for training-related effects on different cognitive domains, while the rest tested the efficacy of the applied training program using self-report scales. Moreover, only half of the studies included follow up assessments to test for gain maintenance over time, while very few of them evaluated the impact of the training in participants' daily functioning. Interestingly, only one study compared the effects of a metacognitive training with a structured cognitive training (McDonald et al. 2017), while the rest provided the control group with discussion sessions or with no intervention at all (waiting list). Hence, there is not enough data that could support claims about whether and to what extent metacognitive training is more effective than traditional cognitive training.

Future research should address the limitations of the available studies in order to gain better understanding on the beneficial effect of metacognitive training. Therefore, use of valid and sensitive neuropsychological tasks, outcome measures for daily functioning as well as follow up assessments after the end of the training are necessary. In addition, it is important for future studies to compare metacognitive training with traditional cognitive training and to recruit large sample sizes. Finally, the use of neuroimaging data could provide some valuable insight regarding the relationship of metacognition, cognition and neural mechanisms, which is still an area of research with very limited data.

To conclude, even though research on this topic is still in its infancy, there is significant evidence for the contribution of metacognitive training in cognitive rehabilitation. Even though metacognitive training in most of the cases did not have a significant effect on cognitive tests, this should not be interpreted as if it is not worth implementing such training. The interventions presented in this chapter clearly suggest that future attempts should combine training that aim to enhance metacognitive knowledge as regards memory and flexible use of cognitive strategies with training to improve self-efficacy about cognitive functioning and promote well-being. Given the promising evidence from the age-related differences research in metacognition, it is important to include metacognitive processes that have been found to remain intact in older adults in order to compensate for memory declines (for reviews see Castel et al. 2016; Hertzog 2016). Older adults have shown, under certain conditions, intact metacognitive monitoring and self-regulatory flexibility, that is, they act strategically by purposefully and selectively allocating their limited attention and effort resources in order to effectively recall interesting and important for them information. Further, future interventions should incorporate possible affective and motivational factors that can facilitate the optimal employment of metacognitive monitoring and control processes. McGillivray (Chap. 12 in this volume) presents and discusses evidence for possible motivational and emotional influences in older adults' metacognitive functioning. The evidence suggests that performance on memory tasks, metamemory judgements and control decisions is affected by motivational and emotional factors, such as interest, the value and importance of to be remembered information or its emotional content. The evidence also shows systematic interrelations between metamemory and affect, which can't be explained by the processing of fluency or disfluency mechanism. Stimulus emotionality, mood states, metacognitive knowledge about the self in specific tasks as well as self-concept seem to play a critical role in metamemory awareness (for a review see Efklides 2016). The above factors may play an even more critical role in activating insight in young patient adults' who suffer from cognitive and metacognitive deficits.

The more we understand the complex interplay of cognition, metacognition and affect in adults' daily functioning, the more able will be to identify the mechanisms that facilitate or hinder self-regulatory behavior in groups of adults with cognitive deficits either due to aging or neurological deficits, and the more able will be to design interventions that help them to maximize the use of their resources for optimal cognitive and metacognitive functioning. A coherent theoretical framework, such as Efklides' Metacognitive and Affective Model of Self-regulated Learning (MASRL model) (2011), would be very helpful for understanding this interplay between cognition, motivation and affect while the person is working on real life tasks or goals. Her emphasis on the affective and motivational character of metacognitive feelings, such as the feeling of difficulty (see also Efklides 2006), in the person *x* task level of functioning could be helpful in explaining some of the intriguing findings in older adults' metacognitive processes. Namely, older adults' metacognitive beliefs about memory in aging, or their feelings about their memory and cognitive functioning in various daily tasks may influence the accuracy of their judgments. Further, the role of self-concept and personal goals would be critical factors for either activating or de-activating their attempts to meet the demands of tasks in various situations. The question of the next decade should be under which conditions we could ensure the optimal benefit for the quality of life of older or younger adults with cognitive deficits. Metacognition and affect are to play a very promising role in any future attempt.

Acknowledgments This research is co-financed by Greece and the European Union (European Social Fund—ESF) through the Operational Program "Human Resources Development, Education and Lifelong Learning" in the context of the project "Strengthening Human Resources Research Potential via Doctorate Research" (MIS-5000432), implemented by the State Scholarships Foundation (IKY).

References

Aben, L., Busschbach, J. J. V., Ponds, R. W. H. M., & Ribbers, G. M. (2008). Memory self-efficacy and psychosocial factors in stroke. *Journal of Rehabilitation Medicine, 40*, 681–683. https://doi.org/10.2340/16501977-0227.

Aben, L., Heijenbrok-Kal, M. H., Ponds, R. W. H. M., Busschbach, J. J. V., & Ribbers, G. M. (2014). Long-lasting effects of a new memory self-efficacy training for stroke patients: A randomized controlled trial. *Neurorehabilitation and Neural Repair, 28*, 199–206. https://doi.org/10.1177/1545968313478487.

Acevedo, A., & Loewenstein, D. A. (2007). Nonpharmacological cognitive interventions in aging and dementia. *Journal of Geriatric Psychiatry and Neurology, 20*(4), 239–249. https://doi.org/10.1177/0891988707308808

Bailey, H., Dunlosky, J., & Hertzog, C. (2010). Metacognitive training at home: Does it improve older adults' learning? *Gerontology, 56*, 414–420. https://doi.org/10.1159/000266030.

Bandura, A. (1986). *Social foundations of thought and action: A social cognitive theory*. Englewood Cliffs, NJ: Prentice-Hall.

Beaudoin, M. (2018). Memory performance in older adults: Experimental evidence for the indirect effect of memory self-efficacy on processing efficiency through worry. *Motivation and Emotion, 42*, 885–895. https://doi.org/10.1007/s11031-018-9703-5.

Berg, I., Konning-Haanstra, M., & Deelman, B. (1991). Long term effects of memory rehabilitation: A controlled study. *Neuropsychological Rehabilitation, 1*, 97–111. https://doi.org/10.1080/09602019108401384.

Bottiroli, S., Cavallini, E., Dunlosky, J., Vecchi, T., & Hertzog, C. (2017). Self-guided strategy-adaption training for older adults: Transfer effects to everyday tasks. *Archives of Gerontology and Geriatrics, 72*, 91–98. https://doi.org/10.1016/j.archger.2017.05.015.

Carretti, B., Borella, E., Zavagnin, M., & De Beni, R. (2011). Impact of metacognition and motivation on the efficacy of strategic memory training in older adults: Analysis of specific, transfer and maintenance effects. *Archives of Gerontology and Geriatrics, 52*, e192–e197. https://doi.org/10.1016/J.ARCHGER.2010.11.004.

Castel, A. D., Middlebrooks, C. D., & McGillivray, S. (2016). Monitoring memory in old age: Impaired, spared, and aware. In J. Dunlosky & S. K. Tauber (Eds.), *Oxford handbook of metacognition* (pp. 519–535). New York: Oxford University Press.

Cavallini, E., Dunlosky, J., Bottiroli, S., Hertzog, C., & Vecchi, T. (2010). Promoting transfer in memory training for older adults. *Aging Clinical and Experimental Research, 22*, 314–323. https://doi.org/10.3275/6704.

Cicerone, K. D., Langenbahn, D. M., Braden, C., Malec, J. F., Kalmar, K., Fraas, M., et al. (2011). Evidence-based cognitive rehabilitation: Updated review of the literature from 2003 through 2008. *Archives of Physical Medicine and Rehabilitation, 92*, 519–530. https://doi.org/10.1016/j.apmr.2010.11.015.

Ciurli, P., Bivona, U., Barba, C., Onder, G., Silvestro, D., Azicnuda, E., et al. (2010). Metacognitive unawareness correlates with executive function impairment after severe traumatic brain injury. *Journal of the International Neuropsychological Society, 16*, 360–368. https://doi.org/10.1017/S135561770999141X.

Duncan, J. (1986). Disorganisation of behaviour after frontal lobe damage. *Cognitive Neuropsychology, 3*(3), 271–290. https://doi.org/10.1080/02643298608253360.

Dunlosky, J., Kubat-Silman, A. K., & Hertzog, C. (2013). Training monitoring skills improves older adults' self-paced associative learning. *Psychology and Aging, 18*, 340–345. https://doi.org/10.1037/0882-7974.18.2.340.

Efklides, A. (2006). Metacognitive experiences: The missing link in the self-regulated learning process. *Educational Psychology Review, 18*, 287–291.

Efklides, A. (2011). Interactions of metacognition with motivation and affect in self-regulated learning: The MASRL model. *Educational Psychologist, 46*, 6–25.

Efklides, A. (2016). Metamemory and affect. In J. Dunlosky & S. K. Tauber (Eds.), *Oxford handbook of metacognition* (pp. 245–267). New York: Oxford University Press.

Ferguson, R. J., & Mittenberg, W. (1996). Cognitive behavioral treatment of postconcussion syndrome. In V. B. Van Hasselt & M. Herson (Eds.), *Sourcebook of psychological treatment manuals for adult disorders*. New York: Plenum.

Flavell, J. (1976). Metacognitive aspects of problem solving. In I. L. B. Resnick (Ed.), *The nature of intelligence* (pp. 231–235). Hillsdale, NJ: Erlbaum.

Hanssen, K. T., Beiske, A. G., Landrø, N. I., Hofoss, D., & Hessen, E. (2016). Cognitive rehabilitation in multiple sclerosis: A randomized controlled trial. *Acta Neurologica Scandinavica, 133*, 30–40. https://doi.org/10.1111/ane.12420.

Hertzog, C. (2016). Aging and metacognitive control. In J. Dunlosky & S. K. Tauber (Eds.), *Oxford handbook of metacognition* (pp. 537–558). New York: Oxford University Press.

Hertzog, C., Price, J., & Dunlosky, J. (2012). Age differences in the effects of experimenter-instructed versus self-generated strategy use. *Experimental Aging Research, 38*, 42–62. https://doi.org/10.1080/0361073X.2012.637005.

Kelly, M. E., Loughrey, D., Lawlor, B. A., Robertson, I. H., Walsh, C., & Brennan, S. (2014). The impact of cognitive training and mental stimulation on cognitive and everyday functioning of healthy older adults: A systematic review and meta-analysis. *Ageing Research Reviews, 15*, 28–43. https://doi.org/10.1016/j.arr.2014.02.004.

Kiresuk, T. J., & Sherman, R. E. (1968). Goal attainment scaling: A general method for evaluating comprehensive community mental health programs. *Community Mental Health Journal, 4*, 443–453. https://doi.org/10.1007/BF01530764.

Kit, K. A., Mateer, C. A., & Graves, R. E. (2007). The influence of memory beliefs in individuals with traumatic brain injury. *Rehabilitation Psychology, 52*, 25–32. https://doi.org/10.1037/0090-5550.52.1.25.

McDonald, B. C., Flashman, L. A., Arciniegas, D. B., Ferguson, R. J., Xing, L., Harezlak, J., et al. (2017). Methylphenidate and memory and attention adaptation training for persistent cognitive symptoms after traumatic brain injury: A randomized, placebo-controlled trial. *Neuropsychopharmacology, 42*, 1766–1775. https://doi.org/10.1038/npp.2016.261.

McDougall, G. J., Becker, H., Pituch, K., Acee, T. W., Vaughan, P. W., & Delville, C. L. (2010). The SeniorWISE study: Improving everyday memory in older adults. *Archives of Psychiatric Nursing, 24*, 291–306. https://doi.org/10.1016/j.apnu.2009.11.001.

Nelson, T. O. (1996). Consciousness and metacognition. *American Psychologist, 51*(2), 102–116. https://doi.org/10.1037/0003-066X.51.2.102.

Ownsworth, T. (2010). A metacognitive contextual approach for facilitating return to work following acquired brain injury: Three descriptive case studies. *Work, 36*, 381–388. https://doi.org/10.3233/WOR-2010-1041.

Ownsworth, T., Quinn, H., Fleming, J., Kendall, M., & Shum, D. (2010). Error self-regulation following traumatic brain injury: A single case study evaluation of metacognitive skills training and behavioural practice interventions. *Neuropsychological Rehabilitation, 20*, 59–80. https://doi.org/10.1080/09602010902949223.

Reijnders, J., van Heugten, C., & van Boxtel, M. (2013). Cognitive interventions in healthy older adults and people with mild cognitive impairment: A systematic review. *Ageing Research Reviews, 12*, 263–275. https://doi.org/10.1016/j.arr.2012.07.003.

Robertson, I. H. (1996). *Goal management training: A clinical manual.* Cambridge: PsyConsult.
Schraw, G., & Moshman, D. (1995). Metacognitive theories. *Educational Psychology Review, 7,* 351–371. https://doi.org/10.1007/s10648-017-9413-7.
Vranic, A., Špani, A. M., Carretti, B., & Borella, E. (2013). The efficacy of a multifactorial memory training in older adults living in residential care settings. *International Psychogeriatrics, 25,* 1885–1897. https://doi.org/10.1017/S1041610213001154.
Wiegand, M. A., Troyer, A. K., Gojmerac, C., & Murphy, K. J. (2013). Facilitating change in health-related behaviors and intentions: A randomized controlled trial of a multidimensional memory program for older adults. *Aging & Mental Health, 17*(2013), 806–815. https://doi.org/10.1080/13607863.org/10.1080/13607863.2013.789000.
Youn, J. H., Lee, J. Y., Kim, S., & Ryu, S. H. (2011). Multistrategic memory training with the metamemory concept in healthy older adults. *Psychiatry Investigation, 8,* 354–361. https://doi.org/10.4306/pi.2011.8.4.354.
Zucchella, C., Capone, A., Codella, V., De Nunzio, A. M., Vecchione, C., Sandrini, G., et al. (2013). Cognitive rehabilitation for early post-surgery inpatients affected by primary brain tumor: A randomized, controlled trial. *Journal of Neuro-Oncology, 114,* 93–100. https://doi.org/10.1007/s11060-013-1153-z.

The manufacturer's authorised representative in the EU is Springer Nature Customer Service Centre GmbH, Europaplatz 3, 69115 Heidelberg, Germany. If you have any concerns regarding our products, please contact ProductSafety@springernature.com

Printed and bound by CPI Group (UK) Ltd, Croydon, CR0 4YY
30/09/2026
02225690-0013